CONTENTS

SECTION 3   Common Allergy-Causing Foods

ALLERGIES

and

holistic healing

Skye Weintraub, N.D.

WOODLAND PUBLISHING
Pleasant Grove, UT

SECTION 4   Allergies and the Environment

8   Contents

FOREWORD

Reviewing books is an arduous task at best and I have always relegated this task to the last hour in bed before I fall asleep. So, with weary eyes at 10:00 p.m., I started to read Dr. Weintraub's latest book on allergies and environmental disease. At 3:00 a.m. my wife, with an irritated voice, told me to go downstairs to the guest bedroom if I wanted to continue reading. I could hardly put the book down because the information was so concentrated, current, and clinically useful.

The book is written in an easy-to-read, no-nonsense style with short, to-the-point introductions to each chapter. The subject matter is discussed in a practical way so that the concepts are easily understood by doctor and patient alike. The treatment protocols are described in plain language with well-annotated resources and useful contacts.

The chapters concentrate on the deleterious effects of our environment, both external and internal on the human body. Extensive information is provided on foods, diets, food allergies, chemicals in the environment, the purity of our water and air, and ways and means of protecting ourselves and family from the onslaughts of "civilization." Patient handouts are extensively used to educate and change poor lifestyle patterns. These handouts represent many hours of thoughtful hard work and research. The information provided is quite invaluable as it enables the busy practitioner to have an instantaneous resource without having to page through multiple articles or books.

I enthusiastically recommend this book to any practitioner or patient who is serious about their health and needs instantaneous and factual information to make informed decisions about a healthy lifestyle for themselves, their patients, and loved ones.

John Diamond, M.D.

AUTHOR'S NOTE

One of my roles as a naturopathic physician is to educate people concerning wellness and illness. It is important that everyone have information about healthy ways to live, not just what drugs to take for an illness. In a busy medical practice there is never enough time to educate people. Each condition may require its own unique nutritional program, lifestyle changes, or other needed therapies. Since I regularly use hundreds of reference books, articles, and notes, I began to find that there wasn't time to discuss every detail a patient needed to know. And even if there were, it would be very hard to remember everything discussed during our time together. I wanted to have complete and detailed information available for each person to take home so I started writing handouts with this information. Over the years my files grew until I had a handout about most of the conditions that I treated in my practice.

When I began my medical practice in 1989, there was a lack of well-written and reliable information on the subject of allergies and sensitivities. It is probably because most practicing health professionals just don't have the time necessary to do research and writing. This book is the product of years of research, reading, attending seminars, writing, and personal observations and experiences. I have tried to fill each section with practical information. If you are interested in a more natural way of treating illness, this book is intended as a reference manual or as a simple guide for healthy living. I hope it will be of use both for the general public and the physician interested in natural therapies.

GOOD ADVICE

Improved nutrition training of physicians and other health professionals is needed. Training should emphasize basic principles of nutrition, the role of methodologies and their interpretation, therapeutic aspects of dietary intervention, and behavioral aspects of dietary counseling.

Qualified health professionals should advise persons with food allergies and intolerances on the diagnosis of these conditions and on diets that exclude foods and food substances that induce symptoms. Diseases of dietary excess and imbalance now rank among the leading cause of illness and death in the U.S., and generates substantial health care costs.

C. Everett Koop, M.D., 1988
U.S. Surgeon General's Report

Two-thirds of all deaths, including those caused by coronary heart disease, strokes, atherosclerosis, diabetes, and some types of cancer are related to lifestyle choices, including what we eat.

Dr. Bernadine Healy
Director of the NIH

We now have food that keeps indefinitely which means that germs cannot live on it, and that, in turn, means that we would be well advised not to try to do so either.

The simple goal of vibrant health was rarely attained because of the worst human habit of all: the daily adventure to see how near to disaster we can go without being caught. Surely if we get rid of a bad thing, it is unnecessary to put anything in its place.

James C. Thomson
20th-Century nature cure philosopher

The doctor of the future will give no medicine, but will interest his patients in the care of the human frame, in proper diet, and in the cause and prevention of disease.

Thomas A. Edison

Introduction

When it comes to diet, there is a direct relationship between a person's level of health and their ability to digest and assimilate nutritious foods. Often people feel deprived if they have to eat a simple and healthy diet. They crave and want to eat all the things that originally made them sick. Extensive dietary restrictions are probably only temporary, but the most toxic foods may need to be eliminated completely. Changes can be hard, but the results of good health can last a lifetime.

Health comes from and is maintained by digested foods. After digestion, food goes through a process of assimilation that converts it into nutrients. Circulating blood carries these health-producing nutrients to every part of the body, repairing damage done to cells, tissues, and organs. Undigested food ferments and putrefies in the intestinal tract. This leads to a state of intestinal toxemia and slowly poisons the body. There is not a drug yet invented that can rectify the damage done by failure of the digestive tract.

It takes some time for someone to reach a state of unhealth, whether it be allergies or some other ailment. Recovery from most illnesses is enhanced by removing certain foods from the diet and improving digestion. A state of wellness and good health takes more than wishful thinking or the use of synthetic drugs—it takes commitment and dedication. The best results come after changing your diet and lifestyle. Eating is often associated with "what I want" instead of what is right or important for the body. Even taste is a matter of conditioning and habit. As you eat healthier and healthier, you will find yourself liking "good" foods every bit as much as the overly-processed, sugar-laden, chemical- and additive-containing, and nutritionally deficient foods that used to be your choice.

Along with poor food choices, we are also adversely affected by thousands of synthesized chemicals. Few of these chemicals are sufficiently investigated for their effects on human health. In addition, radioactive, electromagnetic, and other harmful environmental agents are responsible for further serious influences. As a result, the total burden of harmful substances that we are currently being subjected to increasingly threatens to exhaust the capabilities of our bodies. It is important to develop and implement a holistic medical concept for relief from these burdens.

Keep an open mind and a positive attitude. A person's attitude can be one of the most important factors in healing any condition. Your new lifestyle can be a wonderful journey or it can be an awful, heavy burden; it depends on you. If you decide to begin this journey, it can lead you to a wellness and vigor you never knew possible. It's your choice.

Section 1

WHAT ARE ALLERGIES?

CHAPTER 1

Types of Allergies

AN ALLERGY VERSUS A SENSITIVITY

When a person is exposed to a substance that is perceived by the immune system to be foreign or harmful, the body produces an antibody specifically against that substance. Antibodies, also known as immunoglobulins, are proteins that detect the presence of foreign substances and then initiate the process of neutralizing and eliminating the substance from the body. In doing so the antibodies trigger a series of reactions. When talking about such reactions, it is helpful to keep in mind that there are different types. Some are true allergies and some are sensitivities.

It is the IgE antibodies reacting with an allergen (pollen, mold, dust, etc.) that cause the release of histamine from cells in the body resulting in the typical symptoms we know as allergies. A food allergy may also be the result of producing an excess of immunoglobulin E (IgE). Some food allergies, on the other hand, are the result of immunoglobulin G (IgG). IgG is produced when there is incomplete absorption of digested food protein from the digestion tract. IgG forms complexes with absorbed food and this initiates a series of reactions that can affect many tissues and organs and results in symptoms.

Sensitivities are similar to allergies. Both are bodily reactions to environmental agents such as pollens, molds, dust, as well as foods. A sensitivity is a condition that may come and go with environmental changes, but allergies may be more permanent conditions. An allergic condition implies that an altered protein (an antibody) forms either in the blood or the tissues of the allergic person. A sensitivity does not imply the formation of an antigen-specific antibody in the sufferer, but may result from some other circumstance. A food-derived peptide can escape digestion and be absorbed intact into the bloodstream. In cow's milk it is called Beta-caso-morphine-7. When this happens, a food reaction occurs, but it won't show up on a standard lab test that measures the classical type of allergic reactions that looks for IgE or IgG antibodies. Most types of sensitivity reactions discussed in this book do not show positive on blood tests, skin scratch tests, or other immunologic tests, because these reactions are associated with digestive problems or a toxicity reaction. In either event, the final expression in the patient is a reaction that may range from unpleasant to dangerous in severity when this person is exposed to the offensive substance.

The most common allergy tests available are RAST (radioallergosorbent test), ELISA (enzyme-linked immunosorbent assay), the skin test, or any other immunological test that shows a positive response to report that an allergic problem exists. By clinical standards, if there is no positive response to these types of tests, what is being tested is not an "allergy." However even these tests are not perfect and frequently miss the diagnosis of a true food allergy.

It is often the person with symptoms who gets caught in the middle. It is frustrating to spend money on allergy tests only to have the results show nothing conclusive. It becomes easy to believe that the substances being tested are not causing any problems. Nothing could be further from the truth. The majority of people who have reactions to foods have food sensitivities, not allergies. You can have several major food sensitivities that are causing symptoms and they will not show up on a conventional allergy test.

This may explain why the conventional allergy tests are not adequate to test this type of food reaction. Perhaps 10-30 percent of the food reactions are of this type. Since there is no evidence of the allergic reaction (IgE, IgG) in many people with food sensitivities, doctors often conclude that these people are suffering from an emotional disorder. The doctors just don't know what to look for and don't do the correct tests. Instead of being treated for the actual problem of food sensitivities, these people may end up on drugs used for treating emotional problems.

Considerable evidence exists that food sensitivities occur when the digestive system does not function properly. Most people are unaware of the association of foods with reactions because of the delayed symptoms. They may not appear for several hours up to several days. Typically, food sensitivities are temporary and disappear when the reactive foods are eliminated from the diet for a short time and when dietary habits are improved.

People may have reactions to a specific substance, such as a dog or a plant, but other individuals seem to be highly reactive to a wide variety of substances. There are two major types of allergic reactions we are concerned with when dealing with true allergies: Type-I immediate reaction, and Type-IV delayed reaction.

Type-I: Immediate Reaction

WHEN DOES THIS TYPE OF REACTION OCCUR?

Ten to twenty percent of the general population develop symptoms within minutes of eating certain foods or within several hours after contact with an allergen. These types of reactions are usually obvious since they are immediate. The symptoms are often very violent, and sometimes even life-threatening. Variability in reaction time is caused by differences in the absorption of food allergens from the intestinal tract. Consequently, several hours may pass between eating and the appearance of symptoms.

WHAT ANTIBODY IS THIS REACTION ASSOCIATED WITH?

A Type-I reaction is often associated with the antibody IgE. High levels of IgE antibodies reacting to specific antigens causes this immediate type of reaction. After allergens are absorbed into the blood through the lungs, skin, or intestines, they cause the B-lymphocytes cells (white blood cells) of the allergy sufferer to produce billions of molecules of the allergic antibody IgE. The IgE molecules then travel through the bloodstream until they combine with mast cells or basophils. Mast cells, which line many blood vessels, and basophils, a type of white blood cell circulating in the blood stream, are the storage sites for histamine and serotonin. The IgE allergic antibody then causes the cell membranes of the mast cells and basophils to become "leaky," allowing their storage load of histamine and serotonin to pour into the surrounding blood and tissues. The IgE-released histamine and serotonin produce the familiar allergic symptoms.

WHAT ARE SOME OF THE SYMPTOMS?

Immediate Type-I reactions include rashes, hives, headache, intestinal disorders, allergic rhinitis (hay fever), allergic asthma, and bronchial asthma. Such a reaction increases vasodilation, capillary permeability, and smooth muscle contraction, thus manifesting itself as sinus congestion with watery discharge, sneezing, itching eyes, rashes, digestive upset, and other breathing difficulties. Usually, each time the offending food is eaten, the symptoms occur. The most common foods causing this type of reaction are dairy, fish and shellfish, nuts, corn, wheat, peanuts, strawberries, green peas and eggs.

WHEN IS IT BEST TO USE THIS TYPE OF TEST?

Allergy tests using IgE antibodies are often used in the diagnosis of inhalant allergens, such as pollen, dust, and mold. This test is not very accurate for food testing.

Do you ever outgrow this type of reaction?

Food allergies indicated by IgE tend to be permanent and remain reactive throughout life. Total avoidance or desensitization to these allergens is the best treatment, especially if the allergic symptoms are severe.

Type-IV: Delayed Reactions

When does this type of reaction occur?

Food allergy reactions believed to be cell-mediated by IgG are produced in response to absorption of incompletely digested food proteins from the digestive tract. IgG forms complexes with absorbed food and this initiates a series of reactions that can affect many tissues and organs resulting in symptoms. They occur between 12 to 48 hours after exposure. This type of reaction is difficult to discover since they can occur as late as 72 hours after eating the food making it very difficult to diagnose which food is the offender. In delayed reactions, it is believed that the products formed during the digestive process are responsible for the reaction. This type of allergy is often called a masked allergy or hidden food allergy.

What antibody is this reaction associated with?

In Type-IV reactions the blood levels of antibodies known as IgG4 are often elevated. These high levels usually indicate frequent exposure to specific foods. Adverse reactions may occur if one continues to eat these foods.

What are some of the symptoms?

Common symptoms include chronic fatigue, arthritis, hives, eczema, and many other chronic symptoms such as migraine headaches, bronchial asthma and cerebral allergies.

When is it best to use this type of test?

Most hidden food allergies are revealed by using a test specific for the detection of IgG4.

What if the test does not reveal any allergies?

Food-derived peptides can escape digestion and be absorbed intact into the bloodstream. When this happens, a food reaction occurs, but it won't show up on lab tests that measure IgE or IgG antibodies. We call these types of reactions sensitivities.

Some authorities believe specific food sensitivities are a metabolic toxicity resulting from an intestinal disorder. Symptoms may result from reduced enzyme concentrations either inherited or acquired, and from intestinal bacterial endotoxins. Specific food residues are broken down by the colon's microflora resulting in the production of toxic chemicals. In susceptible individuals with low concentrations of relevant liver enzymes these toxins then pass into the general circulation to produce distant symptoms.

HOW LONG DO FOOD SENSITIVITIES OCCUR?

Food sensitivities are usually temporary and disappear with the elimination of the reactive foods from the diet along with improved dietary habits. These foods can be reintroduced without reoccurrence of symptoms by the process of rotating foods in the diet and properly cooking and combining foods. This process is the most effective way of preventing food sensitivities from developing.

WHAT FOODS CAUSE THE MOST REACTIONS?

Any food can cause a reaction, but some foods are more likely to cause problems. Eating the same food frequently can create sensitivities. In Japan, rice is the most common allergen. In Scandinavia, fish is the most common allergen. In the United States the most common allergens are dairy, beef, wheat, corn, eggs, chocolate, peanuts, and sugar.

WHAT ARE SOME SYMPTOMS RESULTING FROM SENSITIVITIES?

It is not uncommon to see symptoms such as fatigue, headaches, stomach pain, itching, digestive upsets, sinus congestion, flu-like symptoms, aching muscles and joints, bedwetting, hyperactivity, and irritability. Symptoms can also manifest as mental or emotional disturbances. Food sensitivities may also cause a person to be more reactive to other allergens such as to molds, dust, pollens, chemicals, and pollution. Adverse responses to foods can deeply disturb various delicate balances in the body.

HOW RELIABLE ARE FOOD TESTS?

The first step in the treatment of any allergy or sensitivity is to determine the major offenders. Tests are only clues, so interpret them cautiously. There are several methods of testing for allergies and sensitivities, but no one method is ideal for all groups of allergens. Skin or blood testing for food allergies is often inaccurate. The most dependable skin tests for food allergies give accurate results only 30-40 percent of the time. More than half the tests turn out to be false positives—they tell you you're allergic, but when you eat the food you feel fine. Some people never learn whether they have allergies or sensitivities to foods. If you want to test yourself, the elimination diet may be the best way to detect which foods are really causing the problems. Some other less conventional tests involve a great deal of time and attention to detail. These tests can have drawbacks with conclusions based more on subjective, rather than objective criteria. Nevertheless, they can and do pick up environmental and food sensitivities missed on the IgG or IgE tests.

Regardless of the classification scheme used, these reactions are representative of an improperly functioning body. The failure of the immune system or the digestive tract to function properly can present some of the most challenging clinical problems.

POOR DIETARY HABITS

Foods can also cause problems other than allergies and sensitivities. Some people have low blood sugar reactions, especially from the over consumption of sugar and white bread. There are also enzyme deficiency syndromes that could be causing symptoms. These enzymes include the intolerance of alcohol in North American Indians, intolerance to gluten in people with celiac disease, or a lactose intolerance in those who do not have the enzyme to digest the lactose in milk.

Different Types of Reactions

CYCLIC

This describes a variable state in which a small or medium portion of food or exposure to another allergic substance can be tolerated at one sitting. But if a large portion is eaten or exposure occurs two or three days in a row, a reaction occurs. About 80 percent of all sensitivities are cyclic. With the avoidance of the foods for six months or more, most of the sensitivity is lost. However, eating the foods frequently again will renew the sensitivity.

Food sensitivities are much more common than fixed allergies, but they are harder to recognize and often go undetected. Since they are usually caused by an inability of the body to handle the foods in the amount or frequency eaten, eating the food less often decreases the chance of a reaction.

CROSS-SENSITIVE

Foods may be categorized into families. An intolerance to one member of a food family may cause or predispose an individual to react to other members of that family.

CUMULATIVE

Symptoms occur when exposed to two or more substances at the same time, but do not occur if exposed to each substance individually.

FIXED

A few substances may exist that provoke reactions no matter how infrequent they are eaten or how much is consumed at a time. These fixed or permanent food allergies cause obvious allergic reactions every time they are eaten. Avoid the food until desensitization takes place.

ALLERGY TESTS

One of the most perplexing problem confronting some doctors today is the fact that people suffer from symptoms of unknown origin. Allergies and hypersensitivities fall into this category. There is much confusion about food allergies and food sensitivities, as well as the reasons why people have problems with airborne and environmental substances. Many highly qualified professionals devote their entire professional lives to determining and treating problems caused by the foods and additives we eat, as well as by the chemicals and other toxins in our environment. It is their belief that these substances are the source of the majority of illnesses.

Commonly Used Tests for Allergies and Sensitivities

The following are the types of tests you might come across when looking for ways to detect food, chemical, and airborne allergies and sensitivities. These tests are as controversial as the whole field of food allergies and sensitivities. The most commonly available tests for determining reactivity to specific substances are listed below. Each method has its limitations and the particular test you take can make all the difference in the results you get.

ELISA (ENZYME-LINKED IMMUNOSORBENT ASSAY)

Current state-of-the-art technology provides the most accurate and affordable testing for people with immediate (IgE) or delayed (IgG4) allergies. There are panels available covering most of the foods, spices, and environmental allergies. The ELISA test alleviates the stress of elimination/challenge diets in trying to determine which foods are causing the problem. It is probably the best laboratory guideline for the therapeutic treatment of allergies today.

IgG and IgG complex mediators are involved in 80 percent of all food allergy reactions. IgG also has a circulating half life nearly 20 times longer than that of IgE. ELISA is used to identify delayed reactions that cannot be detected using conventional tests such as RAST or skin prick testing.

Using the highly sensitive ELISA technology, a single blood sample is assayed to detect both IgE and IgG mediated allergies. Results reveal the likely causes of immediate anaphylactic reactions, as well as the sources of delayed reactions (hidden allergies). This approach allows the doctor and patient to see the different immune reactions of the body toward a particular substance.

RAST (RADIOALLERGOSORBENT TEST)

RAST is a conventional allergy test. It is performed in a test tube and evaluates IgE elevation in response to specific antigens. Some say it is very good for airborne allergies, but not very accurate for food allergies. This is especially true if someone is on prednisone, has been fasting, or has avoided a particular food for a long time. The test will not detect other types of immune responses or food sensitivities caused by a digestive problem.

If you are looking for an IgE-mediated allergy, this test may be helpful, but it is expensive and limited to only one type of reaction with many false negatives. This means that a food could be causing problems and not show up on this test. Few food allergies are considered immediate or (Type I) IgE mediated. It is also limited in scope and not a cost-effective way of testing.

Another problem with this test is that you must already have a good idea of what the allergy is. It can quickly get expensive to have substances tested at random. Initially, only test common foods such as milk, eggs, wheat, yeast, and citrus. It is also best to test for any favorite foods since these are frequently the problem. For best results, eat the foods for three days before testing.

Food allergies produced by IgE tend to be permanent. Total avoidance of these foods is the best treatment, especially if the symptoms are severe. Some physicians provide immunotherapy to desensitize patients to these foods. This way the person can again enjoy their favorite foods.

CYTOTOXIC TEST

This is an IgG-mediated test. Cytotoxic testing is a laboratory procedure that observes the reactions of living white blood cells, red blood cells, and platelets when exposed to different foods and chemicals. This test checks the immune response of the body in relationship to different foods. It is based on the principle that extracts of foods will induce damage to white blood cells in the test tube. With one blood sample, a lab can test hundreds of foods quickly for their intolerance potential. After interpretation of the test, diet recommendations are useful. Usually it is best to rotate the foods or avoid them to eliminate any adverse reaction. This enables a person's immune response to return to normal.

There are advantages of IgG testing for delayed-onset allergies. Since the person does not need to be present, this test can't cause a reaction to the person being tested. Cytotoxic testing is also more convenient since technicians test many items at once. It is highly sensitive, reproducible, safe, and easy to transport. Some say it could be the best food allergy test done with blood, but it is expensive and the results depend on the experience of the technician. This makes it subject to more errors in interpretation. There are many false positives and false negatives.

The results from the RAST and Cytotoxic tests are rarely the same when compared to each other. You can have a positive reaction to wheat on the RAST test and find it negative on the Cytotoxic test. This is because we are dealing with different types of immune responses. The results of these two types of tests may also differ with the results of sensitivity testing done by electro-dermal machines. It does make for much confusion.

ELECTRO-DERMAL TESTS

There are devices used to detect food sensitivities, but they are not used by most mainstream doctors. This is indeed unfortunate. Qualified and licensed health practitioners, such as naturopathic physicians, can give you more information on this type of testing and what kind of results you can expect. Just because a testing method has not been proven to be "scientific" doesn't mean that it doesn't work or provide reliable information.

Electro-dermal testing for food sensitivities has developed over the last thirty years. It is a technique derived from Oriental acupuncture theory to gain information about a wide range of diseases and deficiencies. The process is painless, rapid, and precise. No needles or invasive methods are used. The technique involves the use of an electronic instrument with a hand-held electrode that applies a weak direct current to the person's body. By measurement of this current at certain terminal points of the acupuncture meridians (hands and feet), the therapist can gain valuable information about the influence of different substances on the person's body. Various substances to be tested (food, chemicals, etc.) are placed in an electrical circuit. It is possible to test most substances with an electro-dermal machine, including inhalants, foods, chemicals, vitamins, medications, and heavy metals. This procedure for measuring changes in skin resistance can be compared to an EKG (electrocardiogram).

Germany and other parts of Europe commonly use this type of testing. Currently, this type of testing is gaining credibility as similar machines are being developed in the United States. The findings obtained by electro-dermal testing are verified by data gained independently from a patient's case history or by improvement in the patient's overall situation.

ELIMINATION-THEN-CHALLENGE DIET

The elimination-then-challenge diet is one way of removing dietary stress and allowing the body to heal. This test involves completely removing a suspected food, or several foods, from the diet and closely observing if symptoms improve. Later, the food is reintroduced to see if the original symptoms reappear. In this way you can determine what foods cause allergies. This is one of the most simple and economical methods, but it is not always successful because most people have problems with several unsuspected foods. The test is also very subjective, time-consuming, and only useful to people who have noticeable symptoms. See the chapter "Diets Used To Detect & Treat Allergies" for more information.

JAR TEST

This is usually a good test for inhalant or brain allergies caused by perfumes, cleaning products, fabric, carpet, flowers, house dust, animal dander, or mold. Put the allergen suspected of causing the problem in a jar. Leave the jar in the sun for a short time. Take off the lid and smell the substance. Note any reaction that may occur. It can take thirty minutes after exposure before there are changes in the brain and symptoms begin. It can take minutes, hours, or days before the symptoms disappear. This test will easily verify any suspected inhalant allergies. Being exposed every day to the same substance can cause continuous symptoms.

PULSE TEST

This test is based on the reactions of two closely spaced feedings after a period of avoidance. Absolutely avoid any form of the food for at least four days before testing, but not more than ten days. When omitting many of the basic foods such as corn, wheat, yeast, egg, milk, beef and pork, be aware that many commercially prepared products contain these ingredients. During a period of food avoidance, it is common to have withdrawal symptoms that usually clear by the end of the third day.

Before starting this test, write down all the symptoms experienced, such as stuffy nose, cough, throat clearing, sneezing, tiredness, fatigue, headache, itching any place, nausea, vomiting, diarrhea, abdominal cramps, urinary frequency and behavior problems. The types of symptoms will vary according to the problem. During the middle of the day on the fifth or sixth day of avoidance set aside two hours for performing the test. During this two-hour period avoid other activities.

Take and record your pulse (or the pulse of the individual being tested) for one full minute before eating. Place two fingers over the artery just inside the wrist of the opposite hand, but don't use your thumb because it has a pulse of its own. Then eat an ordinary serving of one specific food at the designated time, within a five-minute period. Make sure to eat only the test food. Do not add anything to the food, not even salt. If the food needs to be cooked, then use glass or stainless steel pans and utensils. Use only distilled water during cooking.

Now, take and record the pulse for one full minute after finishing eating, and again twenty, forty, and sixty minutes following the meal. If the pulse goes above eighty-four beats per minute, or if there is a variation of more than ten beats per minute, this would suggest an offending food. Observe any symptoms during these intervals and write them down as they occur.

A pulse increase without symptoms indicates a probable sensitivity. If definite symptoms do occur, the test is positive for that particular food. Observe any symptoms that occur over the next 30 minutes. If you do not observe any symptoms, include the test food with the next meal. Watch for delayed symptoms during the night or the next day.

The main disadvantage of this test is that only one body function is being considered, a change in heartbeat. One-third of allergy-prone people will have an increase in pulse rate while another one-third will experience a decrease. The other third will experience no change. This response may differ at various times depending on what foods are consumed. The pulse test is valid only if there is a definite, consistent change in the pulse rate. Another confusing factor is that you can have a reaction to a food for as long as three days after eating it. The pulse test is not 100 percent reliable for a diagnosis of an allergy or sensitivity, but it is a good place to start. It gives you one possible way to determine a food reaction.

If any food test is positive and the symptoms are especially uncomfortable, it is advisable to take a natural laxative to clear the intestinal system of the offending food. You may want to contact your physician before starting any self-test so you will have something on hand to neutralize any possible food reaction.

Skin Scratch Test or Intradermal Testing

A small amount of the allergic substance is injected either near the surface of the skin or between skin layers and any reaction is noted. Scores of tiny scratches made on the person's back or arms should indicate which foods are the problem. This type of testing for food allergies or sensitivities is a waste of time. There is at least a 50 percent chance of false positives and negatives. Skin tests are more valid for determining certain inhalant allergies such as dust, mold, grasses, weeds, cats, and dogs.

The scratch test is also time-consuming and invasive. Often, one reaction will mask another, or the test will fail to pick up a powerful sensitivity to a certain food. This test has become obsolete by most informed physicians because of its inaccuracy, especially to foods.

SUBLINGUAL TESTING

Various concentrated extracts are placed under the tongue, one at a time. These potent extracts are absorbed quickly and any reactions are observed. This test has become obsolete because of the possibility of a severe reaction by the person being tested.

WHITE BLOOD CELL ANALYSIS

A laboratory test, called a complete blood count (CBC) measures the level of a white blood cell called an eosinophil. This particular blood cell can elevate above normal when having an allergic reaction or if there is a parasitic infection in the body. If this eosinophil cell is elevated and you also have chronic health problems, then explore the possibility of hidden allergies.

WITHDRAWAL SYMPTOMS

This test is based on the reactions that occur after the avoidance of a food. Withdrawal symptoms suggest a probable positive reaction to the particular food being avoided.

Blood tests for allergies, especially for foods, have their limits. Few studies have been performed on the incidence of false positives and false negatives concerning these different tests, but it appears that the incidence may be quite high. Many people bring in food allergy reports that do not correlate with the foods causing problems detected by an elimination diet. Relying only on blood tests may not be a good idea, especially if you are not getting results from the information provided. If you don't know what the test is really testing for, you will not be able to correctly interpret the results. When considering any test, it is important to have some idea of their accuracy.

CHAPTER 2

What Causes Allergies and Sensitivities?

O ver the last hundred years, our world has undergone drastic changes. The biggest changes in the food industry have been the refining of food, the use of food additives, and the increased consumption of animal products. We also have many more atmospheric pollutants. This additional burden on the body contributes enormously to the prevalence of allergic-type symptoms. The incidence of allergies and sensitivities may be greater than the incidence of any other type of illness affecting people.

A person who suffers from various unrelated symptoms that produce a multitude of minor, chronic complaints is a prime candidate for allergies. Besides food, one should consider chemical, pollution, and other environmental sources as possible causes. The following is a list of factors that make the body susceptible to allergies and sensitivities:

- adrenal insufficiency, exhaustion
- stimulants (coffee, tea, etc.)
- poor bowel elimination
- excessively acidic diet
- bad diet in infancy
- digestive enzyme deficiency
- toxic chemical exposure
- environmental toxic overload
- food additives, preservatives
- increased intestinal permeability
- pollution inside/outside home
- toxic overload
- not chewing food adequately
- pesticides
- improper cooking of foods
- liver congestion
- food addiction
- hypoglycemia (low blood sugar)
- drug use and abuse
- eating same foods
- immune deficiency
- eating during an illness
- junk-food diet
- *Candida albicans* (yeast)
- vegetable and fruit deficiency
- heavy-metal poisoning
- stress and emotional conflict
- refined carbohydrates and sugar
- vitamin and mineral imbalances
- overeating or undereating
- parasites
- abnormal gut flora
- histamine release
- vaccines

Certain people develop sensitivities to normally harmless substances, resulting in symptoms affecting any part of the body. Such sensitivities could affect digestion or breathing, they might have the pain of arthritis or headaches, or they may suffer from depression. The list is endless. Symptoms usually occur only after repeated exposure to the offending substance. Some of the most common conditions and symptoms are:

- aches and pains
- colitis
- eczema or skin rash
- fatigue, headaches
- hyperactivity
- menstrual disorders
- sinusitis

- arthritis
- cramps
- edema
- heart palpitations
- itching ears/throat/skin
- nausea
- psoriasis

- acne
- ear infections
- being emotional
- hives
- learning problems
- runny nose, sneezing
- stomach pains

The following is a list of some of the more common causes of allergies and sensitivities.

DIET OF AN INFANT

Until about four to six months of age, a human infant cannot digest any food except breast milk About that time the intestines become lined with a substance that produces the digestive enzymes necessary for the proper digestion of starches. A food introduced to infants too early in their development will not digest properly and can leak through the lining of the intestine into other parts of their bodies. The immune system doesn't recognize this undigested food as a "normal" part of the body and treats the foreign food particles as an enemy, and attacking them as if they were unfriendly germs. The child's immune system never gets a chance to develop fully. As a result, this immature, struggling system weakens, gets confused, and develops an intolerance for prematurely eaten foods.

Children who are breast fed usually eat fewer starches and get a better diet than those who aren't. This gives them a healthier start in life. If the mother is also watching her diet and not eating the wrong foods, the baby's risk of illness is significantly reduced. Unfortunately, many infants usually start out life with the wrong diet. What foods do we feed an infant who is not breast fed? Commonly, a baby is given cow's milk sweetened with corn syrup or dextrose-maltose (both from grain), pabulum (also from grain), dry toast and teething biscuits (more grain), egg yolk, and soy milk. What are the most common food sensitivities? Not surprisingly, they're milk, wheat, corn, egg, sugar, and soy. It is essential that the first foods given to an infant are introduced at the right time in their development and in as close to a natural state as possible.

Some infants are highly sensitive to foods the nursing mother is eating. The food's allergic properties can come through the breast milk to affect the baby. About the time children are weaned from breast milk, their diet increases in allergy-causing foods. Most adverse reactions from eating these new foods go unrecognized. An intolerant food eaten by a child often continues to be eaten into adulthood. The child usually recovers from any acute symptoms, but as an adult will have chronic problems that may persist. Additional symptoms start to develop and worsen if the food sensitivity goes unrecognized. The symptoms that were minor at the beginning may develop into conditions such as arthritis, hives, irritable bowel, or migraines.

The Incomplete Digestion of Protein

When foods, particularly their protein components, do not completely digest they act as allergens. When these components absorb into the body, the immune system does not recognize them as nutritional and beneficial. It responds protectively by producing antibodies to that food and starting a series of reactions affecting many tissues and organs. The results can be allergies and sensitivities to various foods.

If a food only partially breaks down, especially the protein content from gluten (grains) and casein (dairy), the result could be the production of toxins in the digestive tract. If absorbed into the blood and transported across the blood-brain barrier, these proteins could also produce behavioral abnormalities. The proteins could come from any food that does not break down adequately in the digestive tract. Technically, we are not really sensitive to foods, but to incompletely digested foods. Consuming sugar, caffeine, alcohol, and taking drugs can upset the body's chemistry causing undigested foods to get into the bloodstream resulting in more food allergies and sensitivities.

The Detoxification System

Being hypersensitive depends on a person's hereditary predisposition, environmental vulnerability, individual biochemistry, and the toxic load at a particular time. The causes of hypersensitivity are different for each individual because everyone has their own unique total toxic load. If an individual's detoxification system works efficiently, then a fair amount of these toxic agents do not cause a problem. If there is a large toxic burden, even the best system does not work well enough and the individual gets sick. If the system is impaired due to genetic or nutritional defects, the body will simply store large amounts of these toxic agents. Then the detoxification system cannot function at its optimum and becomes overloaded and intolerant to new irritants.

It is interesting that modern medicine tries to treat everyone with allergies as if they all had the same problem. They ignore the fact that once the body becomes overloaded and unable to handle the incoming toxins, further exposure causes a back-up of toxic metabolites that damage regulatory enzymes and proteins. Due to the over processing of foods and poor dietary choices, there is a decline in the consumption of nutrients that are necessary for these pathways to function correctly. It's hard for our body to work properly when it is being fed industrialized, excessively processed, and chemically-laden foods.

CELIAC DISEASE

In some cases there is so much damage to the intestinal lining that a disease called "sprue" or "celiac disease" develops. A person has an intolerance to gluten-containing grains. This causes malabsorption of any grain containing this protein. Because of the damage to the intestinal lining, other foods may not be tolerated either, such as foods that are raw or rich in fiber. The digestive tract becomes irritated and the intestinal villi lose their normal ability to function, resulting in decreased absorption. The bowel walls become thin and allow toxic substances into the bloodstream resulting in allergic reactions.

PARASITES

A parasitic infection in the intestinal tract can cause symptoms that are hard to diagnose. Warning signs include constipation, diarrhea, gas and bloating, irritable bowel syndrome, muscle aches and pains, anemia, allergies, skin conditions, nervousness, peptic ulcers, sleep disturbances, chronic fatigue, and other immune dysfunctions. Low stomach acid is thought to predispose people to the bacteria overgrowth of *Helicobacter pylori*. It is also thought that *H. pylori* may be one cause of food allergies, ulcers, and yeast overgrowth. Sensitivity to organisms that inhabit the gastrointestinal tract has long been thought to be a cause of allergic reactions. Laboratory tests can determine if parasites are present.

IMPROPER DOSAGE OF VITAMINS AND MINERALS

Supplementing with the improper dosage of vitamins and minerals can unbalance the body's chemistry and cause reactions. Common examples of incorrect usage would be giving high doses of B-complex vitamins to fast oxidizers and giving copper to a slow oxidizer. A particular nutrient in a food such as the high copper levels in soybeans can cause a reaction to that food if there is already excessive copper in the body.

COSMETICS

Eliminate cosmetic sensitivities simply by avoiding products that provoke a reaction. Be aware that many chemical substances absorb through the skin directly into the blood stream. The chemical ingredients in cosmetics are the cause of many problems on or near the areas they touch. Symptoms such as headaches, sinusitis, or sore throats may not even seem related.

DRUGS AND VACCINES

Another common cause of allergies is the use of drugs and vaccines. It is common to see skin diseases such as eczema and psoriasis occur soon after a vaccination or repeated vaccinations. The cells providing us with a normal immune function can be damaged by many vaccines, some drugs, and massive chemical exposure. The thymus gland that supplies these cells is also damaged. Antibiotics are famous for allergic skin reactions that can be difficult to resolve. Once a foreign substance enters the body, whatever the route, the possibility of allergic reactions increases.

It is hard to tell what comes first: the deficient immune system, the allergic child, or antibiotic overuse. Is the child born with undiagnosed food allergies and sensitivities causing symptoms such as ear infections that are treated with antibiotics? Could it be that the overuse of antibiotics causes an immune deficiency and allergies? Does it really matter which came first? The important thing is to treat the underlying cause and not just suppress the symptoms.

THE IMPROPER COOKING OF FOODS

There is good evidence that the longer food cooks the more difficult it is to digest and metabolize. Foods cooked at high temperatures stay in the gut longer, making them more difficult to digest. We have been eating foods for centuries with certain chemical configurations. Food heated past a certain point will change in its configuration so much that the body does not understand the new chemical makeup of the food. Our bodies do not have the enzymes to digest these new chemical structures easily.

Processes that drive up the temperature to the point of change are deep-frying, pasteurization, and barbecuing. If food is cooked past 112 degrees, the enzymes in the food will not be available and you have to use your body's enzymes to digest the food. The body's enzymes certainly help to digest foods, but becomes taxed if overused. The immune system becomes activated when these over-cooked foods are eaten. It should be keeping foreign evaders away, not having to deal with undigested food. If the immune system is capable, it will do what the digestive system cannot. It will treat the undigested food as a foreign invader and try to rid the body of these particles by escorting them out of the body. When the immune system is called on continuously to repeat this action, it becomes exhausted and unavailable to protect us from infection and illness.

Some people find they cannot tolerate foods raw, but can eat them cooked. Others find they cannot tolerate foods cooked twice. An example would be to not have a reaction to the roast beef on Sunday, but the roast made into Shepherd's pie on Monday causes indigestion. You might find that you tolerate certain foods in small amounts, but not large amounts. Sometimes it may be the frequency with which you eat a particular food.

Do not use aluminum utensils or cookware when preparing food. This toxic metal can get into the food and cause various toxic side effects in the body. Do not use microwave ovens to prepare your meals. It may be the latest in technology, but it disturbs chemical bonds found in food. These bonds are necessary for the proper recognition and assimilation of food.

FOOD-CHAIN TOXINS

The chemical diets and drugs given to animals contribute to allergies. When we eat animal products we also eat everything the animal consumes. Antibiotics and hormones used in raising and treating animals end up in our food. A few years ago a certain allergy outbreak was traced to fish meal that was fed to pigs. The problem was a result of the fish having been treated with several chemicals and antibiotics. The widespread use of such toxins in the food supply has increased faster than our bodies can handle the toxic load. A string bean grown in Mexican soil and contaminated with several pesticides can cause a much different reaction to our body than a green bean grown on an organic farm. Which green bean is being tested when you have allergy tests?

GUT PERMEABILITY

The gut lining was thought to be an impermeable barrier to food proteins and large polypeptides. There is now evidence that these large molecules can and do pass through the human gut intact into the bloodstream, even in normal conditions. This intestinal permeability, known as "leaky gut syndrome," may help explain the effectiveness of enzyme therapy in the management of some food allergies and sensitivities.

Permeability changes occur as a result of several factors besides eating the wrong foods. These could include imbalances of the intestinal flora, chronic nutritional insufficiencies, and various bacterial and viral intestinal infections. The body depends on the natural barriers of the skin, lungs, and gastrointestinal tract to protect itself from toxic substances, a refined diet, medication, allergens, and a stressful lifestyle. Additional stressors such as eating food with low levels of fiber or having malabsorption and malnutrition problems also cause this permeability to change.

The inability to digest foods or derive adequate nutrition from them will weaken a growing child. The child then gets an antibiotic for an infection, often resulting in the colonization in the bowel of a yeast called *Candida albicans*. Yeast grow quickly in the intestinal tract and irritate the lining, causing it to become inflamed and less efficient in handling food. The walls of the intestines become even more permeable and start to allow more allergens through the intestinal lining which triggers more sensitivities.

A study that evaluated children for the effect of cow's milk on intestinal permeability found that most of the children had an increase in intestinal permeability. This means that more pathogens and antigens pass through the gut membrane into general circulation. The increased burden of toxic substances escaping from the intestinal tract places a big demand on an immature immune system. Such studies show that a child's early diet can lead to the development of food sensitivities.

People using chemotherapy and nonsteroid anti-inflammatory drugs such as ibuprofen and aspirin have a higher rate of intestinal permeability. Alcoholics also have elevated permeability that can persist in some cases for up to two weeks after drinking stops. Age is another factor that causes the intestinal barrier to become less efficient.

Why Do Sensitivities Vary?

Have you wondered how sensitivities can vary from day to day or month to month? The reason is that nutritional status, stress, and environmental factors all change constantly. These changes affect the immune response to any substance. A body that has a chronically stressed defense mechanism becomes increasingly susceptible. One of the most frustrating experiences is having repeated tests for allergies or sensitivities. Several months or years after one test, you discover that another test reveals a whole new set of substances. It makes sense to eliminate the allergens found in food, chemicals, drugs, and cosmetics, but if you do not strengthen your body's immune system, there will be other allergies and sensitivities.

Someone is more likely to react to a food, inhalant, or chemical if more than one allergen is present. People who avoid their food allergens tend to become less reactive to inhalants and vice versa. The desensitization against a tree pollen can also reduce the severity to food sensitivities. Reducing the total toxic load on the body is the key to decreasing symptoms.

Most people understand the concept of pain thresholds. There are people who can tolerate a lot of pain and there are also people who can't tolerate much pain at all. Individuals with allergies and sensitivities also have a threshold. There are people who are so sensitive to some foods that even smelling them causes a reaction. This is considered a low threshold for allergies or sensitivities.

Nutrition and Behavioral/Mental Disturbances

Today's food supply makes it easy to choose poor diets. Even in 1987 the *Journal of Applied Nutrition* suggested the connection between food and behavior. It is finally being accepted in some conventional medical practices as it has always been with holistic health practitioners. Vitamin deficiencies and the chemical contamination of food may be just as important as emotional stress in the development of mental and functional disorders. This relationship is being slowly accepted by the average medical doctor. They usually just dismiss nutrition-caused illnesses as irrelevant.

When Greece faced a starvation period during the Nazi occupation, there was a marked improvement in mental disorders among the population. Interestingly, many of their favorite foods, such as wheat and other gluten-containing grains, were unavailable. A sensitivity to gluten is thought to be linked to some forms of schizophrenia and paranoia. Following this idea, Russian researchers have used controlled fasting to treat patients with schizophrenia and other mental and physical illnesses. Only patients who did not respond to other treatments elsewhere were treated. The fast involved total abstinence from certain foods for twenty to thirty days. This treatment for chronic schizophrenia was effective in more than 84 percent of the cases.

California has recently approved legislation allowing studies to see if there is an association between nutrition and criminal behavior. This will include the use of a trace mineral analysis as a tool to determine the benefit of improved nutrition. Certain mineral patterns appear to be present in the criminal population. Type-A episodic criminal individuals have low zinc levels, high copper levels, and high manganese levels. In excess, these metals become toxic. Cadmium and lead are also highly toxic to the brain. It seems that the levels of lead and cadmium are in the 90+ percentile in the Type-A criminal.

Children who have behavior problems are often just put on a drug, such as Ritalin, instead of searching further for the source of the problem. One example is that of a young boy who lived near a smelter that was a source of many toxins. His copper levels were off the chart but his zinc levels were quite low. The zinc-copper ratio was one to one where ideally it should be eight or twelve to one. A deficiency of zinc helps copper become toxic. Copper is highly irritating to the body at high levels and can cause hyperexcitability and irrational behavior. His manganese levels were also in the ninetieth percentile. He was charged with attempted murder at the age of nine. In the past he had been on eight different medications to control his behavior and was presently on Ritalin. After a year of treatment to reduce his toxic metal levels, the boy returned to normal behavior without having to take any drugs.

Researchers have found an association between recurrent ear infection in infancy and later hyperactivity. Children with a history of ear infections usually receive repeated and prolonged courses of broad-spectrum antibiotic drugs. These drugs cause alterations in gut flora including the proliferation of *Candida albicans*. Changes in the gut's permeability promote the absorption of food antigens (allergies) that play a major role in causing hyperactivity and related behavior and learning problems.

Over the last decade similar conditions have manifested such as chronic fatigue syndrome and multiple chemical sensitivity. Attention deficit disorder (with or without hyperactivity) and other behavioral problems are epidemic in our children. Allergy problems such as asthma increase yearly in both frequency and severity. Cancers unrelated to smoking seem to be everywhere when compared to twenty years ago. Are these illnesses directly and indirectly the result of a toxic environment? Large segments of the population now seek alternative approaches for these problems, because the conventional drug-oriented medical system has few answers and may even contribute to the problem.

ALLERGIC-ADDICTIVE SYNDROME

Another major cause in the onset of allergies is that of a food becoming addictive. Consuming a food too frequently is usually what leads to food addiction. People crave the very food that worsens, or maintains, an abnormal body chemistry. Then, if they don't get a "fix" of that food, the withdrawal symptoms start, including depression, anxiety, and irritability. Most people begin craving the food and want to eat it often. It relieves the emotional symptoms and makes the sufferer feel better for the moment. This is why it is so easy to become addicted to your food sensitivities. Seldom is it realized that the food is harmful until the disturbance becomes quite advanced. The foods a person craves and eats most often, or consumes in large amounts, are the most likely ones to cause an adverse response.

One major reason it is so hard to let go of addictive substances is that they serve as survival tools over the years. For those who do not express their feelings easily, foods can blot out reality and insulate. They allow a person to cope with unpleasant situations and help them feel safe. An addictive food acts as a tranquilizer. It can be responsible for "brain fog," sleepiness, lethargy, and mood alteration. Some people discover at a very early age that they feel better after eating or drinking certain foods. In times of stress people seek out these very foods, not consciously knowing that they can alter moods and produce a sort of stupor. When a person is unhappy with life, it is not uncommon to use a particular food to maintain a comfort zone. Psychologists call these "comfort foods."

Why is it so hard to avoid these foods, so hard to kick the habit? When someone tries to get off the foods used to anesthetize their feelings, the old emotions emerge so rapidly that they are hard to deal with all at once. The person feels uncomfortable and unconsciously begins to eat again. Sometimes, it starts with a small quantity, then escalates to larger amounts. Others just binge uncontrollably. Then guilt begins to emerge for not being able to resist the food and some people eat even more to bury the guilt.

Some foods, especially milk, cheese, wheat, sugar, corn, and eggs act as our "friends." They are the coping mechanisms used to bury unrecognized and repressed emotions. This can be particularly unpleasant for the addicted individual. At first there may seem to be no connection between various foods and why a person suddenly becomes so emotional. It can even look as if they are losing their mind with symptoms such as frequent crying, feeling sullen, increased anger, having tantrums, or experiencing extreme fatigue. There seems to be no apparent reason to feel this way. Most people don't realize that it is really old emotional feelings needing expression.

Addiction-prone people often progress from sweets to alcohol and cigarettes, and sometimes stronger drugs. The process can reverse as an alcoholic sobers up and kicks the habit. Then they commonly switch addictions from alcoholic to "food-a-holic." Many people have non-sweet addictions such as for cheese, milk, and bread.

Once a person decides to eliminate from their diet the addictive food, they might feel worse for the first week, but then the old complaints begin to disappear, one at a time. Often, people don't know that they were depressed, experiencing fatigue, or that their symptoms were connected to food sensitivities until they quit eating their addictive foods. They are usually surprised to find themselves feeling much better emotionally and physically, with an increase in energy and well being.

Food addiction is treated like any food sensitivity, by avoiding the intolerant food until all symptoms disappear. At a later time, reintroduction of the food is usually possible without the reoccurrence of the previous symptoms. A favorite food is usually the one responsible for the symptoms. It is called the allergic-addictive syndrome.

Certain nutritional supplements and homeopathic medicines can help overcome the ill effects and the misuse of these foods. Support groups are important in this healing process. We need others to talk to, to discuss how we feel. Codependency groups are everywhere. Check out ACOA, Co-dependents Anonymous, The 12 Steps of Alcoholics Anonymous, or Overeaters Anonymous.

CHAPTER 3

Brain Allergies

To understand what a brain allergy is, it is helpful to discuss what happens with a "normal" allergy. An allergy or sensitivity to a specific substance can cause inflammation of the tissues resulting in swelling and tenderness. When an allergic reaction occurs in the brain, the swelling and inflammation happen inside the skull. The brain can't produce a rash and can't sneeze or wheeze, but it does reacts through changes in thought, mood, and behavior. Brain allergies may cause a wide variety of symptoms that look like mental disorders. Thousands of people find themselves labeled neurotic and psychotic simply because doctors don't know what to look for or take the time to do the correct tests.

At first, brain allergies usually act like regular allergies or sensitivities. They make you feel sick or give you hives, asthma, or diarrhea. After a while you start to crave the food that triggers the allergy. The foods involved are usually the ones that a person craves and eats in large amounts over a long period of time. Once the craving for the food becomes strong, it can trigger other reactions of the nervous system such as depression, confusion, and the inability to function normally. A change in behavior and attitude are often early signs of a reaction. Brain allergies may also be related to heavy metal toxins, imbalances in the blood sugar, adrenal insufficiency, additives, odors, and of course, foods.

In 1971, the first mental illness program was established to detect brain allergies. These doctors found that 90 percent of the patients admitted to institutions had this problem. Wheat and milk proved to be major factors triggering allergic brain responses. Any food, inhalant, or environmental chemical could provoke these severe mental symptoms. Fifty percent of the schizophrenia patients who did not respond well to the traditional therapy were found to have brain allergies. Research continues to support the involvement of wheat and dairy as problems for schizophrenics.

When a child complains at school of various symptoms such as headaches, dizziness, or feeling feverish, what does the school nurse do? She takes the child's temperature. If it's normal, the nurse returns the child to class labeled as a "troublemaker." The most common symptoms of brain allergies in children are fatigue, aggression, irritability, tantrums, mood swings, sleeplessness, depression, hyperactivity, learning disorders, and the inability to concentrate. Since the mind and body are connected, the child may also have physical symptoms such as intestinal problems, a runny nose, swollen glands, glassy eyes, restless legs, facial pallor, or allergic shiners (red or purple coloration below the lower eyelid). It is common to hear complaints about odors, or that the child is experiencing some muscular aches and pains.

In adults, brain allergies frequently manifest themselves as manic-depressive disorders, hyperactivity, anxiety, and various phobias. It is also common to see symptoms such as headaches or migraines, lethargy, loss of appetite, decreased sex drive, and insomnia. Brain allergies can also result in physical symptoms such as arthritis, skin and nerve problems, ulcers and other stomach disorders. Any reaction to foods, inhalants, and chemicals can trigger a response within the brain. Someone can have several major food sensitivities without knowing it. It is thought that for every food sensitivity found there may be at least two hidden. Ordinary foods such as milk, eggs, and wheat can cause some people to act drunk, suffer epileptic seizures, seem confused, and even attempt suicide.

In the majority of central nervous system allergies a copper imbalance plays a vital role. High levels of copper are toxic and may be a principal cause of brain allergies. Hair mineral analysis can identify this imbalance. Excess copper can cause a zinc deficiency which may result in a rise in tissue sodium levels. A high sodium level is responsible for many of the symptoms associated with brain allergies. In adults, high sodium levels frequently manifest themselves as an emotional disorder. The way to handle central nervous system allergies is the same way as handling other allergies. Identify and treat any imbalances in the body's chemistry and avoid the offending substance.

People may think you're crazy when you tell them that a brief exposure to someone's perfume ruins your whole day. Changes in brain chemistry can occur after exposure. It can take up to thirty minutes from the time of substance exposure before there is a change in the brain's chemistry. Some people have trouble thinking and concentrating, or they behave very emotionally. The time to get over the reaction can sometimes take weeks. This is really a problem if there is daily exposure. As houses become tighter and people have increased chemical exposure, the risk factors increase. Houses formerly exchanged their air at least once each hour, but now they are airtight.

When something is smelled, the signal travels up the nose by the olfactory nerve and the odor affects the brain. Sensitive individuals, when exposed to common chemicals, can have brain changes so severe that they cause brain injury. Glutamate and aspartate compounds that have fewer than four to five carbon units tend to set off these reactions. Some common substances that cause reactions are formaldehyde, methyl ketone, ethyl ketone, and acetone. The smelling of something that releases the aspartate and glutamate molecules can have a powerful reaction inside the brain, causing a reduction in thinking, concentration, and memory. Symptoms may also include fatigue, depression, muscle weakness, and the inability to exercise. If a child's handwriting, drawing, or behavior show signs of uncharacteristic deterioration, teachers are likely to call the problem psychological. They label the child as hyperactive or as having attention deficit syndrome. Then, they often recommend that the child be put on one of the current drugs for this condition. What if the inappropriate activity and behavior are not psychiatric, but due to food, chemical, or environmental toxins? School officials need to be more attentive to all complaints and recognize that children's symptoms may be telling us important clues about what is really going on with their health.

There are several ways to isolate the allergic or intolerant substance—both testing and treatments are available. One method of testing used by many naturopathic physicians is the electrodermal method of determining sensitivities. It does not use needles or electric shock. Instead, it involves the measurement of changes in skin resistance using certain points on the hand. This method can test virtually any substance, including pollens, foods, chemicals, vitamins, and medications.

People get bounced among many doctors without success. They receive a variety of diagnoses, ranging from depression to hyperactivity. With the identification and removal of specific substances from the diet or environment, their moods improve, their emotions level out, and their minds clear. Tension, stress, and sleeplessness will simply disappear. These sufferers feel like completely new people. So, the next time you feel depressed, anxious, irritable, or too emotional, look for the solution as close as your grocery shopping cart or the odors around you. If you suspect your health problems may be allergy related, don't just give up. Call your holistic-minded health practitioner for more information.

CHAPTER 4

Hyperactivity, Behavior Problems and Attention- Deficit Disorder

I t's hard to recall even one hyperactive child or anyone having the symptoms of attention deficit syndrome back in the 1950s. Now, you find many of them in every classroom, as any teacher will confirm. One child out of every five suffers from varying degrees of behavior problems. Presently, there are about four million children taking Ritalin, or a similar drug, to control difficult behavior. Surveys show a greater incidence in boys than girls with onset usually by the age of three, but diagnosis is generally after the child starts school. Something is seriously wrong when so many children must be drugged to control their behavior. No responsible person can feel comfortable about giving powerful drugs to children, especially a young child. Instead of treating a child with drugs first, try diet management and other alternatives suggested in this book and in my book *Natural Treatments for ADD and Hyperactivity.*

This explosion of disorders involving learning difficulties and behavior problems are becoming one of the most important health factors in otherwise intelligent children. Many a child's school performance improves drastically by balancing his or her body chemistry as well as nutritional levels. Attention deficit disorder (ADD), with or without hyperactivity, can be the result of food additives (artificial flavoring, synthetic food dye, and preservatives) or allergies and sensitivities, nutrient deficiencies, sugar consumption, over activity or exhaustion of the adrenal glands, copper imbalance, reactive hypoglycemia, heavy-metal toxicity, or chemical sensitivities.

Symptoms may include brief attention span, poor concentration, increased emotional liability, distracted easily, failure to finish things, not listening, being more impulsive, disorders of memory and thinking, specific learning disabilities, disorders of speech and hearing, and hyperactivity inappropriate for the age group. Other signs are constant fidgeting and restlessness. Such behavior can be exasperating and a source of great distress to the parents. The child is often troublesome and violent. At worst, they can wreck the house; at best, they are clumsy, uncoordinated, tearful, and difficult. They may need little food and little sleep and sometimes possess an abnormal thirst. Hyperactive children are more likely than other children to suffer from headaches, asthma, bed wetting, and eczema.

Some symptoms of hyperactivity in adults include: constant talking, fidgeting and nervousness, inability to relax, inability to concentrate or finish a thought, excessive irritability, excitability, and insomnia. Delinquency, violent behavior, and other anti-social behavior may be manifestations of a hyperactive condition.

ADD AND DIET

Little attention is paid to the nutrition of children as the cause of hyperactivity. The hair trace-mineral analysis commonly reveals biochemical factors that contribute to this condition. Often, the results of the test disclose an excessively fast oxidation rate along with low levels of the sedative minerals: calcium, magnesium, and zinc. Many children have low calcium levels despite drinking plenty of milk daily. If there are also high mineral levels of sodium and potassium, the child can have excessive irritability and inflammation. This mineral analysis can reveal if there is also toxic metal poisoning causing neurotoxic effects, especially of copper, lead and cadmium.

A British group, Hyperactive Children's Support Group, conducted a large study that led to the conclusion that children with hyperactivity might have a problem with the conversion of essential fatty acids to prostaglandins (hormones that control all bodily functions at the cellular level). It seems there is a high incidence of improper fatty acid conversion in hyperactive children. Many of these children also have eczema and asthma.

Almost all the substances included in the Feingold diet that could cause hyperactivity also can inhibit this conversion of essential fatty acids to prostaglandins. Another possibility is that they are chemically related to such known inhibitors and called salicylates. (see the chapters "Salicylates and the Feingold Diet" and "Food Additives and Phenolic Compounds").

It is becoming more evident that parents that are hyperactive have children with the same problem. It appears that mineral imbalances can pass from the mother to the child during pregnancy. Since this imbalance is not in the child's inherited genes, but in the body's chemistry, it is usually easy to correct with nutritional therapy. There may be a correlation between children who are very sugar sensitive and a family history of alcoholism, sugar cravings, diabetes, or all three. This history is so common that it suggests a strong genetically determined possibility.

Major medical journals in the United States are blind to the link between food sensitivities and hyperactivity. The conventional medical establishment maintains its contemptuous attitude about this possibility. Conventional allergists will use "allergy shots" to reduce reactivity, yet they consider using a similar practice to treat food sensitivities as quackery. I highly suggest that you read and consider for yourself the different information available. Also consider that conventional medicine does not use diet and nutritional treatments because they are not trained in these areas.

Food Additives

Food additives include a wide range of chemicals with over 5000 additives available for use in the U.S. alone. The daily consumption is more than fifteen grams. According to Dr. Ben Feingold, M.D., the developer of the Feingold diet, more than 50 percent of hyperactive children are sensitive to artificial food colors, preservatives, flavors, and to naturally occurring salicylates and phenolic compounds. He based his claims on over 1,200 cases of learning and behavior disorders that improved significantly when there was the elimination of food additives from the diet.

Food additives are receiving more attention as a cause of adverse reactions. Tartrazine (yellow dye), BHA, BHT, and monosodium glutamate (MSG) are included in the additive category. Due to adverse effects, the artificial sweetener aspartame is receiving more attention.

In 1979, the public schools in New York City ranked in the thirty-ninth percentile on standardized achievement test scores. They reduced the sugar content of foods served in school programs and banned two synthetic food colorings. The achievement test scores soared to the forty-seventh percentile nationally. They further removed all synthetic colorings and flavorings from the food program. The test scores increased to the fifty-first percentile. With the removal of BHA and BHT, the test scores rose even further up to the fifty-fifth percentile. Just by changing the food program in 803 public schools there was an academic improvement of 16 percent.

A study conducted at the Royal Children's Hospital, University of Melbourne, Australia, determined the effect of synthetic food coloring on behavior in hyperactive children. Two hundred children were included in a six-week trial of a diet free of all synthetic food coloring. The parents of 150 children reported behavioral improvement with the diet. They noted deterioration of behavior on the introduction of foods containing artificial colors. These results once again support the Feingold hypothesis.

Children with behavior disorders usually experience significant improvement with a low allergen diet. Many even achieve a normal range of behavior. World-renowned, retired pediatrician and author, Lendon

Smith, M.D., reports that 80 percent of children get better just by changing their diet and taking vitamins. He is a pioneer in the field of food sensitivities and child behavior. Dr. Smith believes that food sensitivity is the key factor for many of the children with attention deficit syndrome. He says that these children are also more susceptible to blood sugar fluctuations. Children with food sensitivities and blood sugar problems are the "Jekyll and Hyde" type kids who experience drastic mood swings. The children will usually get better when they eliminate the offending food(s), stabilize their blood sugar, and consume more nutritious foods.

Dr. William Crook, M.D., a pediatrician from Tennessee, has used a natural approach to hyperactivity for twenty-five years. In a study reported in the *Journal of Learning Disabilities* (May 1980), he published the observations of parents of 182 hyperactive children. A majority of them said that their child's hyperactivity was definitely related to specific foods. Sugar was the worst offender, followed by food additives, and then common foods such as milk, corn, wheat, and eggs. Dr. Crook says that 94 percent of the hyperactive children he sees are sensitive to foods or food colors of some sort. With a healthy, organic diet there is a good chance that a child's behavior problems can be controlled without the use of drugs.

The most common foods and additives to cause reactions are cane sugar, chocolate, corn, cow's milk, eggs, fish, grape, oats, oranges, peanuts, soy, tomato, wheat, and red and yellow dye. Foods bearing phenolic rings in their structures, such as salicylates, coumarin, phenylalanine and uric acid were frequently the cause of hyperactivity reactions. In one study, 57 percent of the people tested with phenolic compounds showed a sensitivity and had some immunity abnormalities in the blood. The immune system became dysfunctional when continuously exposed to phenols. The following is a list of phenolic compounds and other food substances and inhalants tested in a large study. The relative frequency of hyperactivity reaction induced by these compounds is listed below:

SUBSTANCE TESTED	FREQUENCY OF REACTION TO SUBSTANCE
Acetyl salicylate	80%
Ethanol	70%
Dopamine, Norepinephrine, Histamine	50%
Coumarin	40%
Indole	36%
Malvin, Ascorbic acid, Gallic acid	33%
Sugar, Phenylisothio, Phenylalanine	30%
Corn, Beef, Eggs, Uric acid	25%
Cat hair, House dust	25%
Dog dander	10%

There appears to be an interrelationship between sugar consumption and artificial food dyes. Studies have shown that destructive, aggressive, and restless behavior significantly increases with the amount of sugar consumed. Refined carbohydrates found in junk food and high sugar-containing products appear to be the major factor in promoting unstable blood sugars.

Nutritional Deficiencies and ADD

A common mistake made by parents is to give their children sweet-laden foods or drinks either because children ask for them or as a reward for good behavior. This seems to aggravate many problems such as hyperactivity, anxiety, nervousness, poor concentration, and irritability. You may not see changes in behavior merely by giving a child some sugar, because the exposure to sweets may take some time before the symptoms of hyperactivity occur. If a child has mood swings, inappropriate behavior and is mean and surly, he is usually sensitive to sugar or some food in the diet. If a child gets into fights on the school grounds just before lunch and 3 to 4 hours after a breakfast of sweet rolls and juice, there may be a blood sugar problem. Some get headaches after this type of breakfast, others get stomach aches, and still others become hyperactive or mean.

Modern diets are often deficient in trace minerals and vitamins. Any nutrient deficiency can result in a stress on the body influencing learning and behavior. Iron deficiency is the most common in American children. Symptoms of iron anemia may markedly decrease attentiveness, narrower attention span, decrease persistence and activity, but usually responds to supplements. Some studies have shown that individual B vitamins may keep other vitamins from working properly such as megadoses of vitamin B6 inducing a significant folic acid deficiency. Keep this in mind when taking large doses of vitamin B6 or large doses of any vitamin or mineral.

Dr. Nathan Masor's *The New Psychiatry* cites many examples of the effectiveness of treating mental symptoms with high doses of vitamins and no psychotherapy. Dr. Linus Pauling blamed the deficiencies of vitamins B1, B6, B12, as well as nicotinic acid, biotin, vitamin C, and folic acid for disorders of the brain, the nervous system, and mental illness. A vitamin B12 deficiency may cause severe psychiatric symptoms that vary in severity from a mild disorder to paranoid behavior.

According to researchers Mefford and Potter, most of the hyperactive children receiving drug therapy in the United States are actually suffering from low adrenaline levels. They found that low levels of adrenaline in children create the same hyperactive symptoms of difficulty focusing attention, restlessness, and difficulty understanding and solving problems. This manifests itself through excessive activity in the part of the brain that regulates many aspects of attention and sleep. The use of Ritalin and similar drugs relax low-adrenaline anxious children by helping produce adrenaline or mimicking its effects, resulting in a calming effect. In people with normal adrenaline amounts, these amphetamine-like drugs can raise levels too high and create anxiety. Wouldn't it be better to find out why all these children are having symptoms from low adrenaline levels when this condition did not exist to any great extent even twenty years ago?

There have been promising improvements in behavior and function by using essential fatty acids, such as evening primrose oil, that contain a prostaglandin called GLA. In some children there are better results by rubbing the oil into the skin than by giving it orally. Many children improve significantly from hyperactivity when on evening primrose oil. This therapy did not help all the children, especially those without a history of asthma, allergies or eczema.

It seems that when essential fatty acids are low in the body the reaction to additives, such as yellow dye, is more intense. Once the amount of essential fatty acids in the body is adequate, the child is not as susceptible to the various food additives that block prostaglandin formation. Use evening primrose oil or another fatty acid called quercetin as a safeguard for times when the child breaks the diet and goes to parties and outings. Food sources of essential fatty acids are: flax seed oil, safflower oil, tofu, avocados, barley, cashews, garbanzo beans, peanut butter, rice, and corn. Fish such as cod, salmon, mackerel, albacore tuna, and halibut are also sources of essential fatty acids (also see the chapter "Fats and Oils").

There were examples of families where only one child in a family was hyperactive while other siblings eating the same diet were normal. There may be a defect in essential fatty acid absorption in only the one child, so he or she needs a much larger amount of dietary essential fatty acids than others. There may also be a defect preventing these children from converting the fatty acids to GLA.

Behavior studies in school children show that normal lighting can be a factor in hyperactivity and inattention. In school settings standard cool-white fluorescent lighting increases hyperactive behavior while full-spectrum lights with radiation shields decrease hyperactivity. Our bodies are adapted to full-spectrum white light. This type of light is important to normal brain function and can stop hyperactivity in some children.

Other factors in the environment may also be responsible. Many people are also sensitive to air-borne chemicals, especially in urban and industrial areas that contain a phenolic component or a hydrocarbon (petroleum by-product) that can provoke chemical sensitivities.

Numerous studies show a strong relationship between childhood learning disabilities and body stores of heavy metals, particularly lead, mercury, cadmium, copper, and manganese. Correction of these minerals and nutritional imbalances often causes dramatic improvement in concentration, behavior, and social interaction. Poor nutrition and elevation of heavy metals usually go together. Foods that pull the heavy metals out of the body or decrease their absorption are usually missing or certainly reduced in the diet. Some copper-sensitive children are unable to properly eliminate or regulate copper levels in their body. The copper becomes toxic in their body causing dramatic violent changes. This was discovered shortly after some children took copper-containing multivitamins.

Hair analysis is a test used to indicated storage levels of toxic heavy metals and minerals. A small bit of head hair is used because trace elements accumulate in hair at concentrations that generally appear higher than those present in blood or urine. Deficient or excessive levels of minerals as well as toxic metals store in the hair and become a long term record of these substances in the body. Certain patterns are common in the studies of the criminal population with the most common ones being low zinc, high copper, and high manganese levels.

Brain toxicity from an overload of manganese causes a depletion of the neurotransmitter, dopamine. The first symptoms of manganese overload are fatigue, hypnotic-like state or trance, irritability, and erratic behavior. An individual suffering from "manganese madness" may exhibit various antisocial or compulsive acts, irrational violent behavior, and involvement with impulse crimes such as domestic violence. There may also be emotional instability typified by easy laughter or crying, acting drunk, muscular weakness, headaches, impaired equilibrium, and slurred speech.

Lead affects brain function. Studies done on the criminal population found levels of lead and cadmium in the 90+ percentile during their crime periods. Prison populations commonly have higher heavy metal levels when compared with the general population.

Cadmium is also a highly toxic neurotoxin and concentrates in the kidney, liver and blood causing symptoms that could include high blood pressure, decreased fertility, enlarged heart, serious vascular disease, arteriosclerosis, cerebral hemorrhage, and kidney disease. Cigarettes are the major source of cadmium in our society. This first exposure to the fetus gets into the placental tissue from the smoking mother. Cadmium interferes with zinc absorption and utilization by the fetus. Exposure continues after the child is born by being exposed to air levels of cadmium. This can be the beginning of a learning and behavior disorder in the child. Sources of contaminants include refined foods, industrial contaminants in the air, soft water, coffee and black tea, cigarette smoke, and many processed meats. Coffee is the second largest source of cadmium and white refined flour is another high source. A study indicated that children with learning disabilities had significantly higher cadmium and lower zinc levels than children without learning disabilities.

Many children exhibiting personality swings and appearing hyperactive or violent may be suffering from reactive hypoglycemia (low blood sugar). This is one of the most common food-mood connections and creates a wide array of psychological symptoms including behavioral changes. See the chapter on hypoglycemia for more information. A low blood sugar can also occur in those with under active adrenal glands. This usually results in a craving for sweets and can directly influence behavior. Inadequate adrenal gland function can be inherited from the parents, especially the mother. She can pass it to her child during pregnancy if she was over stressed, had a poor diet, or suffered from copper or other toxic metal poisoning.

The Adrenal Glands and ADD

Children already have a fast metabolism rate and combined with overly stressed adrenal glands can result easily in low blood sugar. Other symptoms are various degrees of anxiety, nervousness, mental confusion, and fatigue. Eating sugar only fuels the fire. Most stimulants, such as caffeine, act directly or indirectly by increasing adrenal gland activity. Some personality types have a more difficult time handling stress appropriately. They are very emotional and high-strung children who go into the "fight or flight" response at the slightest provocation. Excessive exposure to any stress or noise just further stimulates the adrenal glands. The overuse of prescription drugs and exposure to pesticides and other environmental toxins can also deplete the adrenal glands to exhaustion and cause hyperactive behavior.

One of the effects is an increase in adrenal hormone secretion that increases the speed of the nervous system while also causing a reduction in the sedating minerals: calcium, magnesium, and zinc. This lowering of minerals results in increased nervous excitability and irritability. More activity occurs if the sodium and potassium levels are also elevated. Another adrenal hormone causes the body to pour sugar into the blood, like pouring gasoline on a fire. This increase in blood sugar levels contributes to hyperactivity. These children may even be aggressive and violent, especially when tired or feeling threatened. Sleeping may be a problem. They can wear out parents and teachers who try to discipline them. Quick solutions often do not reveal the real cause of the behavior problem.

With the correction of these mineral levels, the child can get well. Some children seem normal at home, but have troubles in school when they are placed in a stressful situation where they are more reactive to stress and have difficulty remaining calm. Increasing sedative minerals is often an important part of the nutritional correction of attention deficit disorder and hyperactivity disorders. These minerals help to slow the adrenal glands, and reduce the fight-or-flight reaction.

Fast oxidizers require more fat and oil in their diet. They feel worse on carbohydrates, particularly simple carbohydrates such as fruit, fruit juices, and all sweets. Many children are eating precisely the wrong diet for their body type. Parents are being told that all fats and oils are bad and discourage giving the child adequate amounts. This only aggravates the symptoms and speeds up the oxidation rate. Correcting the diet can decrease the symptoms.

Environmental Toxins and ADD

It has to be more than coincidental that the present epidemic of hyperactivity and behavioral problems among school children has coincided with steadily increasing levels of volatile organic chemicals found in modern buildings. Behavioral problems may be the earliest sign of chemical toxins according to standard texts on neurotoxicology. Toxins can be absorbed easily through the skin and the fumes inhaled. The organs most affected are the brain and nervous system. Common symptoms include the inability to think, impaired memory, poor concentration and coordination, and drowsiness. A list of organic solvents is: toluene, xylene, acetone, benzene, chloroform, carbon tetrachloride, trichloroethylene, and others. The potential of these substances for causing brain and neurologic damage is well documented in the medical literature.

Organophosphates are now the most widely used pesticides in the United States. They poison the nervous systems of unwanted pests. Children may have continual or repeated exposures to these pesticides through pesticide residues in fruits and vegetables and through their use in or about the school buildings and homes. Research indicates that this pesticide causes behavior and learning deficits that may be irreversible. Symptoms include impairment of intellectual functioning, abstract and flexible thinking, and simple motor skills. A study conducted on the effects of pesticides on the nervous system concluded that it is possible that organophosphates may be another cause of brain dysfunction so frequently demonstrated in our younger population.

Much has been said about pesticides as a major cause of what appears to be a food allergy. Even very low levels have been shown to cause learning and memory impairment, hyperactivity, and aggressive behavior. The possible effects of pesticide residues in human milk on an infant's behavior surely deserve investigation. It may be beneficial to test for common pesticides such as diazinon, because of its common use on crops.

Most organic solvents and pesticides in use today are fat-soluble and have an affinity for the fatty tissues of the body. The brain and nervous system are more than 25 percent fat in content and are especially vulnerable because of the rich blood supply to these areas. These chemicals may attack the cell membranes of the body made up almost entirely of fats. Children and developing fetuses are much more vulnerable to the damaging effects of these toxins because of their rapidly growing tissues and because of the immaturity of their detoxification systems. On a more positive note, children have great recuperative powers so they recover from injury more rapidly and completely than adults.

With hyperactivity and behavior problems epidemic in today's schools, perhaps one of the most urgent questions needing an answer is whether toxic chemical exposure is capable of causing personality and behavior changes? If the answer is yes, we need an immediate reduction of organophosphate pesticides. It could be very important to the health and welfare of our youth.

In one study, there was an association between recurrent ear infections in childhood and later hyperactivity. A sensitivity to dairy and its ability to create mucus also contributes to the cause of ear infections. Almost 70 percent of the children being evaluated for school failure, who were also receiving medication for hyperactivity, gave a history of more than ten ear infections. These children received repeated and prolonged courses of broad-spectrum antibiotic drugs that caused alterations in gut flora, including the proliferation of *Candida albicans*. These changes promote the absorption of food antigens and put the child at risk for food sensitivities. This may play a major role in causing hyperactivity, attention problems, and related behavior and learning problems.

Other Factors Linking ADD and Allergies

Hypothyroidism in childhood severely limits development of the brain and may be an important component of hyperactivity and attention deficit syndrome. The cells need thyroid to produce enough energy to become quietly relaxed. For many years, some physicians have known about the quieting effects of thyroid hormone and have prescribed it for hyperactive children. This condition has increased since the mid-1950s as the use of unsaturated vegetable oils (proven to cause brain damage in rats) has also increased. The more unsaturated an oil, the more it interferes with the function of the thyroid gland. An iodine deficiency may also be the cause of thyroid dysfunction causing personality changes in individuals on iodine-deficient diets. Symptoms may include irritability, sluggish memory, slow reaction time, depression, a tendency to be quarrelsome, as well as a lack of cooperation.

At least three studies of asthmatic children show a relationship between learning and behavioral problems and the use of theophylline. This is a common medication used for asthmatics. When the children took approximately ten to twenty micrograms, adverse effects in school behavior and performance resulted. Many children, especially asthmatics, are also low in hydrochloric acid. This deficiency seems prevalent in children below the age of seven, but hydrochloric acid tends to rise in production as the child gets closer to puberty.

There has been a parallel increase in behavior difficulties such as hyperactivity, attention problems, and learning disabilities in children after receiving vaccinations. There is a known interaction between the nervous and immune systems. Injuries to one system affect the other. Stories abound of parents who observe changes in the personality of their children following immunizations. Some children are just never the same. These observations by parents deserve some notice by the medical community.

We have a million children who have mental and emotional problems. A large number of children with learning disabilities can benefit from nutritional treatment. In one experiment in a school for "impossible" children, they had their lunch boxes checked when they arrived in the morning. Their behavior improved under a treatment that incorporated food and vitamin therapy. It startled the teachers who were not knowledgeable about the role that nutrition plays in health and behavior. This study was based on a book called *The Orthomolecular Approach to the Treatment of Children with Behavior Disorders and Learning Disabilities,* published in 1977 by Dr. Allan Cott, a New York psychiatrist who disclosed the biological and chemical basis for learning disabilities and their treatment. It seems really sad that this information has been available since 1977, and now almost 20 years later it is barely being considered. Nearly every issue of the *Journal of the International College of Applied Nutrition* from 1980 to 1983 contained at least one article showing the relationship between nutrition and some behavior disorder. So many children continue to suffer when this information has been available, but not used by doctors in conventional medical practices.

As many as a million American children take Ritalin (methylphenidate) to control hyperactivity and attention deficit disorder. Lately, Ritalin is being publicized as a drug that can "unlock" a child's potential compared with the supposed limitations of the dietary approach to hyperactivity. The drug view espoused by Ritalin promoters is that this drug, an amphetamine, works by correcting biochemical imbalances in the brain. No evidence exists to support that view or evidence that Ritalin makes any lasting change. No long-term studies have been performed on the safety and effectiveness of this drug. *The American Textbook of Psychiatry* shows a 75 percent improvement with Ritalin, but a 40 percent response with just a placebo.

Ritalin suppresses growth, makes a child more prone to seizures, and could cause visual disturbances, insomnia, anorexia, nervousness, and toxic psychosis. This is a class II category controlled substance similar to barbiturates, morphine, and other drugs with high potential for addiction or abuse. Careful supervision is required during drug withdrawal because numerous suicides have occurred after drug withdrawal due to severe depression. The effects of chronic over activity can be unmasked during this time.

This drug is regulated by the Drug Enforcement Administration (DEA). It is the treatment of choice by many pediatricians for attention deficit disorder and hyperactivity. There were shortages of Ritalin in 1993. We should be asking ourselves what is wrong with a society that is unable to keep its young population supplied with enough of a drug that in actuality is an amphetamine.

In 1991 *Toxic Psychiatry* stated that the long-term use of Ritalin causes irritability and hyperactivity. These are the very same problems that Ritalin is supposed to cure. In a 1986 study cited in *Psychiatric Research,* evidence of brain atrophy was shown in more than half of the twenty-four adults treated with psychostimulants. In another study of fourteen children, only two responded to Ritalin. One child showed significant deterioration and another marked deterioration.

Before putting any child on a drug for hyperactivity, attention deficit disorder, or other behavior problems, have him or her checked for reactive hypoglycemia, allergies, or food and environmental sensitivities. There are often alternatives to experiencing a lifetime of problems, antisocial behavior, and an inability to learn even simple tasks. It is well worth the time and effort. The easy way out is to just put the child on drugs. It is important to discuss any treatment with a physician who has training in nutritional therapy.

Section 2

ALLERGIES AND NUTRITION

CHAPTER 5

It Could Be Something You're Eating

Most physicians rarely ask what you eat or what you are feeding your children. If they did, how would you reply? Do you think that part of being a good parent is having your child drink milk, eat bread, cheese, peanut butter, or pop tarts? Do you believe that your children couldn't live without cookies or sugar-containing cereals? Reactions to some common foods have become alarmingly familiar.

Even "good" food may not be best for a person with food allergies or sensitivities. Examples could be a baby who is "allergic" to mother's milk or an adult who suddenly develops a sensitivity to corn or bread. Because allergies and sensitivities are commonly due to delayed reactions, it makes the offending foods, chemicals, or inhalants not so obvious. These foods may be so enmeshed in the diet that it is difficult to discover the cause of the symptoms. Even with all the available evidence, many doctors refuse to accept that widespread food allergies and sensitivities exist.

Symptoms that occur in children in response to foods usually go unrecognized as parents attribute a rash, diarrhea, irritability, or constant crying to other causes. The child may appear to "outgrow" the original condition, but what may be happening is that the response has changed as the child grew older and the symptoms just became masked. For example, the infant who reacts to drinking milk with diarrhea or colic may later have eczema. At age two there is a constant runny nose, ear infections, and dark circles under the eyes; at age four there is hyperactivity and bed-wetting; and at age twenty there is asthma. By that time, other foods, inhalants, or chemicals have complicated the original milk sensitivity.

Some food problems are more difficult to track down because the problem originates in the combination of foods consumed at a given time and their effect on the digestive tract as they are digested and assimilated. The foods are often favorites or an integral part of the diet. Many parents insist their child does not seem to crave or be sensitive to a particular food, but they have not considered the many available forms. Foods can cause almost any symptom imaginable, and possibly appear within seconds or minutes after consumption, or be delayed for twelve hours or longer. The sensitivity response can also take on different forms and intensities. Relating these responses to a specific substance can be difficult because we eat so many kinds of food in so many combinations.

The response to a food intolerance depends on individual susceptibility and constitutional strength. Each person's specific food sensitivity is so unique that it is somewhat of a biochemical fingerprint. Even siblings raised together eating the same foods develop different food problems. But unlike fingerprints, these patterns usually change over time.

The foods eaten most frequently are often the chief sources of the problem. Large amounts in the diet of a single food, such as wheat and milk, are not recommended for this reason. A sick person usually craves the food that makes them sick. In contrast, healthy people rarely eat their sensitivities. It seems that at first the person has a natural repulsion for their food intolerance, but if its use is further encouraged, then they become addicted to it. The body tries to reach a balance by first adapting and then developing a dependence on any substance that is reintroduced again and again.

Since today's progress in food production makes most foods available year round, it is possible to eat the same food daily. This wonder of modern civilization is the reason allergies and sensitivities are skyrocketing. According to some recent studies, the incidence of food sensitivity is greater than that of any other type of illness. By some estimates, 60 percent of the American population have unknown food sensitivities and about 95 percent of those go undiagnosed. This problem can be the most puzzling and frustrating cause of illness with vague symptoms usually dismissed as neurotic in origin. A person who suffers from a multitude of minor, chronic complaints is a candidate for the diagnosis of food sensitivities.

Food reactions easily masquerade as many illnesses and conditions. There may be occasional or continuous symptoms that become worse after certain meals, or better when not eating. If you are experiencing a constant, resistant illness, you should consider hidden food allergies or sensitivities as the underlying cause. It is important to emphasize that the symptoms are not necessarily traditional allergic disorders. In the strictest sense, adverse responses to foods are not usually true allergic reactions but digestive problems that deeply disturb various delicate systems in the body. Any body system can be affected, but it is commonly the cardiovascular, digestive, immune, and nervous systems. The weakest part of a person's body is the first to show dysfunction. Manifestations of symptoms may result in one or more of the following responses:

- *Blood sugar:* diabetes, hypoglycemia
- *Cardiovascular system:* heart palpitations or fluttering, numbness, arrhythmia, poor circulation, high-blood pressure, racing pulse
- *Ear, Eye, Nose, Throat:* ears stop up, ring, buzz, or hurt with repeated bouts of ear infections, impaired hearing, vertigo or dizziness; dark circles under the eyes, discoloration or lines under eyes, itchy eyes, blurred vision, discharge from eyes or nose; bleeding or stuffy nose; hoarseness, swollen, dry, or tickling throat; sneezing or coughing. Meniere's disease is sometimes the result of food allergies or sensitivities.
- *Gastrointestinal tract:* indigestion, cramps, hemorrhoids, cold sores, constipation, vomiting, gas, diarrhea, irritable bowel syndrome, Crohn's disease, ulcerative colitis, or other types of colitis or gastritis. There could also be stomach ulcers, malabsorption, or celiac disease (an extreme intolerance to a fraction of wheat called gliadin that produces crippling diarrhea and weight loss).
- *Genitourinary tract:* itching, burning, or frequent, urgent, or painful urination. There could be bedwetting, chronic bladder infections, kidney disease, fluid retention and bloating.
- *Immune system:* chronic sinus infections, frequent colds and flu, autoimmune diseases, allergies or sensitivities
- *Lymph system:* chronic enlargement of lymph glands especially in the neck.
- *Musculoskeletal system:* muscles aches, spasm, stiffness, cramps, twitching, joint problems, low back pain, arthritic-like symptoms or bursitis
- *Nervous system and brain:* mood and personality changes, frequent headaches, migraines, anxiety, fainting, insomnia, depression, irritability, psychoses, hyperactivity, attention deficit syndrome
- *Respiratory system:* asthma, chronic bronchitis, respiratory infections, wheezing, sinusitis, congestion, post-nasal drip, and frequent stuffy or runny nose
- *Skin:* hives, rash, itching, acne, sweating, hot or cold flashes, rough-red cheeks, earlobes red and warm to touch. Different types of eczema may be induced that are dry or weeping, itchy, thickened, or reddened patches of skin usually on the face, wrists, and inside elbows and knees. Some people have an allergic wrinkle on the nose from constantly wiping.
- *Miscellaneous:* inflammation, mouth breather, a low-grade fever (99 to 99.8 degrees Fahrenheit), swelling of different parts of the body, heavy sweating not related to exercise, fatigue not helped by rest, marked fluctuations in weight, anemic appearance

If a child has a rapid pulse, low-grade fever, body aches, and a pale complexion, it could be a mild case of rheumatic fever, but the chances are not likely. If enlarged lymph glands occur in the neck along with paleness, fatigue, and a low-grade fever, this could possibly be infectious mononucleosis. More often it is a food sensitivity.

Chronic stomach aches and bloating after eating may be an indicator of a hidden food intolerance. The stomach can hurt so much it appears to be an ulcer. Often, children and adults have physical exams, blood and urine tests, and even x-rays only to find nothing wrong. When the tests come back within normal ranges, it appears that the person has an emotional problem. If other causes of abdominal pain have been rules out, consider the possibility of food sensitivities. Removing the offending foods from the diet will usually clear the symptoms completely.

Yeast in food is another common allergen that can alter moods. It is present in a huge range of foods and drinks consumed daily such as alcoholic beverages, vinegar, pickled or fermented foods, most cheeses, dried fruits, and baked goods. Many people who complain of irritability, fatigue, and depression are affected by these products.

The widespread use of nonsteroid anti-inflammatory drugs in recent years may contribute to many health problems. There is evidence that people who use them develop an increase in intestinal permeability leading to food reactions. The intestines usually provide an effective barrier against the excessive absorption of large molecules, food antigens, and bacteria. When this barrier becomes ineffective, food antigens enter the system in excessive amounts. This leads to food sensitivities in some individuals. This is especially true with cow's milk.

There are now one million cases of Crohn's disease with children making up 15,000 new cases each year. Ulcerative colitis has reached a figure of one million cases and children total 100,000 of these. There are millions who are suffering from related intestinal disorders often caused by the foods they eat. Eating the wrong foods may irritate the bladder causing frequent urination and the symptoms of bladder infections. A sense of urgency is likely with a burning sensation. Many parents and doctors rarely think of food sensitivities when a child wets the bed, shows protein in the urine, or suffers from repeated urinary infections or any other disorder of the urinary tract.

If a person gets one cold after another, or if it persists for days and weeks at a time, the cause may be foods rather than infection. The "bug" is probably an opportunistic organism finding a weakened host to prey upon. These types of reactions were unheard of a few years ago. So what caused this sudden change? The environmental pollutants certainly contribute to the picture, but they are only part of the problem. Various preservatives, dyes, fillers, sweeteners, and other toxins in the food have shocked the immune system, and a high level of stress adds the final insult. A combination of things has beaten down the body's resistance resulting in a compromised immune system.

A food allergy or sensitivity can be an important triggering factor for many autoimmune diseases. All people suffering from diseases that have an autoimmune component should consider an elimination diet and investigate the different types of food testing. Many people benefit from dietary intervention.

Nervous system symptoms can be food related and make an adult or child excessively active, irritable, restless, or clumsy. It can interfere with sleep and even disturb the personality. More serious symptoms may include depression, numbness, tingling, and an inability to concentrate. Perhaps half of the hyperactive children who are unruly and unable to learn in the classroom may be suffering from hidden food sensitivities.

Iron anemia is not the only cause of a persistent pale complexion. Food sensitivities can also cause circles under the eyes and the skin of the face to be puffy, pale and pasty in appearance. Irritability and a lack of enthusiasm may be present as well as fatigue and lethargy, but taking iron supplements and vitamins have no effect. Improvement is usually swift and complete by removing the guilty foods from the diet.

People show a reaction to cow's milk more often than any other food. Products made from cow's milk are not readily digestible and stay in the digestive tract much longer than other foods. It is difficult to manage dairy sensitivities with a rotation diet, but it usually works well for other foods.

Sending a child to school for the first time can be of a great concern. It puts a food intolerant child into an environment where these foods predominate adding enormous stress to the body. The Food Allergy Network is a nonprofit organization established to help families cope with food allergies and to increase public awareness. They created a two-booklet guide to help make the transition from home to school easier. Parents seeking advice on how to handle children with food allergies can send a stamped, self-addressed envelope to the Food Allergy Network, 4744 Holly Avenue, Fairfax, VA, 22030.

Several options remain open for treatment. You may benefit from eliminating the offending foods, using a rotation diet, or be desensitized to the problematic food. Discuss what treatments are available with your health-minded physician. Keep in mind that no elimination diet will work unless you remove all forms of the suspected food from your diet. Multiple food sensitivities require the elimination of various foods.

Introducing genetically altered and cross-species transferred foods into the marketplace makes the job of identifying food sensitivities even harder.

The public is probably not aware of all these foods that have been developed and sold to consumers. This information is not on labels so you are probably eating them without knowing it. What does this have to do with food allergies or sensitivities? The proteins from the donor plant or animal might transfer the allergic properties to the host plant you are eating. This makes the detection of food allergies and sensitivities more complicated.

Symptoms mentioned as food related may have other causes. This is why it is important to be thoroughly checked for any other medical problem. If you suspect that hidden food sensitivities may be the cause, the first step in treating a food sensitive person is to test which foods are the major offenders by a physician trained in this area. Join the many thousands who now live healthier, happier lives because they discovered which foods were wrong for them.

CHAPTER 6

The Importance of Good Digestion

As the old saying goes, "You are what you eat." But actually, there is more to it than that. Not only what you eat is important, but what you digest, what you assimilate, and what you eliminate. The way you eat can also influence your digestion. When you eat quickly, without chewing your food adequately, digestive enzymes have a hard time breaking down the food into absorbable, essential nutrients. You can also swallow a great deal of air with your meal when you eat in a hurry and swallow frequently. Additional air ends up in your digestive tract and can cause discomfort. Digestion is a complex process and we can either help or hinder by what we choose to eat and how we eat it.

THE STAGES OF DIGESTION

The first stage of digestion occurs before eating even begins. The first stage involves cooking and processing of food. If food is cooked or processed for too long or at too hot a temperature, there may be substantial nutrient loss, which can lead to a variety of problems, including allergic reactions or sensitivities.

The next stage of digestion begins when chewed food breaks down in the mouth and mixes with saliva. Chewing food slowly and thoroughly breaks it up into small particles allowing the digestive process to work efficiently and properly. It is essential for saliva to mix with the food, allowing enzymes a chance to work. Proper digestion depends on this process. If a person hurries through meals, bolting their food or eating without careful chewing, as well as drinking too much liquids, they are washing down partly chewed food and diluting the digestive enzymes responsible for proper digestion. With adequate chewing, almost 50 percent of starch digestion takes place in the mouth and stomach. Starch digestion continues in the small intestine with the aid of amylase, an enzyme released by the pancreas.

Swallowing pushes food into the stomach and the next stage of digestion begins. Digestive enzymes from the mouth continues to break down starches. Stomach cells begin to release chemicals that break down proteins. Two of these chemicals are pepsin, which begins protein digestion in the stomach, and hydrochloric acid. After mixing with these chemicals, food moves from the stomach into the small intestine.

Once food moves into the small intestine it mixes with more digestive enzymes from the pancreas and gall bladder. One of these enzymes, bile, is produced in the liver and stored in the gall bladder. Pancreatic enzymes complete the breakdown of any large proteins into amino acids, of starches or complex carbohydrates into simple sugars, and of fats into smaller fatty acids. Some of the larger hormone proteins are absorbed whole, but most are broken down into their smallest and most easily digested forms as amino acids.

As food passes through the entire length of the small intestine, nutrients are absorbed into the blood stream. These nutrients circulate throughout the body to nourish the body or to be stored in appropriated tissues. Water and important minerals are reabsorbed in the large intestine. Fiber, microorganisms, and other indigestibles and wastes are eliminated. Adequate fiber and fluid in the diet ensures a healthier function of the large intestine.

GUIDELINES FOR GOOD DIGESTION AND GOOD HEALTH

The 1988 U.S. Surgeon General's report on nutrition and health indicated that two-thirds of all deaths in the United States are linked to dietary choices. We need to change out eating habits if there is to be any chance of reaching optimum health. After being told for decades to eat lots of meat and dairy products to grow up big and strong, now we are being told just the opposite. Everyone, adults and children alike, should eat a wide variety of foods. Most people would benefit from eating more fresh fruits and vegetables, seeds, cereals, beans, and whole grains. These foods provide necessary fiber and fluid, high-quality fats, proteins, and the vitamins and minerals necessary for optimum health. The following guidelines outline some suggestions for a healthful, balanced diet. I hope this information will bring you new ways of understanding food. Changing lifelong eating habits can be confusing and difficult at first, but there are so many good reasons for trying. Here are some ideas to get you started.

Making the Change

Changing one's dietary habits can be a very difficult process. Start today and move at a comfortable pace for yourself. Think of this change as a new adventure, not just another burden to endure. Get your family involved; support is wonderful. You may find yourself struggling against years of deeply ingrained bad habits. I encourage you to stick with it and focus on your successes. In cases of overwhelming physical or emotional changes, a naturopathic physician or other nutritional expert can offer advice, treatment, and guide you to success.

The idea of eating well is a simple one. Buy, prepare, and serve foods in their whole state, when possible. Use whole grain flour instead of white, refined flour. Unrefined oils are healthier than the refined kind. Prepare vegetables such as potatoes, squash and carrots with their skins, unless they have been sprayed with harmful pesticides. This takes advantage of the valuable nutrients in the skin of the plant. Whenever possible, buy meat free of steroids, antibiotics, and pesticides. Completely avoid white sugar, bleached white flour, highly salted snacks and junk foods. You have a lot of control over the quality of food you buy and eat. Another way to start is to use a diet diary and record what you eat every day. Gradually substitute healthy foods for the ones you want to eliminate. In this way you can change as slowly as you need to or as quickly as you can. Another way is to buy a cookbook with healthy recipes and use their ideas for menus. As you become familiar with healthy foods, your choices for putting meals together will be much easier.

It's important to experiment with what is best for you and your particular lifestyle. You will find the widest selection of natural and organic foods at health-food stores. Food co-ops offer similar fare at lower prices. If you have limited resources to acquire healthy foods, then consider ordering from the mail sources included in this book. However, if you must shop at the local large chain grocery store, you can still use common sense in your selections.

Eat Foods as Fresh as Possible

All foods begin to decompose immediately after harvesting. Besides losing nutritional value, there is an increase in potentially harmful bacteria. The development of chemical preservatives helps retard these natural processes, but it is becoming a major health concern that we are ingesting these potentially toxic and nutrition-robbing substances. Whenever possible, eat fresh foods. Frozen foods are the next best if fresh is not available. Canned and packaged foods are the least desirable. Shopping for smaller quantities and cooking fewer meals in advance insures freshness. Store foods that do not need refrigeration in cool and dark places. Find an organic produce shop and buy local meat or fish from a chemical-free store. Such changes in shopping and eating habits will lead to not only fresher foods, but more nutritious and better tasting ones. It will also reduce waste and this reduces the cost of foods.

Are You and Your Foods Compatible?

Just as we must adapt our lives to the climates we live in, so must our food sources adjust their genetic make-up to survive and flourish in their environment. Plants have developed over thousands of years. They work to have their water content, vitamins, minerals, and nutrients compatible with their surroundings. An orange grove would not last long in New England; an apple tree cannot flourish in the deep South. Spinach and lettuce do well in the spring and fall, but not in the hotter summer months. Foods adapted to the same climate that we live in fill us with the characteristics that serve us best. This is a great argument for supporting your local food growers.

Children Need Nutritious Foods

Small children eat small amounts of food and are dependent on very little food to obtain the nutrients they need. Eating foods that have little nutritional value adversely affects their appetite and decreases nutritional intake. With the elimination of candy, cookies, sugared cereals, soft drinks, food additives and preservatives, many children improve both physically and mentally.

Good Elimination Is Important

With billions of cells being replaced daily, the body must eliminate the nonreusable parts of these spent cells along with toxins and by-products from the foods we eat, the air we breathe, and the water we drink. If we eat biologically correct foods, our eliminative process is usually up to the task of maintaining an acceptable internal environment. If we consume foods not suited to our digestive capabilities, the internal waste products increase past the toleration point. If the total burden is too large, our whole elimination process may be incapable of removing the toxins from our bodies and this results in illness.

The body's need to eliminate toxins has many different disguises: colds, diarrhea, acne, sinusitis, allergies, or asthma. The name usually isn't important, because they all indicate that the elimination process is trying to cure a toxic condition. Since most people are unaware of what the body is really trying to do, they take even more poisons in the form of drugs and over-the-counter medicines to stop the process. These poisons are not usable in building or maintaining healthy cells or tissues so the body must expend more energy, vitamins, minerals, and other important substances trying to eliminate these added toxins. The best treatments are the ones that support the body during this time by aiding the elimination process.

Water Is Part of Good Nutrition

Adequate water intake during the day is important for flushing out the body's toxins. As a result of not drinking enough water, many people have problems such as poor muscle tone and size, decreased digestive efficiency and organ function, increased toxicity in the body, joint and muscle soreness particularly after exercise, and water retention. If the body does not get enough water, it starts retaining water to compensate for this shortage. One of the ways to eliminate fluid retention is to drink more water, not less.

Heavy metals, chemicals, pesticides, and other toxins are absorbed into the blood-stream along with the normal metabolic waste products and need to be eliminated from the body. Some wastes are excreted by the kidneys, some move through the skin and other tissues, some go out through the large intestines, and some pass through the lungs. If a person does not drink enough fluids, especially water, they will not be able to eliminate these harsher chemicals through the kidneys.

How much liquid is consumed during mealtime can influence digestion. It is best not to drink too much when eating because excessive fluids may dilute your valuable digestive enzymes. The most disruptive beverages are milk and soda pop because they can interfere with digestion in the stomach by neutralizing the acid. Drink adequate pure water between meals, but drink water with your meals only if necessary. Many people use liquids as a way of washing down unchewed food.

There is a difference between pure water and other beverages that contain water. Drinks containing water often contain substances that are not healthy and contradict some of the positive effects of the water. Beer contains alcohol; coffee contains adrenal-stressing caffeine; fruit juices contain natural sugar and often have added sugar which stimulates the pancreas; and soda contains phosphorus that pulls calcium out of the bones. Such drinks may tax the body more than cleanse it and they contribute little to the elimination process. Another problem with these beverages is that you lose your taste for water. The recommended daily water intake means just that, drink water! If you find this hard to do, the next best thing to drink is herbal, noncaffeinated tea.

Proper water intake is the key to weight loss. The body can't metabolize fat if there isn't enough water. A healthy person should drink six to eight eight-ounce glasses a day. Drink more if you're overweight, exercise a lot, or live in a hot climate. Overweight people should drink an extra glass for every twenty-five pounds they exceed their ideal weight. Spread your water intake throughout the day, including the evening. Dark-colored, cloudy urine often suggests you are not drinking enough water. The following is a list of general information and hints of proper water consumption.

• Water eases digestion and regulates body temperature.
• Water bathes the cells of our body and accounts for about 60 percent of our body weight.
• Water can help us exercise longer and more efficiently. It reduces cardio-vascular stress and improves performance. Be sure to drink water after exercise so you will not suffer from dehydration.
• Drinking water can ward off constipation and maybe even crankiness.
• It is a natural appetite suppressant and may help in losing weight.
• It helps the skin to stay healthy.
• Adequate water helps prevent urinary tract infections.
• Sufficient water can be helpful for people with a history of kidney stones.

Drinking tap water may be a health hazard. Impurities that are in tap water may be a contributor toward ill health. Use purified or distilled water for all cooking and drinking purposes, never tap water. It is wise to install a purification system for your drinking and bathing water. The skin absorbs toxins and chlorine very readily during bathing and showering. Water softeners are particularly hazardous, as sodium is added to the water as a part of the softening process. For more information see the chapter "Water Filters."

Basic Building Blocks for the Body

Carbohydrates, fats, proteins, vitamins and minerals provide the fuel our bodies need to function and perform. Carbohydrates are our main source of quick energy. Fats, whether solid or liquid, are our primary slow-burning energy sources. For proper brain development, infants need adequate fat in their diet until the age of two. Proteins are the body's chief building materials. Obtaining the right proportion of nutrients is critical to good health. Eating the right number of calories is just as important. Keeping your body healthy is a personal balancing act. The goal is to get the essential nutrients you need, while eating no more calories than your body expends.

Proteins

Nine essential amino acids cannot be stored in the body and so must be obtained daily through diet or supplementations. These amino acids are a critical component of dietary protein. Adequate protein is essential to the growth and development of organ tissue, blood, and builds and repairs muscles. If even one essential amino acid is missing, the necessary protein cannot be made. It will be used for fuel instead. It is wasteful to use all this protein just for energy when burning carbohydrates is more efficient and less stressful for the body. See the chapter "Protein" for more information.

Complex Carbohydrates: The Body's Source of Fuel

Carbohydrates are the principle fuel of the body and needed for the continuous and repeated muscular contractions that occur during prolonged exercise. Ideally, they should be the most plentiful substance in a properly balanced diet. They are stored in the muscles and liver in the form of glycogen. Carbohydrates are present in the diet in two forms—simple carbohydrates and complex ones. Due to misconceptions by the public, carbohydrates have received a bad reputation. People think of them as only high-calorie sweet foods. They neglect to distinguish between natural, unrefined complex carbohydrates (whole grains, legumes, fresh fruits and vegetables) and refined, processed, simple carbohydrates (sugar, white-flour products, candy, soft drinks, and potato chips).

Complex carbohydrates digest and absorb slowly. This is because they contain fiber and other materials that slow down digestion so that starches can slowly convert into sugars. The body usually stores them efficiently. This natural form of food is the major energy source for metabolic function, physical activity, growth, digestion, and as a regulator of protein and fat metabolism. Natural (unrefined, complex) carbohydrates provide the necessary bulk for a healthy digestive system. Without complex carbohydrates, you would not get the full value from your protein nor would you be able to properly break down fats. Complex carbohydrates also contain the vitamins and minerals that allow the carbohydrates to "burn clean" into carbon dioxide and water. Examples of complex carbohydrates are: brown rice, whole wheat, oats, rye, millet, and other grains, lentils, tofu, fresh corn, apples, buckwheat, barley, beets, chard, onions, carrots, berries, melons, bananas, potatoes with their skins (white and sweet), beans, and peas.

Finding refined, simple carbohydrates (refined sugars) in the marketplace is easy. This includes white, refined, or brown turbinado sugar, and corn syrup. They are fattening and contribute to the development of hard-

ening of the arteries, heart disease, high-blood pressure, dental caries, peri-
odontal disease, and other major health problems. Refined carbohydrates
such as white bread, cake mixes, most national brand pastas, and grains are
of an inferior quality. Look for unrefined sweeteners that are more wholesome and nutritious such as organic, raw unfiltered honey, barley malt,
blackstrap molasses, and real maple syrup free of formaldehyde.

Fats

Fats provide the most concentrated source of energy in the diet and help
digest fat-soluble vitamins. Certain fats also provide the important essential fatty acids. Bad press has characterized fats and oils as unhealthy substances responsible for a wide range of disorders. But quality fats and oils
are necessary for good nutrition and health when taken in the proper quantities. They should provide about 15 to 20 percent of the total diet. A typical meat-eater's diet usually far exceeds this amount. For those who eat
smaller amount of meats and have a high quality diet, a limited intake of
fats poses no problem. It is best to include unsaturated cold-pressed oils
such as safflower or flaxseed. Many parents today withhold fats and oils
from children because they think that they are helping them keep their
weight and cholesterol levels down. The truth is, however, that a growing
child needs adequate levels of healthy fats and oils to grow. Fatty acids are
essential to the well being of the growing body. Children often crave more
sugar if they are deprived adequate protein, complex carbohydrates, fats
and oils in the diet. See the chapter "Fats and Oils" for a more complete
overview of fats, oils and their importance in avoiding food allergies and
sensitivities.

Vitamins and Minerals

Vitamins and minerals are essential to human growth and metabolism.
The arrival of the modern diet and lifestyle has led to a wide range of "deficiency" diseases and their side effects. The amount of minerals vary in the
body from somewhat large amounts to "trace" elements. They are essential
in maintaining physiological processes, especially digestive and neurological functions. Even in a seemingly well-balanced diet, it is possible to be
lacking one or more of the essential vitamins and minerals.

The efficiency of a mineral depends on the proper amount being balanced within the body's orchestra of other minerals. Sometimes a key mineral is not actually deficient, but its function is just being interfered with
by toxic levels of other minerals. The mineral ratios get out of harmony
when activities involving minerals are overused or inhibited by lifestyle

choices or diet. Vitamins are vital constituents of enzymes that help regulate metabolism, convert fats and carbohydrates into energy, and form bone and tissue. Use vitamin and mineral supplements if certain nutrients are lacking in the diet, or when there is a condition that requires special nutritional attention. Supplements available in health-food stores are usually superior to the "multi-vitamins" found in most supermarkets and drugstores. Laboratory-made synthetic vitamins, minerals, or amino acids can never be quite the same as the energy in living food. The food industry and the National Research Council, funded and controlled by the food industry, would like us to think otherwise. They maintain that synthetics and natural vitamins are identical, but research shows they are not. Take supplements with care. Excessive use can result in waste or in undesirable symptoms. It is important to remember that vitamins and mineral supplement but do not replace a well-balanced, quality diet. Anyone who takes megadoses of vitamins and minerals should be under the care of a health practitioner trained in nutrition.

Living food is imprisoned sunlight. How can laboratory-made vitamins, minerals, or amino acids ever be quite the same as the energy in living food? The food industry and the National Research Council, funded and controlled by the food industry, would like us to think that they are the same. They maintain that synthetic and natural vitamins are identical, yet research shows that they are not. Distress on the body (pain, exhaustion, severe burns, hyperventilation, extreme cold or heat) can all upset the body's chemistry and cause a depletion of vitamins and minerals. The body uses more nutrients when exposed constantly to environmental, chemical, and food toxins. If nutrients are not replaced with a good diet and supplements, the body will become deficient and more symptoms will occur.

Nutrient Deficiencies

Undiagnosed nutrient deficiencies, like a vitamin B12 deficiency, can cause psychiatric disorders or can mimic the symptoms of multiple sclerosis. Any single vitamin or mineral deficiency may cause one or more of the following symptoms: depression, anxiety, attention deficiency syndrome, insomnia, hyperactivity, mood swings, autism, delusions, premenstrual syndrome, lethargy, confusion, postpartum depression, euphoria, or schizophrenia. A direct connection exists between nutrition and mental health. How can food that is canned, synthetic, hydrogenated, frozen, freeze-dried, dyed, preserved, emulsified, flavor-enhanced, and aluminum-containing be as healthy as fresh food? The more a fresh food is changed the more likely it will become deficient in nutrients. This increases the risk of developing an illness.

How can you tell if your diet is working for you and you are getting all the nutrients you need? Some of these symptoms may give you a hint: loss of energy, gray or pasty complexion, brittle and dry hair, dry and scaling skin, fingernails easily break, sugar cravings, a general lack of interest in things, a dragging feeling, depression, abnormal weight loss or gain, feel sick frequently, no or irregular periods, premature menopause, insomnia, skin breaks out or feels rough, and frequent colds. The addition of vitamins, minerals, and supplements to the diet may be of vital importance today. The prime importance of supplements is to fill in the nutritional gaps produced by faulty eating habits and by nutritionally inferior foods.

Weight Control

In order to lose weight many people disregard proper nutrition. A familiar cycle of temporary weight loss followed by weight gain has proved the ineffectiveness of many quick-loss diets. Weight control often requires supportive counseling, lifestyle changes, and exercise, as well as careful attention to proper nutrition. Each individual needs a specially tailored nutritional plan to insure successful and permanent weight control.

Snacks and Desserts

Contrary to what most people believe, snacks and desserts can be nutritious and pleasing. The same principles that apply to other foods are important here. Most snacks and desserts available in supermarkets and restaurants today contain large amounts of sugar, salt, white flour, MSG, artificial preservatives, flavors, and colors. Try to eliminate these products. Many natural-food stores sell packaged chips, pretzels, cookies, and candies that are wholesome, tasty and nutritious. Nuts, seeds, and fruits are good choices for snacks. Carob is a healthful replacement for chocolate. Natural fruit juice (diluted) is a great improvement over juice drinks and highly synthetic, chemical-laden soft drinks.

Fast Foods

Fast foods are mostly high in sugar, salt, refined carbohydrates, fats, and calories, but very low in fiber and certain vitamins and minerals. Depending on fast foods as the major component of your diet can have serious nutritional consequences. One fast food meal can easily supply half of your total daily calorie needs. A three-piece fried chicken dinner with mashed potatoes and gravy, coleslaw and a roll can contain 950 calories, without the drink included. With a 12-ounce soft drink, the total can come to 1,100 calories. The salt content may be 75 percent of the day's recommended 2,200 milligrams of salt. A burger or pizza can have around 1,100 or more milligrams of salt, and shakes and pies probably contain at least 400 milligrams.

Fat is usually the main source of calories in a fast-food meal, and this doesn't mean just the fried parts. This includes the addition of any cheese and sauce. Fast-food shakes are also high in fat with saturated vegetable oils such as coconut oil. A typical fast-food meal can easily contain around 46 grams of fat. On average, most fast foods do not provide the body with the proper nutrients it needs.

Exercise

Regular exercise can help everyone. It increases metabolism and also helps nutrients get to every cell in the body. In addition, it helps create a valuable feeling of well-being and accomplishment. Include vigorous physical exercise in your life routine at least three times weekly. Exercise is an excellent tonic that improves circulation, enhances digestion, strengthens the heart, tones the muscles, firms up the waistline, and helps to overcome constipation. It also normalizes appetite levels and regulates blood sugar and cholesterol. If possible, get your exercise in the open air. If you're overweight or in poor health, begin slowly and gradually increase activity. Walking is a good beginning exercise.

Sweating due to moderate exercise, a wet sauna, or a steam bath will aid in the elimination of toxins. While in a steam bath, drink a minimum of 1/2 liter of water before and after the activity. For those who are unable to exercise or endure a sauna or steam bath, soaking in a tub with hot water may be helpful. If your pulse increases fifteen or more beats over your initial heart rate, you should exit the heated area.

Relaxation and Stress Reduction

Generate a relaxed atmosphere around meals. Have a peaceful, leisurely mealtime to provide a healthful relief from the stress and fast pace of daily routine. Meals can be a focal point for togetherness and sharing. Their role in improving personal and family relationships is valuable. Do not use mealtime to discuss problems. Instead, have a relaxing conversation and avoid arguments or stressful topics when eating. Try to avoid reading or watching TV with your meals. Sit and eat slowly, chewing your food well. This will aid the digestive process and improve both digestive functioning and overall nutrition, and reduce digestive stress.

Reducing stress through exercise, meditation, biofeedback, yoga, martial arts, or hobbies is often helpful. It is especially useful for those who are tense and have difficulty resting, relaxing, or sleeping. Stress increases the body's needs for nutrients and interferes with proper digestion. Excessive stress is often the culprit behind many illnesses. When the stress in our lives becomes distress, the body no longer is in balance.

High-Stress and Low-Stress Foods

Our need for different foods can depend on our individual biochemistry. One food can be low stress for a certain person and high stress for another. This may result from a toxic liver, poor digestive enzyme production, poor chewing habits, improperly combining of foods, or many other reasons. Low-stress foods are those that digest quickly and easily, leave little residue for the liver to detoxify, and do not cause toxic build-up for the bowel and vascular system. They provide your system with extra supplies to rebuild, strengthen reserves, and increase resistance and endurance.

All vegetables and vegetable juices are low-stress foods. They digest easily and quickly providing concentrated sources of minerals as well as vitamins and enzymes. Vegetables have an alkalinizing effect on the entire system. Raw vegetables aid in detoxifying the body rapidly and their high-fiber content aids in keeping the intestinal tract swept clean. Steamed vegetables are good to have at the evening meal. It is best to steam them at the lowest heat needed.

Gas-forming vegetables have a high sulphur content, making them difficult for some people to digest. Eat sparingly of cabbage, cauliflower, Brussels sprouts, broccoli, mustard greens, and radishes if there is a problem. Over cooking vegetables will destroy the enzymes, making them harder to digest, and putting them in the high-stress category. You can heat vegetables completely, but allow them to remain crisp.

Sleep

Sleep is necessary for all bodily processes. The degree of restfulness and ease in arising in the morning can be an indicator of proper sleep. Eating before bedtime can cause poor sleep and lead to a feeling of drowsiness or irritability in the morning and contribute to weight gain. Yet, some people who tend to have low blood sugar may need to eat later in the evening in order to sleep well.

Awareness

As you get healthier it will be more obvious when you eat something wrong. The symptoms may come right after eating or maybe the symptoms will come in the form of moodiness, headaches, cloudy thinking, or other behavior changes. If you're paying attention, you will discover that your digestion is affecting every part of your life. Now, instead of being told what you should and shouldn't eat, you can get that information directly from your own body, but you have to listen.

Other Guidelines for Good Health

• Three servings (1/2 cup per serving) of fresh vegetables should be eaten daily. One of these should be a dark green vegetable, one orange in color, and another choice could be a raw vegetable.

• It is important to get adequate calories each day. Females age 15 to 50 need approximately 2100 calories; over the age of 51 is 1800 calories. Males age 15 to 22 need approximately 3000 calories; age 23 to 50 need 2700 calories; and over the age of 51 need 2400 calories.

• Choose foods that produce a diet that is about 60-70 percent complex carbohydrates, 15-20 percent fats, and 15-20 percent proteins. This is optimal.

• Complex carbohydrates should be eaten daily. Examples are: most whole grains, lentils, tofu, vegetables, buckwheat, whole fruits including berries, potatoes with their skins, beans and peas.

• Eat only moderate levels of protein, limiting animal protein to no more than two servings per day. Limit servings of meat to six to eight ounces with any visible fat removed. Proteins from meat sources are high in fat. Most American diets are already too high in protein causing stress on the kidneys as well as other health problems. Include turkey, fish, or eggs in your diet rather than red meats, if you eat animal products. Eat more protein from combined vegetable sources.

• Eat a low amount of fat in the form of cold-pressed vegetable oils, especially containing essential fatty acids. Fat should only make up approximately 15-20 percent of the daily calories. The average fat intake in this country is about 40-50 percent of total caloric intake. Nuts and seeds are high in fat and their intake should be in moderate amounts.

• Combine fruits properly. Do not eat them with other types of food. Eating fruit and other simple carbohydrates at the same time you eat protein interferes with the completion of protein digestion. Eat fruit at least 1/2 hour before a meal or at least two hours after a meal. Eat two to three servings of fresh fruit daily.

• Substitute organically raised animals and organically grown fruits and vegetables whenever possible.

• Eliminate foods suspected of containing heavy metals (swordfish, tuna, or canned foods).

• Avoid vinegar in salad dressings. It is a fermented product that suspends salivary digestion and retards the digestion of starches. Instead, substitute lemon juice for vinegar.

* Avoid the excessive consumption of raw onions and garlic. They pervert the taste buds and cause you to crave more concentrated foods.
* Taking *Lactobacillus acidophilus* and *Lactobacillus bifidus* helps with digestion. Take 1/2 hour before meals, on an empty stomach, to keep it from being destroyed by the hydrochloric acid in the stomach. These organisms are now being added to dairy products, but most are killed during digestion. That is why they have to be taken by themselves on an empty stomach.
* Be creative in your food selections.
* Eliminate food intolerances and sensitivities, if known.
* Balance acid and alkaline foods.
* Avoid milk and sodas, especially at mealtime. They can interfere with digestion by neutralizing stomach acid.
* Drink 6 to 8 ounces of pure water daily, but try not to drink with meals.
* Do not eat when tired, anxious, or if excessively stressed.
* Eat most of your food earlier in the day and smaller meals at evening.
* Chew all foods well while relaxing in a peaceful atmosphere.
* Stop eating before feeling full or when no longer hungry.
* The diet should have adequate total calories, but be low in total fat and refined carbohydrates, food additives, stimulants (salt, teas, coffee, and tobacco), and processed foods.
* Avoid foods that have a long shelf life. Use chemical- and pesticide-free foods whenever possible.
* The best way to replace the important nutrients that are lost in our current diets is to eat a greater variety of foods, but not the same foods two days in a row. Shop organic produce, cook foods less and at lower temperatures, and perhaps add a home garden.
* Get adequate sleep.
* Minimize prescription and over-the-counter medications. Do not use recreational drugs.
* Do your best to develop a regular schedule of fluid intake, meals, rest, and exercise, including breathing and relaxation exercises..

Our environment usually influences us more than heredity. Nutrition is an environmental factor and the lack of proper nutrition is a major stress. Many reports from many sources indicate that acute diseases and senile degeneration are all cellular diseases. The basic condition that makes cells vulnerable is inadequate nutrition. Little by little we are eating ourselves to death, not to life. Following these guidelines to proper nutrition will increase a healthy person's chances of staying healthy. A diet and lifestyle adjustment along with appropriate therapies used in holistic medicine can help the sick person to recover and experience optimal wellness.

FOOD COMBINATIONS AND RULES FOR GOOD HEALTH

Proper food combining is one of the most important things you can do to enhance your good health and well being. It is every bit as important as drinking enough water each day, eating the correct balance of acid and alkaline foods, decreasing the wrong type of fats in your diet, and getting enough vitamins and minerals.

Proteins, starches, and fats require different types of digestive enzymes. Proper food combining at the same meal requires less time and energy for their digestion and absorption. The most energy is required by protein and fats. Vegetables, cereals and grains require less work. Fruits and juices require the least amount of work.

Combining these types of foods at the same meal may interfere with proper digestion and allow a significant amount of food to reach the large intestine undigested. Undigested food in the large intestine will cause toxic by-products; the proteins will putrefy, the carbohydrates ferment, and the fats become rancid. This can cause food sensitivities, as well as the loss of nutrients normally derived from the food.

CLASSIFICATION OF FOODS

The following charts and text give general guidelines that are designed to enhance your health. This way of eating is usually easy on the digestive system and compatible with the treatment of yeast infections and immune-building diet plans. It is common to feel worse during the first week because of all the toxins leaving the body. This is especially true in people who use alcohol, coffee, sugar, and an excessive amount of refined carbohydrates.

PROTEINS	CARBOHYDRATES/STARCHES	FATS
Almonds	Barley	Avocado
Brazil nuts	Beans (dried)	Butter
Beans (dried)	Bread	Canola oil
Cashew nuts	Buckwheat	Corn oil
Cheese	Chestnuts	Cottonseed oil

PROTEINS	CARBOHYDRATES/STARCHES	FATS
Coconut	Corn	Cream
Eggs	Millet	Meat fat
Fish	Oats	Nut oils
Hazelnuts	Peanuts	Sesame oil
Hickory nuts	Peas	Soybean oil
Macadamia nuts	Plantain	Sunflower oil
Meats	Potatoes	
Milk	Rice	
Olives	Rye	
Peanuts	Sweet potatoes	
Pecans	Wheat	
Pine nuts	Winter squash	
Poultry	Yams	
Pumpkin seeds		
Sesame seeds		
Soybean		
Sprouts (mung, lentils, alfalfa, radishes)		
Sunflower		
Tofu		
Walnuts		

FOOD COMBINING CHART

If you can't separate proteins from carbohydrates then at least separate fruit from other foods in the diet. This speeds up digestion and makes it more efficient. If you would like to read more about how and why to combine foods, read *Eating Alive* by John Matsen, N.D., and *Fit for Life* by Harvey & Marilyn Diamond.

Carbohydrate	Non-starch Vegetables	Protein	Fruit		
			acid	subacid	sweet
grains	asparagus	beans	grapefruit	apple	banana
pastas	broccoli	soybeans	lemon	papaya	date
rice	Brussels sprouts	fish	lime	pear	raisins
corn	cabbage	poultry	orange	berries	apple
potatoes	cauliflower	wild game	pineapple	cherry	fig
turnip	celery	meat	currant	plum	prune
squashes	cucumber	seafood	tomato	grape	dried
parsnip	kale	seeds	sour plum	mango	peach
carrots	leafy greens	nuts	tangerine	pineapple	apricot
avocado	zucchini	dairy	strawberry	nectarine	
eggplant	green beans	olives	sour apple	guava	
beet	Swiss chard	sprouts		quince	
taro corms	artichoke	eggs		prickly pear	
tubers	sea vegetables			huckleberry	
	endive			persimmon	
	okra				
	onions				
	peppers				
	radishes				
	asparagus				
	parsley				
	garlic				
	mushroom				
	bamboo shoots				

Ratings: GOOD — GOOD — GOOD (Carbohydrate, Non-starch Vegetables, Protein); FAIR — FAIR — FAIR (Protein / Fruit / subacid, sweet); POOR (Carbohydrate and acid fruit combinations).

Fruits

Fruits are our cleansers. They are the best source of pure, naturally distilled and enzyme- and vitamin-active water. How much fruit you eat depends on the climate in your area, as well as physical and emotional conditions. Most people need about twenty percent of their diet in the form of fruit. Fresh fruit is not mucus forming and is the most cleansing of all foods. It supplies vitamins, minerals and enzymes, but the vitamin factor is the most important. Eat properly ripened fruit, because under-ripe fruit contains acids toxic to the body. Fruit is ideal for a small breakfast or between-meal snacks. Allow time for fruit to leave the stomach before the next meal. This is about one-half hour before meals. It is usually best not to combine too many fruits at one time. Eat fresh fruits in season and preferably organically grown.

If you eat fruit first thing in the morning, it should be whole fruit, not juiced or dried. You can continue to eat it as often as you like during the morning. Have at least two servings of fruit in any three-hour period. Never eat fruit with or immediately following anything. Fruit and fruit juices use different digestive enzymes and are best when eaten away from other foods, especially protein. Eating more frequently is better than eating a lot of fruit at one time. Eat whole, fresh, in season, uncooked fruit 20-30 minutes before eating anything else.

The digestive system is at its strongest between 7:00 a.m. and 11:00 a.m. For this reason eating fruits by themselves for the first few hours in the morning is an excellent strategy for cleansing the digestive system. Fruits are easy for most people to digest and do not seem to interrupt the cleansing cycle of the body. If you eat fruit all morning, do not continue eating fruit the rest of the day. Since this process stirs up old toxins, you don't want to continue this all day. Ideally, eat fruit until about 11:00 a.m., following by vegetable juice an hour later. Then have lunch. If you can only handle a fruit diet for one to two hours in the morning that is just fine. Having a rushed meal in the morning with coffee or black tea is a certain path to gastrointestinal dysfunction, disease, and degeneration.

Eat sweet fruits and strongly acid fruits at separate times, especially if feeling sick. Sweet fruits are apples, pears, grapes, blueberries, bananas, and figs; acid fruits are oranges, kiwi, grapefruits, strawberries, pineapples, and pomegranates. It is best to eat sweet fruits when fresh and whole. Juicing and drying tends to amplify their sweetness and sugar content.

The continued use of sweet fruit (or other sweet foods) after eating protein is the worst of the food combinations, and one of the most destructive to your health. This is also true of most fruit juices when combined with protein meals. (*Note:* Melons are not fruit and should be eaten by themselves or with other melons, not at the same time as fruit.) Melons often do not mix well with fruit. They digest in the intestines and decompose very quickly (in 20-30 minutes). When held up in a warm, moist place (the stomach) melons cause gas and discomfort. It is best to have melons 15-30 minutes before having any fruit. Melons are watermelon, honeydew, and cantaloupe.

FRUIT LIST

Acid	*Subacid*	*Sweet*
Dried fruit	Apple (granny smith)	Apple (sweet)
Gooseberry	Apricot	Banana (ripe)
Grapefruit	Avocado	Carob
Lemon	Berries (most)	Date
Lime	Cherry	Figs
Orange	Grapes	Grapes (sweet)
Pineapple	Mango	Litchi
Pomegranate	Nectarine	Papaya
Sour plum	Passion fruit	Persimmon
Strawberry	Peach	Prune
Tomato	Pear	Raisins
	Plum	

Vegetables

Green plants are our healers. They are blood builders and sources of enzyme-rich plant protein. Our diets should consist of 50-60 percent vegetables. They contain more enzymes when eaten raw or mildly steamed. This could mean a salad for lunch and dinner as well as steamed vegetables. Learn the art of sprouting to yield fresh and nourishing shoots.

Since vegetable juice and broth tend to buffer or neutralize toxins, they follow fruit in the morning very well. They are best when drunk an hour or two after eating fruit. A good plan would be to have fruit first thing in the morning, followed one to two hours later by vegetable juice or broth. Get a little hungry before you eat lunch, but don't let the blood sugar fall. If you experience symptoms such as light-headedness, weakness and confusion, you have waited too long to eat. Eating usually relieves these symptoms. To cure low blood sugar problems see the chapter "Hypoglycemia."

Eating vegetables in the morning may be an alternative to eating only fruit. This is important to know if you are diabetic, have hypoglycemia, chronic yeast infections, or just can't tolerate much fruit. Consider having vegetable soup in the morning, as needed.

SLIGHTLY STARCHY VEGETABLES

Beets, Carrots, Jerusalem Artichokes, Parsnip

NON-STARCHY VEGETABLES

Asparagus	Celery	Okra
Anise	Chives	Other leafy greens
Artichoke	Cucumber	Peppers
Beans (green)	Eggplant	Radish
Broccoli	Fennel	Silver beets
Brussels sprouts	Kale	Squash (young, summer)
Cabbage	Kohlrabi	Watercress
Cauliflower	Leafy lettuce	

Proteins

Proteins are our builders and feed the nervous system. Too much protein disrupts digestion and circulation in both the vascular and the lymphatic system. Our diets should consist of about 10 percent high-quality, low stress, and easily digestible protein.

Sweeteners inhibit the digestion of protein and so do most refined carbohydrates such as white sugar. Proteins combine best with non-starchy, succulent vegetables. All foods combine best with vegetables, especially the green leafy ones. It is best to eat most of your protein at the end of the day so it will be used to build collagen, the building material for the body. Those who burn calories extremely rapidly (fast metabolizers, hypoglycemics) may be helped by mixing protein and starches or grains together.

The more concentrated the protein (e.g. red meat) the longer it takes to digest. Eat only one concentrated protein food at a meal. Concentrated foods require complex digestive processes for adequate breakdown and absorption. Try to wait three hours before eating these types of proteins again or having dairy. If you must mix more than one concentrated food at a meal, try to keep them in the same group. Avoid cross-category combinations of concentrated foods. Do not combine concentrated proteins with concentrated starches or fats, if possible.

Protein and Starch

Protein requires an acid medium for digestion, but starch requires an alkaline medium. This is a combination that may be best to avoid when you are under excessive stress or having digestion problems that are not resolving by other methods. When concentrated starches are mixed with protein it can cause fermentation in the stomach and produce gas.

Adequate hydrochloric acid will prevent this to some extent, but the major cause of stomach gas is improper combining of food groups. Too many Americans are accustomed to finishing off a protein meal with a sweet dessert. This is a very poor way to combine foods. Concentrated sweets should be eaten on an empty stomach. This includes fruits as well as fruit juices.

Protein and Acid Foods

The enzyme pepsin breaks down complex proteins in the stomach in an acid medium only. Eating excessive acid foods inhibits the production of pepsin.

Protein and Fat

Fats decrease the secretion of pepsin, hydrochloric acid, and other gastric juices. Don't eat papaya with protein. Papaya does have an enzyme that aids protein digestion, but it will weaken your own ability to digest protein unaided.

Eating Carbohydrates and Proteins Together

The sweeter and the more refined the carbohydrate, such as white sugar, the more it inhibits the digestion of proteins by interfering with stomach acid. The heavier the protein the longer it takes to digest, and eating a carbohydrate will inhibit the protein's digestion. A piece of fruit may take an hour to digest whereas a protein meal of rice and beans may take three to four hours, or longer. Mixing the two groups together greatly increases the production of intestinal toxins. These toxic by-products are what foul up the elimination organs and cause most diseases.

Carbohydrates/Starches

Carbohydrates are our builders and help to balance our body's energy. They are our chief source of energy, promote proper muscular function, and assisting in digestion and assimilation. Our diets need to consist of approximately 60 percent wholesome carbohydrates including 10 percent starchy vegetables.

Diets that contain too many refined or simple carbohydrates feed intestinal yeast especially during cold, wet weather when they are more active. Sweet fruit ripens at the time intestinal yeast are the least active. By eating fruit in the winter we feed the yeast and cause problems with the intestinal flora. In these cases avoid fruit juice completely and limit whole fruit until the intestinal critters can be controlled. Have vegetable juice or broth instead.

Avoid mixing carbohydrates and proteins together if you have excessive yeast growing in your intestinal tract. This will speed up digestion without feeding the harmful flora. Carbohydrates eaten by themselves will burn cleanly and be easily eliminated. Don't eat carbohydrates and protein together if you have chronic digestive problems.

It is best to eat concentrated carbohydrates at least two hours apart. Try to eat carbohydrates without drinking liquids, and remember to chew thoroughly. Light steaming aids in digestion by beginning to break down the food fibers. Avoid eating sugar with other foods because it ends up fermenting quickly in the warm, moist stomach instead of where it is meant to digest. Sugars usually digest in the intestines, not in the stomach.

BOWEL REGULARITY

When the body is cleaning itself and removing toxins, you may feel worse before you feel better. Take something such as psyllium hulls to move the toxins out of the body. They help the bowels without being scratchy like wheat bran. Take a small amount in the beginning and increase the dosage slowly. Start with one teaspoon twice a day before meals and slowly increase the amount so that the intestine gradually gets filled. Bentonite clay can be used along with psyllium hulls.

Exercise regularly to aid proper waste elimination and to stimulate muscles. It is very important to keep the bowels regular. If you experience constipation, it is important to drink plenty of water and eat adequate fiber. Start slowly and stay away from constipating foods such as cheese and bananas. Start the day with soaked or stewed prunes, figs, and raisins.

ROTATE FOODS

Repetitive eating is the major cause of food sensitivities. This is eating the same foods day after day. Wheat, dairy, eggs, and sugar are usually eaten daily and are the most common allergens. Rotate your foods, trying not to eat the same food within 48-72 hours.

VITALITY

If you are a person with average vitality, and a fair number of toxins has accumulated over the years (though you have no chronic disease) you should eat fruit in the morning to continue removing the old built-up debris. You should continue to separate the carbohydrates/grains from the proteins whenever possible. Using small amounts of carbohydrates/grains with protein will not usually cause problems, if done occasionally.

However, if you have weak vitality you may have large amounts of accumulated toxicity and probably some chronic disease. You will need to remain on a stricter diet regimen much longer. The separation of proteins, carbohydrates, and fruits should be maintained as long as necessary. It takes time to chip away at those years of accumulated fat and metabolic debris. Ideally, such a person should be under the supervision of a physician who can suggest treatments to aid the removal of old accumulated toxins.

The Results

Good digestion is one of the most important factors of continued good health. The increasing incident of degenerative diseases should be enough to make us pause and think. The more you use proper food combining the better you will digest your food. Usually, the first sign of progress is an increase in energy and a decrease in digestive problems. Your digestive system will be able to perform its function more efficiently and benefit you with increased assimilation of nutrients. There will be fewer toxins ending up in your intestinal tract making you sick. As your digestive tract gets healthier it will be able to remove other toxins more effectively. Your digestive tract will be able to handle mixing proteins, carbohydrates, and fats much better. As long as there is impaired digestive function it is better to follow the basic rules for food combining. Learning how to combine foods properly may mean changing some old habits and trying some new ways to eat.

Generally, it is preferable to avoid mixing too many varieties of foods at one meal. Try to attain simplicity. This is not to imply that food combining is more important then the wholeness and wholesomeness of individual foods. The quality of food is of prime importance. Many factors can affect the digestion of foods besides how foods are combined. These may include emotional stress, the amount of food eaten at any one time, and the proper balance between acid and alkaline foods, etc.

MORE HELPFUL HINTS

- Do not mix more than four foods from any one group. At one meal it is best not to mix foods from more than two different classifications.
- Tomatoes may be combined with low-starchy vegetables and proteins or avocados.
- Avocados are best combined with acid or sub-acid fruits, or green vegetables.
- Buy fruit and vegetables fresh and organic whenever possible. Buy frozen foods when fresh is not available. Buy meats that are free of chemicals and antibiotics.

• Dairy combines poorly with all foods due to its high fat content. If you must have dairy, eat or drink it by itself, not with other foods.

Food Families

People who have a problem with a particular food may not realize that they could also be having problems with other foods in the same plant family. For that reason the following list will help you identify similar foods that might be causing you problems:

Apple: apple (including cider, vinegar, and pectin made from apple), pear, quince.
Aster: lettuce, chicory, endive, escarole, artichoke, dandelion, sunflower seeds, tarragon.
Banana: banana, plantain
Beech: chestnut
Beet: beets, spinach, Swiss chard, lamb's quarter
Birch: filberts or hazel nuts
Blueberry: blueberry, huckleberry, cranberry, wintergreen
Buckwheat: buckwheat
Cashew: cashew, pistachio, mango
Citrus: lemon, orange, grapefruit, lime, tangerine, kumquat, citron
Dairy: Milk products (consisting of lactalbumin, whey, lactose, casein). Avoid products made from any part of cow's milk including: butter, cheese, yogurt, buttermilk, evaporated cow's milk, half and half, ice cream made from cow's milk, and skim milk.
Fresh-water fish: sturgeon, salmon, whitefish, bass, perch, trout
Fungus: mushrooms, yeast (brewer's yeast, etc.)
Grape: All varieties of grapes and raisins. This includes products made from grapes such as: fruit juices containing grape juice, wines, champagne, and foods containing them. Most baking powders contain cream of tartar or tartaric acid that is a by-product of the wine-making industry. This includes cream of tartar, breads, biscuits, and muffins made with tartrate baking powders.
Grass: wheat (includes graham flour, gluten, bran, wheat germ, kamut); corn (includes cornstarch, corn oil, margarine made from corn, dextrose, corn syrup; cane includes sugar, molasses); other grasses include: rice, wild rice, oats, barley, rye, millet, sorghum, bamboo sprouts
Crustaceans: crab, crayfish, lobster, prawn, shrimp
Ginger: ginger, turmeric, cardamom
Gooseberry: currant, gooseberry
Honeysuckle: elderberry
Laurel: avocado, cinnamon, bay leaf, sassafras, cassia buds or bark
Onion: onion, garlic, asparagus, chives, leeks

Olive: black or green or stuffed with pimiento

Mallow: okra, cottonseed

Melon: cucumber, squash, zucchini, acorn squash, pumpkin seeds, pumpkin, watermelon, cantaloupe, and other melons

Mint: any mint, peppermint, spearmint, thyme, sage, marjoram, savory

Mollusks: abalone, snail, squid, clam, mussel, oyster, scallop

Mulberry: mulberry, figs

Mustard: mustard, turnip, radish, horseradish, watercress, cabbage, Chinese cabbage, broccoli, cauliflower, Brussels sprouts, collards, kale, kohlrabi, rutabaga

Mutton: mutton, lamb

Myrtle: allspice, cloves, guava

Night shade: potato, tomato, eggplant, peppers (red and green), chili peppers, paprika, cayenne, pimento, and tobacco

Oils: soybean oil, peanut oil, cottonseed oil, safflower oil, corn oil

Palm: coconut, date, date sugar

Parsley: carrots, parsnips, celery, celery seed, anise, dill, fennel, cumin, parsley, coriander, caraway

Pea: soy beans, lentils, licorice, peanut, alfalfa

Pedalium: sesame, tahini

Pineapple: juice pack, water pack, or fresh

Rose: strawberry, raspberry, blackberry, dewberry, loganberry, young berry, boysenberry, rose hips, plum, prune, cherry, peach, apricot, nectarine, almond

Salt-water fish: herring, anchovy, cod, sea bass, mackerel, tuna, swordfish, flounder, sole, halibut, snapper

Spurge: tapioca

Sweet potato: sweet potatoes or yams

Swine: all pork products

Walnut: English walnut, black walnut, pecan, hickory nut, butternut

CHAPTER 7

Hypoglycemia

Often an allergy is a symptom rather than a disease; it may only be a sign of a deeper, underlying problem. Many of the allergies I treat in a person often are accompanied by depression, mood swings, lethargy and overall irregular energy levels. Many times I determine that the person has hypoglycemia, or low blood sugar. "So what?" you ask. Often, after treating and effectively controlling the person's hypoglycemia, the original allergy that we were treating also clears up.

Hypoglycemia is a deficiency of glucose (sugar) in the blood. This condition is responsible for a great deal of suffering that most of its victims do not understand. It is also known as "functional hypoglycemia" or "reactive hypoglycemia." Absolute proof of hypoglycemia will not always be revealed with a glucose tolerance test. If the symptoms are present, a trial diet will usually help. Fortunately, in most cases this problem is curable or controllable with proper dietary management, nutritional supplements, and stress management.

All cases of behavioral and emotional problems should be evaluated for blood sugar abnormalities, food allergies and sensitivities, or endocrine imbalances. New medical research supports the view that the effects of hypoglycemia may be behind many mental and emotional disorders, including hyperactivity, antisocial behavior, mood swings, learning problems, criminal personalities, drug addiction, and allergies. Often, a person doesn't require a psychiatrist, but is the victim of a food illness.

In a large-scale study, 200 hyperactive children had low blood sugar often enough that it started or aggravated typical hyperactive behavior. Many of these children also had allergies to common foods. These were usually the foods they favored and ate whenever possible. This set off abnormal behaviors, many of which were the same ones used in the diagnosis of attention deficit syndrome (ADD). In another study with 265 hyperactive children, glucose tolerance tests were abnormal in 76 percent. This suggests that abnormal glucose metabolism may be a factor in the cause of hyperactivity.

SIMPLE AND COMPLEX CARBOHYDRATES DIFFERENCES

Carbohydrates are more efficient and more readily available as a source of energy than either fats or proteins. They digest easily and enter the bloodstream quickly. The least desirable carbohydrates are simple carbohydrates; they rapidly break down to sugar, or glucose and enter the bloodstream too fast, causing rapid elevation in the blood sugar, which is followed by a drop. When simple or refined carbohydrates are the main part of the diet, hypoglycemia (low blood sugar) is usually present.

Complex carbohydrates, found in most vegetables and whole grains, break down more slowly into glucose and do not cause rapid changes in the body's blood sugar. Instead, complex carbohydrates replenish glucose at regular intervals, keeping the body's energy constant. The ideal diet for most people is about two-thirds complex carbohydrates. Because of biochemical individuality, some individuals do not do well on a diet rich in carbohydrates. These are people with fast metabolisms. They burn their foods too fast and seem to do better when additional protein is added to their diet. Also, some people are carbohydrate-sensitive and do not thrive at all on carbohydrates.

SYMPTOMS OF HYPOGLYCEMIA

Low blood sugar creates a wide array of psychological symptoms including behavioral changes. The most common food-mood connection includes symptoms such as the inability to concentrate, mood swings, anxiety, depression, and being more emotional than usual. Other symptoms are asthma, fatigue, headache, hyperactivity, nervousness, insomnia, irritability, restlessness, poor memory, and indecisiveness. Someone exhibiting any of these behaviors could really be the victim of a bad diet.

CAUSES OF HYPOGLYCEMIA

The brain and other body tissues must have a steady supply of glucose (energy) to maintain health. The bloodstream carries this fuel source to all parts of the body. There always must be a certain amount of glucose in the blood to guarantee that each part of the body gets its adequate share. When the level of glucose in the blood drops below normal, the result is low blood sugar.

While all foods contain energy, different foods may affect the blood sugar in different ways. Simple carbohydrates or sugars absorb very quickly from the intestines into the bloodstream. If you continue to eat these foods, the body overreacts and much more insulin is produced than the body needs. This results in a large amount of blood sugar being absorbed in a short amount of time. The blood sugar then drops dangerously low.

Mental, emotional and physical changes may begin as the energy level decreases. Depression, anxiety, fatigue, or other symptoms begin to occur. And what does a person with hypoglycemia do? Reach for sugar. This type of sugar craving begins a vicious cycle. The person eats the sweet and feels revitalized from the quick "up" that a soda or candy bar gives. Soon, the sugar load over-stimulates the pancreas and a burst of insulin comes pouring forth. Promptly, the blood sugar level drops lower than before. What does the person do next? There is only one recourse, eat more sugar. But this is only a short-term solution that ultimately causes the problem it is meant to solve.

How is this ugly cycle stopped? How can blood sugar levels be maintained without abusing the body? The answer is to eat complex carbohydrates—the food group that will positively influence our moods, our ability to think, and our energy levels. Because we want to avoid hypoglycemia, the bulk of our diet should be in the form of complex carbohydrates. Along with unrefined starches from whole foods they can provide the necessary nutrition that the body needs to maintain a stable blood sugar.

Treating Hypoglycemia

If all conditions were as easy to treat as hypoglycemia, the world would be an Eden of wellness. This is not an over-simplification. A change in diet can mean a change in symptoms. The main things required of anyone who suffers from low blood sugar are: to stop eating sugar-containing products, caffeine, refined carbohydrates and junk foods, and to learn how to have a healthy diet. A positive result of treating hypoglycemia is that allergy symptoms will often disappear. The following are steps essential to treating hypoglycemia:

STEP 1. All sugar intake must stop. Most of the people affected with hypoglycemia have a poor diet history. They either don't have breakfast or eat sugared grain cereals and milk. Their lunches and suppers consist of fast foods, and their snacks are filled with sugar and caffeine. They eat foods full of preservatives, dyes, and other chemicals and pesticides. The common drinks are usually milk (with or without chocolate), some sugar-laden soda, or a sugared fruit drink. This type of diet is more than likely deficient in fresh vegetables, whole fruits, and adequate water. (Please note that some people with hypoglycemia do not function well when consuming fruits.) Hypoglycemics should also avoid all fruit juices, dried fruits, and even some vegetable juices. These are concentrated forms of sugar even in their natural states and evoke low blood sugar reactions minutes to hours after eating.

STEP 2. To treat hypoglycemia, the diet must consist of adequate protein and complex carbohydrates. Protein in this case includes moderate amounts of fish, lamb, turkey, and chicken. It is best to avoid the more dubious varieties of meat like hot dogs, chain-store hamburgers, and high-nitrate lunch meats. Other good sources of protein and complex carbohydrates include eggs, green leafy vegetables, dried peas and beans, brewer's yeast, whole grain cereals, soybeans, lentils, bean curd (tofu), sunflower seeds, pumpkin seeds, kefir, almonds, cashews, soy flour and other grains such as spelt and quinoa, wheat germ, fresh fruit, and vegetables. With few exceptions, the high-protein diets advocated in the past for hypoglycemia may make the condition worse.

STEP 3. The ideal approach to overcoming hypoglycemia is to eat several small meals a day rather than three large ones. It is also important to eat only when hungry, not according to the clock, and to not skip meals. Five or six somewhat lean feedings are best, with plenty of fresh food. Try a small breakfast, a good mid-morning snack, a light lunch, a mid-afternoon snack, dinner, and a snack before bed. The point of eating a little food at frequent intervals is to maintain a certain amount of naturally-derived sugar in the bloodstream to maintain proper blood sugar levels.

STEP 4. Children need dietary fats and oils to grow. Especially vital to body tissues are fatty acids. Children who are fast oxidizers need fats to calm them down, provide steady energy, and avoid the energy roller coaster of hypoglycemia. Deprived of healthy foods, children often crave and eat more sugar, leading to sugar addiction. Feed your children regular meals and teach them good eating habits. Adults also need adequate fats especially in the form of essential fatty acids.

STEP 5. The following are guidelines you can employ in managing your child's diet, as well as your own. Eat enough to prevent hunger, but do not persist until stuffed. Don't eat more than two pieces of bread daily; consume only a moderate amount of fats. Avoid foods high in refined sugars and artificial sweeteners. Eat three to five fresh vegetables, steamed or raw, as well as two servings of fresh fruits daily. If you or your child exhibits even a touch of hypoglycemia, avoid refined white flour, dried fruits, soft drinks, caffeine, citrus drinks and fruits, black tea, and salt. Also, beware of foods containing cocoa with a sugar base.

How to Deal with Sugar Cravings

Foods such as walnuts, bananas, and fresh pineapple may help reduce sugar cravings. Usually after a week or so of having no sugar in the diet, the blood sugar will stabilize and the craving for sugar will go away. Pantothenic acid (100 milligrams) may be chewed whenever a craving for sugar becomes strong. Using mineral supplements high in magnesium and trace minerals is helpful to decrease sugar cravings. Bile salts can also reduce craving for sweets in some people. The biochemical cell salts useful for sugar cravings are silica, magnesium phosphate and calcium sulphate. For more information on cell salts read my book, *Natural Healing with Cell Salts*.

Hypoglycemia often occurs after food allergens are consumed, triggering uncontrollable hunger and eating. Any food can trigger hypoglycemic symptoms and any system in the body can be affected, but most sensitive people have a target organ. Once the pancreas has become hypersensitive to sugar over a long period of time, complete recovery is not always possible. In experiments done on rats, it was found that hypoglycemia could be corrected and kept under control with a change in diet. If the rats went back to the old diet, hypoglycemia and the resulting symptoms returned fairly rapidly. Obviously you or your child are not rats, but the lesson is there. A more healthful diet will undoubtedly improve everyone's health, and can undoubtedly assist in overcoming allergies.

CHAPTER 8

Acid-Alkaline Balance

When people hear the term "balanced diet," they usually think of eating foods belonging to all of the basic food groups. There is, however, another aspect of balance in the diet that is essential to health. This balance has to do with the levels of acidity and alkalinity of our food and their proper ratios. If the food metabolized by our body is too acid or too alkaline, it is not properly assimilated. The typical American diet is usually highly acidic. This explains the success of antacid tablets, since they are alkaline and neutralize acidic conditions. They may bring temporary relief, but the stomach needs acid in order to digest the food. Neutralizing stomach acid with pills results in more digestion problems.

Maintaining a proper acid-alkaline balance is essential for health and vitality and is probably the most important thing we can do with our diet. In healthy people, a proper balance is normally maintained through a buffering system. This balance depends on a healthy digestive system as well as a healthy liver. Poor assimilation and elimination, lack of hydrochloric acid, severe infection or illness, heavy smoking and drinking alcohol, or drug consumption all interfere with this buffering system.

It is necessary to realize that all the trillion of cells in the human body are slightly acidic and must exist in a slightly alkaline environment to remain healthy and produce energy. As each cell performs its task, it secretes wastes that are acidic. These wastes are the end product of cellular metabolism and must not be allowed to build up, so the body goes to great lengths to neutralize and detoxify these acids. A diet balanced in acid-alkaline foods is essential for the body to meet this goal. If the body can't detoxify, it puts excessive demands on the immune system. This increases the risk of other immune problems.

The natural ratio in a normal, healthy body is approximately 4 to 1; four parts alkaline to one part acid. With such an ideal ratio, the body has a strong resistance to disease. A person with an acid body chemistry recovers quicker from illness if they begin to eat more alkaline foods. In the treatment of most diseases, the diet should include plenty of alkaline ash foods offsetting the effect of too many acid-forming foods. Once food is digested, it is known as "ash." Generally, meat and cereals yield an acid ash, fruits and vegetables yield an alkaline ash, and fats yield a neutral ash.

Ideally, keep your body in a neutral or slightly alkaline state, neither too acid nor too alkaline. When a body gets too acidic, off-centered, or unbalanced, then unpleasant symptoms are likely to occur such as arthritis, bursitis and rheumatism. The excess acid usually settles in the joints causing inflammation and pain. In addition, an over-acid body inhibits the production of natural cortisone, which feeds the adrenal glands and helps the body metabolize proteins. When the blood becomes acidic, the body is going to pull calcium from the bones to make the blood more alkaline, more in balance. Other symptoms of an acidic diet could be fatigue, allergies, headaches, boils, canker sores, and general malaise. Some other causes of an acid system may be allergies, parasites, high stress, poor diet, a toxic environment, sedentary lifestyle, illness, or a combination of these.

The human body contains several types of pain receptors. One of them can detect chemical changes in the body produced from an acid or alkaline imbalance. For these types of pains, acid and alkaline balancing is especially important. Keep the liver, kidneys, skin, and bowels healthy. This helps the body to balance its chemistry.

In general, it is best to combine acid foods with alkaline foods, not acid foods with acid foods, As a rule, the body needs more alkaline foods. They are necessary for the pancreas to produce enzymes and for the liver to function best. Acid foods include carbohydrate-rich foods, while alkaline foods are mostly fruits, vegetables, herbs, and spices. It is important not to eat excess meat protein, because it can result in excessive acidity. This acidity interferes with the potassium and magnesium balance of the cells and upsets the calcium stores, as well as other mineral balances. It also congests the lymphatic system and decreases its ability to carry toxins from the body.

A healthy body keeps large alkaline reserves to meet emergency demands. A body can function normally and sustain health only in the presence of adequate alkaline reserves and the proper acid-alkaline ratio in all the body tissues and the blood. Eating the wrong type of foods depletes these alkaline reserves. For optimum health and maximum resistance to disease, your diet must have the proper ratio of acid, alkaline, and neutral foods. A slightly alkaline system leaves you with a sense of well being.

Alkaline Foods

The following common foods are more alkaline than acid. The most alkaline foods are those that appear in the left-hand column at the top of the list. Figs and carrots, for example, are very alkaline, whereas asparagus and coconuts have a low alkaline value. Some of the most alkaline foods are molasses, beans, raisins, beet greens, spinach, brewer's yeast, almonds, soybeans, celery and most vegetables. The most alkaline sugars are molasses, real maple syrup, and honey. If you eat excessive amounts of these sweetener then they become acid-formers. Sprouted seeds and grains become more alkaline in the process of sprouting.

ALKALINE-FORMING FOODS

Foods with highest alkalinity start at the top of the left-hand column and move down each column. So figs has the highest alkaline content, cherries have a moderately high alkalinity, while ice cream has the lowest.

Figs	Watercress	Peaches, fresh
Molasses	Rutabaga	Mango
Olives (green or ripe)	Endive	Mushrooms
Lima beans	Cantaloupe	Eggplant
Soybeans	Lettuce	Brussels sprouts
Apricots, dried	Parsley	Garbanzo beans
Turnip or beet greens	Apricots, fresh	Broccoli
Spinach	Potatoes, sweet, white	Red Cabbage
Taro roots	Pineapple	Pears, fresh
Cucumber	Pomegranate	Squash
Dandelion greens	Beans, baked	Grapes
Mustard greens	Nectarines	Strawberry
Raisins	Cabbage	Apple
Beet	Cherries	Bananas
Avocado	Sauerkraut	Watermelon
Kale	Grapefruit	Buttermilk
Chive	Tomatoes	Whole milk
Swiss chard	Radish	Millet
Prune, dried	Currants, dried	Brazil nuts
Almonds	Cauliflower	Coconuts
Parsnips	Lemon	Buckwheat
Carrot	Bamboo shoots	Onions
Beets	Cantaloupe	Green peas
Dates	Blackberry	Asparagus
Chestnuts	Guava	Ice cream
Celery	String beans	

Acid Foods

The following common foods are more acidic than alkaline. The most acid foods are those that appear in the left-handed column and at the top of the list. Egg yolk is one of the most acid forming foods, but lentils are very low on the acid chart. Some of the most acidic foods are wheat germ, animal products, and most sugars. Other acid-forming substances are alcohol, coca-cola, catsup, cocoa, flour products, mustard, and pasta. Dairy products are fairly acidic: these include all cheeses, ice cream, custards, and milk. Prunes, cranberries, and plums are acid-forming fruits, but just because a fruit has an acid taste does not indicate that its reaction in the body is acidic. It may breakdown to being alkaline. Most drugs and coffee are acidic in the body. White or acetic vinegar is very acidic whereas balsamic vinegar is low acid and rice vinegar is the lowest in acidic properties.

ACID-FORMING FOODS

The following list gives a sample of foods in order of their acid-forming ability. The foods with the highest acidity are at the top of the left-hand column, while those at the bottom of the second column have the lowest acidity. So, egg yolks are high in acidity, bacon is moderately acidic and lentils are low in acidic forming ability.

Egg yolk	Bacon
Herring, smoked	Lamb
Oysters	Duck
Crab	Turkey
Duck	Barley
Turkey	Spaghetti
Lobster	Other organ meats
Oatmeal	Rice
Sardines	Haddock
Veal	Crackers in general
Salmon	Bread, white
Perch	Most nuts (not almonds/Brazil nuts)
Swordfish	Egg whites
Most other fish	Corn
Most meats and fowl	Zwieback
Liver	American cheese
Chicken	Natural cheese
Pork	Lentils
Ham, smoked	Peanuts
Goose	
Macaroni	
Most grain (wheat, rye, spelt, quinoa)	

A diet that is overly acidic is more likely to cause excessive mucus. Too much mucus can be harmful in that it may block both respiratory and digestive functions. Children with chronic ear infections and people with chronic post nasal drip and sinus infections usually do not eat enough of the alkaline-forming foods.

HOW TO TREAT AN OVER-ACIDIC STATE

Eating raw potatoes and turnips is excellent for over-acidity. Baked or boiled potatoes are also good, but eat them without toppings (butter, sour cream, salt, etc.). Alfalfa helps to relieve pain from too much acid-forming foods in the diet. Eat fresh sprouts daily, take alfalfa tablets, or make alfalfa tea. To make the tea use one teaspoon herb to one cup boiling water and drink two to three cups daily.

Buffers neutralize an excessive acid condition. Common buffers include Alka-Seltzer Gold, common baking soda, or buffered vitamin C with calcium, magnesium, and potassium. These buffers will neutralize stomach acid, but can interfere with digestion. If you feel awful after a meal, then use a buffer, but don't make a habit of it. Buffers can reduce unpleasant symptoms such as headaches, aches, and pains caused by foods, chemicals, stress, or environmental allergies.

Further reduce an overly-acid condition by avoiding allergens, caffeine, sugar, and animal products and include more alkaline foods in your diet. Learn to breathe deeply. The rate that you breathe affects the acid or alkaline balance of your body. Exercise makes your body more alkaline.

Consuming an alkaline broth will also help relieve over-acidity. Use a stainless steel, enameled, or earthenware utensil. Fill it with 1 1/2 quarts of water. Take two potatoes, one cup carrots, one cup celery (leaves and all), and one cup of other available vegetables high on the alkaline list. Do not peel the vegetables, just clean them well with a vegetable brush. Use seasonings as desired such as cayenne, black pepper, basil, or oregano. Cover and cook slowly for at least 1/2 hour. Let stand for another 1/2 hour then cool until warm, strain, and drink only the broth.

HOW TO TREAT AN ALKALOSIS STATE (OVER-ALKALINITY)

Alkalosis occurs when the body is too alkaline. It is often the result of excessive intake of alkaline drugs, such as sodium bicarbonate for the treatment of gastritis or peptic ulcers. It can also result from excessive vomiting, high cholesterol, an endocrine imbalance, poor diet, diarrhea, and osteoarthritis. Continued alkalosis occurs less often than acidosis. It produces over-excitability of the nervous system and results in symptoms such as being highly nervous and suffering from hyperventilation. Alkalosis may cause calcium to build up in the body causing heel spurs. Other symptoms of alkalosis include sore muscles, creaking joints, bursitis, bone spurs, drowsiness, protruding eyes, hypertension, hypothermia, seizures, edema, allergies, night cramps, asthma, chronic indigestion, night coughs, vomiting, blood clotting and thick blood, menstrual problems, hard dry stools, prostatitis, skin thickening with burning, and itching sensations.

NEUTRAL FOODS

When acid and alkaline ash are in approximately equal quantities in the diet, then the residue will be essentially neutral. Some neutral foods are: butter, margarine, cream, tapioca, cornstarch, fats, arrowroot, cooking fats and oils, lard, and other greases.

CHAPTER 9

Diets Used to Detect & Treat Allergies

The following diets are often used to detect food allergies and sensitivities. It is always better to be guided by a health professional that is trained in nutrition when attempting any of the following diets, especially when fasting. Never fast children without a physician's guidance.

Modified Fast

During any acute illness or times of high internal toxic levels, the appetite naturally decreases even to the point of fasting. Our body automatically knows when to divert its energy from the muscles and digestive tract to eliminate the offensive toxins. The body slows down to complete the cleansing process. This is why we often feel like resting and drinking fluids when ill. It is not a good time to force foods or engage in excess physical activity. Adding more poisons and toxins (drugs) to a body that is already trying to rid itself of toxic material is damaging and often unnecessary.

WHAT FOODS CAN I HAVE?

On a modified fast be sure that the juice or the foods used for juicing are organic. If they are not free of herbicides, pesticides, additives, and chemicals, you may be wasting your time trying to determine what is making you sick. Many times it is the added toxin, not the food, causing the problem. The following are the foods allowed on a modified four-day fast unless you think they are causing some of the symptoms:

- Spring, filtered, distilled, or bottled water stored in glass, not plastic. Don't drink chlorinated tap water.
- You may have lemon or grapefruit juices if diluted at least 50 percent. Buy juices in glass containers without sugar or preservatives. Do not drink cranberry, grape, or orange juice. Drink juices one hour away

from any other liquids other than water. It is best to drink juices derived from fruit or vegetables that are not regular items in your diet. If juice causes any intestinal discomfort, discontinue and drink only water.
• Drink mixed vegetable juices slowly, swishing them in your mouth before swallowing; this increases their digestion. Drink at least 24 to 32 ounces of vegetable juice each day. It is best if the vegetable juice does not contain tomatoes.
• Watermelon is a good melon to eat on a modified fast.
• If you have several different whole fruits at the same time, you should follow the food-combination guide. Eat fruit by itself and don't eat sweet fruit at the same time you have acid fruit.
• Eat rice and vegetables that are steamed or as vegetable soup.
• Drink herbal or noncaffeinated teas.

How much should I eat?

There are no restrictions on the amount of food eaten.

How long do I fast?

This modified fast should continue for four days. (Never put a child on any kind of fast without guidance from a physician.)

What else do I need to do?

Your body will naturally require energy for this cleansing period. To insure this, get plenty of rest. Drink at least eight glasses of pure water a day, but not with food. Avoid being constipated. Skin brushing with a brush or loofah sponge before showering increases your ability to detoxify. Follow with a hot shower and end with a cold or cool shower over your thyroid, liver, abdomen and back. Consider some mild form of exercise while detoxifying such as yoga, stretching exercises, meditation, and walking. Some people benefit from a daily enema, especially after showering. Write down in detail any symptoms that you experience during the fast.

Do I need a laxative?

A food may cause symptoms as long as it is in your digestive system. Depending on your bowel transit time, this could take from one to three days. A laxative taken the night before you start the fast will clean out your digestive tract faster and start the detoxification process sooner. The laxative can be of your choice, but find one that does not have additives, artificially sweeteners, and is sugar- and flavor-free.

SPECIAL INSTRUCTIONS WHEN FASTING

• Do not use fluoride toothpaste, but only water or baking soda.
• It is best to drink 8 glasses of pure water each day (without chlorine), but if you just can't, then drink as much as you comfortably can.
• Do not use tobacco. If you are unable to stop smoking for four days, then try not to smoke two days before being tested for foods, chemicals, or inhalants.
• Do not use any drugs unless discussed and approved by your physician.
• Do not take vitamins or other supplements that aren't necessary.

DETOXIFICATION SYMPTOMS

Since this will be a period when the body releases toxic materials, you might expect some temporary symptoms to begin during the first 24 hours such as headaches, nausea, chilliness, increased heart rate, or fatigue. Symptoms tend to reach their peak during the second or third day of fasting. The initial ravenous appetite usually subsides as the fast advances.

A phenomenon of the second or third day of fasting may consist of flu-like symptoms along with headaches, elevated pulse rate, depression and irritability, nausea, skin sensitivity, backache, and various other aches and pains from muscles and joints. Another common feature is hyper-acute perception, especially the increased sense of smell. Symptoms can be uncomfortable during the fast so stay quiet and rest. Activity will usually increase hunger, fatigue, dizziness, and the pulse.

A body will work hard to remove toxins. If symptoms become uncomfortable, you need to relax more, because stress accelerates these symptoms. Do not breathe rapidly through your mouth. This will cause hyperventilation and greatly increase discomfort. For severe headaches, relax, apply cold compresses to your forehead and put your feet in hot water, and rest quietly. Other ways to get your mind off your symptoms is by reading, watching television, or visiting with family.

Consider planning your work schedule so that during the fast you can rest whenever possible. Doing unnecessary work while fasting may lower your blood sugar too far and cause an accumulation of toxins in your blood that can cause unwanted stress. Various healing crises may occur during the modified fast. The more you need to detoxify the more you may produce symptoms. If symptoms become severe, contact your health-minded physician.

AFTER THE FAST

After finishing the fast, introduce any highly suspicious foods known to produce a sensitivity reaction. Now is the time to do the elimination-then-challenge diet, but you will need to keep a diet diary.

Diet Diary

Foods that trigger symptoms can take anywhere from one to four days to do so. If you eat a food that causes problems on Monday, but don't get symptoms until Wednesday, it's hard to recall what you ate that far back. By using a diet diary, you will be able to recall all the items eaten within the last few days along with your symptoms. You begin to see an association between what you eat and the illness it causes.

If the offending substance is hidden in a form that is hard to recognize, such as potato starch, it will be tougher to figure out without a diet diary. To draw effective conclusions about your present state of health and how to improve it can depend to an extent on your ability to recall your diet accurately. When filling out a diet diary form remember to:

• List all foods and beverages that you eat or drink.
• List the ingredients if you eat a combination of foods such as a salad, casserole, or lasagna. Usually the quantity is not as important unless it is out of the ordinary.
• Write down the time you eat so that you can see if the spacing between meals is causing a low blood sugar reaction.
• Note any symptoms that occur during the time you fill out the diet diary.

If you are interested in the pulse test for food sensitivities, review the section "Allergy Tests" for more information. Taking your pulse can be one way of determining if the foods you eat are making you sick. Each time you eat, record your pulse on the diet diary, before and after meals.

DAILY DIARY

MEAL	DAY 1	DAY 2	DAY 3
Time Morning			
Snack			
Time Noon			
Snack			
Time Evening			
Snack			
Additional Foods			
Water			
Condiments			
Beverages			
Supplements			
Fats and Oils			
Misc.			
Pulse			
Before Meal After Meal			
Symptoms			

Date _____   Name _____

THE ELIMINATION-THEN-CHALLENGE DIET

Start the diet diary three days before beginning the elimination diet, keeping a record of the foods introduced and the symptoms. Continue recording the diet and symptoms during the elimination diet and while reintroducing the suspected foods.

Certain foods commonly cause the majority of symptoms of food allergies and sensitivities. After avoiding the offending foods for a time, symptoms will improve or disappear, but when eaten again the symptoms usually return. In trying to determine what is causing the symptoms, this sort of elimination diet can be useful. Everyone deserves an elimination diet trial, especially before using prescription drugs and more invasive treatments. An elimination diet is very safe and cost-effective for evaluating the effects of various foods and food additives. Before starting, it is important to decide what symptoms you hope the diet will relieve. Otherwise, it will be difficult to decide whether the diet has been effective. Do not become discouraged if improvement does not occur immediately. The foods causing symptoms can stay in the digestive tract for many days. These effects will decrease faster if you add an intestinal cleanser for the first seven days after beginning the elimination portion of the diet.

Part 1

To begin an elimination diet, remove the following foods from the diet for at least seven days, and go fourteen days if possible: milk and other dairy products, wheat, eggs, corn, peanuts, bananas, beef, cheese, potatoes, orange juice and other citrus fruits, sugar, chocolate, coffee and black tea, alcohol, and soy. You should also avoid some or all of the person's "favorite" foods. Avoid packaged and processed foods whenever possible, as well as canned foods. Most people are not as likely to react to foods that are fresh, whole, organic, and without added preservatives and other chemicals.

Wheat and corn are likely causes of unrecognized food sensitivities and are two of the most difficult foods to eliminate in the diet. Other likely allergens are food additives, especially FD&C yellow dyes (found in cheese, butter, and ice cream), pollen, yeast, and spices. Asthmatics should remove avocado from their diet. Eating sugar makes any sensitivity to food additives worse. The following are guidelines for foods that should be excluded and that are allowed during the elimination part of the diet (unless you know they make you or your child ill).

• Include any vegetable except corn. Beets, spinach, cabbage, cauliflower, broccoli, turnips, Brussels sprouts, squash, lettuce, carrots, celery, and sweet potatoes should all be included in the diet.

- Include any fruit except citrus. Cherries, cranberries (juice), blueberries, apples (juice), and fig are all acceptable. Juice should be diluted at least an additional 50 percent.
- Exclude luncheon meats, sausage, bacon, hot dogs, ham, or other foods made with beef or pork. It is fine to include chicken, turkey, lamb, and fish.
- Include any grains except wheat or corn. Include buckwheat, spelt, millet, quinoa, white rice, and oats.
- Include any drinks except milk, coffee, black tea, or soft drinks. Herb teas, mineral water, unsweetened and diluted fruit juice (not citrus), and pure water. The water should be chlorine and fluoride free.
- It is fine to include nuts, except for peanuts. Honey, blackstrap molasses or real maple syrup can be eaten in moderation, if a child is not hyperactive. Oils such as safflower, sunflower, or canola oil are acceptable. It is best if the oils used are cold-pressed and organic.

Part 2

It is best not to start the challenge part of the diet until the symptoms you are addressing have stopped. On day eight, or when you decide to begin the challenge part of the diet, select one food that was eliminated and reintroduce that food into each meal that day. If there is no reaction to that food throughout the day, you may assume that there is no sensitivity to it. On day nine remove the food that was tested on day eight from the diet. Select a new food to test in the same manner as before. Follow this procedure for each food. Sometimes, with delayed-onset food symptoms, it can take three days to trigger a reaction. This is the reason for a diet diary. If the procedure of introducing a new food back into the diet each day does not work, because you cannot identify which food is causing the symptoms, then it may be necessary to introduce a new food only once each week.

After you are finished with the challenge part of the diet, it usually takes about seven days to see improvement. Some children with chronic food sensitivities won't improve for at least ten to fourteen days. When the observed improvement lasts for at least one week, you may begin adding foods back into the diet that you did not think caused any reaction, but only one food at a time. First, add back the food you think is the least likely to be causing any problems. Save any suspected foods until last. If the person being tested is sensitive to any of the eliminated foods, then symptoms should develop when the food is eaten again. If you cannot tell which food is causing the problem, here is a suggested schedule of returning foods to the diet:

Day 1: add oranges
Day 2: add egg
Day 3: add wheat
Day 4: add corn
Day 5: add food coloring
Day 6: add chocolate
Day 7: add sugar
Day 8: add milk

The following suggestions can help make this type of testing more accurate and effective:

• Eat as much of the reintroduced food as wanted for breakfast. If there are no symptoms, then eat more of this food for lunch, dinner, or even at snack time. If there is no reaction to the reintroduced food it must be stopped at the end of that day to get ready to introduce another suspected food back into the diet the next day.
• If you think symptoms developed when a certain food was reintroduced into the diet, but just aren't certain, then eat more of that food until the symptom or symptoms are obvious. Be sure to keep the rest of the diet the same as before. If there is an obvious reaction after eating any food, then do not ingest any more of it. Wait until the reaction stops (this may take up to 48 hours) before adding another food to test.
• When adding food back into the diet, it is always best to use certified organic ones, if possible, or make sure the food is in a pure form. Use whole milk rather than a milk product that contains wheat, sugar, and other possible allergic ingredients. A wheat product, such as Cream-O-Wheat, would be better than bread that contains milk and yeast.
• It is extremely important that no allergic foods be consumed during this test. An accidental or unknown intake of the allergen may precipitate a reaction. This diet must be adhered to exactly. Conclusions derived from this test may be followed for the next several months or years. It won't be helpful if the results of these trials end in false conclusions.
• If a food sensitivity is causing symptoms, there will usually be improvement after eliminating the food. The symptoms usually return on the first day the food is eaten again. In some individuals the symptoms will not return until the food is eaten in quantity for several consecutive days. If a person eliminates a food for several weeks or longer, there may be a tolerance to that food. this means that larger quantities must be consumed for several consecutive days before any symptoms reappear. Since more than one food sensitivity is usually involved, there may not be a significant difference if the other foods remain in the diet.

Part 3

Once you have tested all the foods that you suspect of causing symptoms, you can introduce back into the diet those foods that did not cause any reaction when eaten on a continuous basis. When you test a food that has not been in the normal diet, be sure to eat it in excess. If there are no reactions after several weeks, do not eat that food for four days, and then test it again. If there are still symptoms using the above diet, then continue with the following elimination diet:

- Most vegetables are permitted, but not corn, potatoes, or soy (legume) products.
- Fruits are acceptable, but not apples, bananas, or any citrus fruits; this includes fruit-sweetened products.
- Meats such as lamb and turkey may be eaten, but not chicken, beef, pork, or packaged meats.
- Do not eat grains that are wheat, corn, soy, barley, or rye.
- Have only bottled spring water, mineral water, or distilled water.
- Nuts are permitted, but not peanuts or Brazil nuts.
- Organic oils made of safflower, sunflower, or canola oil are usually non-allergic.
- Avoid sugar or products containing sugar, as well as artificial sweeteners.
- Avoid chocolate, coffee, tea, or alcohol.
- Avoid eggs, food coloring, preservatives, and yeast-containing foods.

Avoid all foods eaten regularly or more than once or twice a week. If the person being tested loves a particular food and wants to eat it all the time, then be sure to eliminate it during this diet. Avoid commercially prepared foods because they usually contain allergic-type additives and hidden ingredients. Eat simply and buy certified organic foods when possible.

Part 4

Begin adding the eliminated foods that cause reactions back into the diet in about six months. Eat the food by itself in the morning, before eating anything else. If there are no symptoms it is probably safe to begin rotating the food back into the diet. If they do react, then wait six months before trying the food again. The reintroduction of sensitive foods can produce a more severe reaction than before. Maintain a carefully detailed record describing when foods are reintroduced and any symptoms that occur. It may be helpful to use the pulse method when you suspect a food sensitivity, since the pulse often changes when a food sensitivity occurs.

A Last-Ditch Effort

If you tried all of the above diets and they do not seem to eliminate the symptoms, then you might want to try one more diet before giving up. You will need to limit the diet to rice, fish, and steamed vegetables for ten days. It usually takes that long for any foods causing the problem to be eliminated from the body. Of course, do not eat these foods if you know they cause problems. After this ten-day cleansing diet, reintroduce foods back into the diet one at a time as you did before.

Foods that cause violent symptoms must be eliminated from the diet completely. You need to learn which food ingredients may be found in unsuspected places. Avoid all forms of the food. Even the smallest amount can cause reactions. Initially, this may be uncomfortable and strong cravings may occur. They usually last only a few days and then the person will begin to feel better.

SYMPTOMS OF ELIMINATION

During the first week of the elimination diet, it is common to feel irritable and tired. A person may become more hyperactive than before or have an increase in symptoms such as headaches, leg cramps, changes in bowel movements, cravings for certain foods, or just not feeling good.

When you eliminate sugar you may encounter tiredness, drowsiness, depression, feelings of alienation, and lack of coordination for the first week. With the elimination of coffee there can be headaches, shakiness, and nervousness for up to 10 days. The elimination of alcohol can cause tension in the body with an inability to relax. The time it takes to eliminate the symptoms depends on the extent of the drinking. Eliminating milk and other dairy products usually cause mucus to be eliminated through the skin, sinus passages, mucous membranes, lungs, and sexual organs. This can continue for several months.

After a person stops eating meats, fats, and excessive protein there can be a foul body odor, coated tongue, toxic feelings, and skin eruptions for several weeks. Sometimes if the body is really toxic, there can be symptoms for months. Signs and symptoms that the body is house cleaning are: general fatigue, abnormal sweating, frequent urination, diarrhea or constipation, fever, chills, coughs, skin discharges, unusual body odors, a decrease in sexual desire, cessation of menstruation, low vitality, mental irritability, minor transitory symptoms, minor hair loss, restlessness, aches and pains, bad dreams, and feeling cold.

Tips to help you succeed

- You need the cooperation of the person being tested and other family members before starting the diet plan.
- Do not try this diet on your child when they are visiting others or during a holiday. It is also a bad idea to start an elimination-then-challenge diet when you do not have the time to give it your full attention.
- If your child is in school during the time you are testing them, you will need the school's and the teacher's cooperation so that they will not get any foods at school.
- You will need medical help before carrying out this diet if your child has a history of asthma or has experienced swelling or other serious reactions. Consult your holistic health-care provider for guidance.

ROTATION DIET

Food sensitivities are usually temporary. Typically, they disappear after you eliminate the reactive food for thirty to sixty days. Most people can then reintroduce the foods back into their diet, one at a time, without the reoccurrence of symptoms. The most effective way of preventing food sensitivities from developing again is to rotate, cook, and combine your foods properly. The most common rotation diet is the four day food rotation plan. This means not eating the same food again for at least four days.

A rotation diet allows for optimal nutrition with minimal risk of allergic reaction or sensitization. The body responds best to natural foods and rotated menus rather than to processed foods eaten repetitively. Since eighty percent of all food sensitivities are cyclic, most people can improve their health by rotating foods in their diet. If a person does not consume a food for several months, it is likely that they will lose any sensitivity to that particular food. If a large number of foods appear to provoke symptoms, it is likely that insecticides or other toxic additives are responsible.

When Will Symptoms Disappear?

When you eliminate the offending food, symptoms usually clear up within one to two weeks. If the food is eaten again after only a short period of elimination, the symptoms return. If the food is not eaten for several months the body will usually regain some tolerance to it. By only eating the food occasionally such as every four to seven days, no symptoms are produced.

If there are obvious reactions after eating a particular food, you can shorten the reaction time by giving one teaspoonful of a soda mixture. Make it with two parts baking soda and one part potassium bicarbonate.

Alka Seltzer Gold (without aspirin) dissolved in a half glass of water can decrease allergic symptoms. The dosage is two tablets for anyone over thirteen years old; one tablet for children ages six to twelve years; 1/2 tablet for children one to five years old. A laxative, such as milk of magnesia, will also help to stop the reaction by removing the food from the intestinal tract where it is causing problems.

Food Families

Foods are classified by families. You may eat more than one food in the same food family at a single meal. If you have a reaction to a specific food, this could mean that other foods in that food family are not safe to eat. You will then need to eat members of the same food family on a rotating basis. If there are continued reactions, you may need to test each complete food family before adding them back into the diet.

Eat different foods from different food families at any time. Do not compromise your health by eating a food simply because you like it when you know that it is causing symptoms. This diet plan is designed to get you well. Remember, some of your favorite foods are the ones that make you ill.

Starting the Rotation Diet

An example is having one salad per day and rotating the salad vegetables used on a four-day plan. For the leaves, use romaine lettuce on day one, spinach on day two, iceberg lettuce on day three, butter lettuce on day four. On day five go back to the day-one menu and go through the series again, unless there are other choices for day five, day six, etc. Also rotate the garnishes and salad dressings used.

Several times per month use something completely different such as a salad without greens, a Greek salad, or a vegetable salad without any lettuce. Rotate cooking oils by using safflower oil on day one, sunflower oil on day two, canola oil on day three, olive oil on day four. Rotate herbal teas in the same manner. Rotate other foods and beverages including grains, vegetables, and meats. Take time to try new foods and spices several times per month.

You will need to plan ahead. Spend the time needed to plan a rotation diet. Set aside extra time to browse through your local health food and grocery stores. Carefully read labels, finding foods that are safe to eat. This will simplify future shopping trips since you will know in advance what foods to purchase.

If you are in the habit of planning dinner on the way home from work, you will need some self-discipline. Try organizing your menu on a weekly basis and buying everything you will need at one time. Even if you spend a little extra time at first, it will reduce time spent in the long run. The reward of feeling better is well worth it.

Prepare whole foods such as fish, poultry, fruits and vegetables. Avoid prepackaged products loaded with allergens. Make extra portions when you cook soups, stews, casseroles, etc., and freeze them. You will have these foods already prepared when you do not have the time or desire to cook.

FOODS TO EAT ON A ROTATION DIET

• Flesh Foods and Eggs: You can have meat, fish, or poultry as long as you rotate them on a four-day plan. Trim extra fat, and do not fry. Eggs can be eaten daily if varied by species of origin.

• Fruits, Juices, and Vegetables: Use unsweetened fruits and juices. People with yeast infection, hypoglycemia, or a weight problem should avoid fruit juices and dried fruits. Eat four or more servings per day (some raw) of vegetables, rotated. Watch for excess salt in canned and frozen vegetables.

• Grains: Eat four servings of grains each day. Try to use whole grains instead of bakery products. Vary the grains so you are not eating the same ones at each serving. See the chapter "Grains" for more information.

• Nuts and Seeds: Use sparingly, once or twice per day, rotated. These contain important fatty acids needed for health, but they are usually high in calories.

• Water: Drink six or more glasses of pure water each day, without chlorine or fluoride. Store in glass containers.

FOODS TO USE SPARINGLY

• Fats: Keep animal fats to a minimum.
• Salt: Everyone can benefit from reduced salt intake.
• Caffeine: Caffeine can aggravate nervous conditions.
• Cheese and other milk products: Use unprocessed, natural varieties of cheese if you must eat cheese. If you have respiratory problems, ear infections, sinus problems, or other mucus-forming conditions, then it is best to avoid dairy completely.

FOODS AND ADDITIVES TO AVOID

• Refined Carbohydrates: Consumed in quantity over long periods these foods dispose you to obesity, diabetes, urinary tract disorders, atherosclerosis, diverticulosis, mental disorders, and other illnesses.
• Hydrogenated Fats: These fats do not contain essential fatty acids and

actively block the normal metabolism of essential fatty acids taken in from other sources. Hydrogenated fats are found in margarine and some cooking oils.

• Nitrates and Nitrites: Preservatives in meats and some other processed foods may be nitrates or nitrites. It is always best to avoid preservatives whenever possible.

• Avoid all artificial flavors and colors.

Basic Rules of the Rotation Diet

1. Eat whole, unadulterated foods. It is better to eat whole, fresh foods rather than highly processed ones. Organic foods have more flavor than those grown with synthetic chemicals. Avoid as many food additives, preservatives, and pesticide residues as possible. They add to the toxic load in the body. If you prepare your own food at home, it is easier to know what ingredients are present in your food.

2. Plain foods are best. With simple unprocessed foods, it is easier to tell what is causing your reaction. It is better to eat a simple piece of steak rather than a hamburger topped with such things as pickles, tomatoes, mustard, and lettuce. If a reaction occurs, the link to one specific food is more obvious.

3. Do not eat any food that you suspect causes a reaction, even if minor.

4. Rotate all ingredients used in cooking, including spices, oils, herbs, sweeteners, and starches. Food mixtures often contain these substances. They must be tested just as any other food. Don't overlook these substances as possible allergens.

5. Do not overeat. Excesses of any food, even if nutritious or wholesome, will add toxicity to your body. Eat slowly and in an unhurried atmosphere and chew the food well.

6. Be sure to meet your nutritional needs. When arranging food combinations, preferences, and tolerances, you must always give the body adequate vitamins and minerals, as well as meet other nutritional needs.

7. Think creatively. Try to prepare your foods in different ways for variety, such as raw, steamed, shredded, as a juice or soup, pureed, fresh, dried, hot or cold. Use recipe books to get your creative juices started.

8. Keep meals simple. The fewer foods used in a single meal, the less chance of having an allergic reaction.

9. Drink safe water. Remember to always use pure water when preparing your food or drinking. Sometimes plastic containers holding the water can be a problem. If you are in doubt, use glass containers.

10. Stock up with necessary foods for a rotation diet in advance so you do not have to deviate too frequently from your planned rotation menus.

11. Avoid stress. Prepare and label snacks ahead of time. Have several days on hand so that a person could help themselves to these foods during the day without you having to prepare something new each time.

12. Listen to your body. Pay attention to how you feel and keep records to verify your perception of events. If allergens or stresses are interfering with your ability to cope on a specific day, don't be afraid to make adjustments to your diet on that day.

OTHER GUIDELINES

• If you have any symptoms during this period, write them down. If this occurs again, there is obviously a food or foods that may be causing problems. Often, it is a close relative of a food you reacted to. A review of the food families will usually reveal the offending food. If you react to several members of the same family, you may have to eliminate the whole family of foods for several months before you can reintroduce them. Some foods will be "fixed allergies." They are the type that will cause a reaction each time you eat them.

• Once you identify the offending foods, it is important to avoid them for several months to one year. During this time, it is important not eat even one bite of those foods in any form. You will begin eating a greater variety of foods on a rotation diet. This means that on Monday you will eat certain foods belonging to certain families. On Tuesday, Wednesday, and Thursday, you will eat different foods that you did not eat on the previous days. This gives the body a rest for at least seventy-two hours before eating the food again.

• Continue eating foods on a rotary basis for six more months. Reintroduce the foods again that caused problems earlier, using the same technique. If you have a reaction to any of these foods, continue to avoid them.

• After the avoidance period has passed, you will reintroduce the previously offending foods to determine their effects on you. Each week introduce one food. Record the time you eat, and anything unusual about the way you feel. Some foods cause delayed reactions seventy-two hours later, or more, after you eat the food. You have to be a detective to catch the clues. If there is a reaction, continue to avoid that food. If you don't react, add that food to your rotary diet sheet and don't eat that food more often than every four days. Eating it frequently may cause a reoccurrence of the sensitivity. Add one food per week until you have exhausted your list.

• If you find the rotary diet difficult to follow, write down everything you eat. Do not repeat any food within a 72-hour period. This requires more record-keeping, but accomplishes the same purpose.

CHAPTER 10

Food Additives and Phenolic Compounds

A dditives comprise a big part of the American diet. In fact, the average American eats about fourteen pounds of additives a year and about eight pounds of salt. The Department of National Health and Welfare defines a food additive as "any substance or its byproducts, the use of which results, or may reasonably be expected to result in, becoming a part of or affecting the characteristics of food." Additives do not include spices, seasonings or flavorings. Approximately 75 percent of the foods we consume undergo some sort of chemical alteration. Consumers use more than 100 million pounds a year of approved food additives. In the United States, there are over 10,000 food and chemical additives legally allowed into our food supply.

It is true that food additives provide us with a greater selection of food throughout the year. They add variety and convenience to shopping. Yet, scientific discoveries indicate these "approved" additives can and do cause reactions. It appears that young, developing nervous systems are particularly prone to the damage or irritation that many food additives can cause. One effect is hyperactivity. There may be difficulties with speech, balance, and learning, even if the child has a high IQ. Studies corroborate the theory that food dyes can affect behavior and learning in some children. According to Dr. Ben Feingold, more than 50 percent of hyperactive children are sensitive to artificial food colors, preservatives, flavors, and to naturally occurring salicylates and phenolic compounds. He based his claims on over 1,200 initial cases of learning and behavior disorders that improved significantly when food additives were eliminated from the diet.

Additives are receiving more attention from scientists on a world-wide basis as a cause of adverse reactions. A recent study conducted at the Royal Children's Hospital, University of Melbourne, Australia, determined that synthetic food coloring had an effect on behavior. In a six-week trial, 200 children were given a diet free of all synthetic food coloring. The parents of 150 children reported significant behavioral improvement. They noted that children's behavior worsened when foods containing artificial colors were introduced back into the diet. The more synthetic food coloring the children consumed, the longer the undesirable behavior lasted.

In this study, behavioral changes associated with the intake of yellow dye included irritability, restlessness, and sleep disturbances. The more dye ingested, the longer the reaction time lasted. Younger children, ages two to six, experienced constant crying, tantrums, irritability, restlessness, and severe sleep disturbances. The older children, ages seven to fourteen, were irritable, aimlessly active, lacking in self-control, whiny and unhappy. Although other dyes were not studied, their effects are probably similar because most dyes are chemically derived from coal tars and have related chemical structures. Interestingly, the children who reacted to yellow dyes had allergies of some kind: asthma, eczema, allergic runny nose. They also tested positive for one or more of eight common food allergens. Most of the children studied had members of the family who also had allergies.

In 1979, the public schools of New York City attempted to improve student performance by reducing or eliminating common colorings and flavorings in the school's feeding programs. Soon after, the achievement test scores soared to the 47th percentile nationally. With the removal of the preservatives BHA and BHT, the test scores rose even further. By changing and improving the food program in 803 public schools, there was an academic improvement of 16 percent.

Consumer Information

In order to avoid the problems often associated with food additives, consumers need to be better informed. What we really need is better label information concerning specific naming of additives in foods. Because a label says a product is "pure and natural" doesn't mean that it is additive-free. White sugar looks bright and pure because it's bleached. Meat looks healthier and sells better with the addition of red dye. Most of the coloring in food comes from artificial chemicals. Smoke flavor is actually pyroligneous acid, but the FDA allows food manufacturers to call it "smoked." Less formidable names of chemicals are substituted whenever possible. People have a misconception that additives are safe just because the FDA approves them as GRAS (Generally Recognized As Safe). Did you know that the FDA offers no guarantees for the safety of additives in our foods?

Beware that unintentional additives such as pesticides and herbicides remain on plant crops and that hormones and antibiotics given to animals are present in milk and meat. You will never find these pesticides, herbicides, hormones, and antibiotics on any food label. Don't forget the most popular food additives, sugars and salt. They should always be consumed with discretion.

Categories of Food Additives

Additives fall into two categories: those that prevent food from going bad, and those that make food more appealing. The following is a list and description of some commonly found food additives that cause reactions.

ARTIFICIAL COLORINGS

Artificial food colors alter the functioning, either permanently or temporarily, of the nervous and muscular systems. Food dyes reduce the ability of nerves and muscles to respond to signals from other nerves. At the same time the intensity of signals sent spontaneously from nerves to muscles is greatly increased. Animal studies indicate that certain food dyes interfere with chemical communication in the brain and normal development. This adds further support to the theory that artificial colorings cause hyperactivity and behavioral disturbances in children.

The only purpose of artificial colorings is to add color to our food. There are no claims made that they do anything else, and as a result, are not essential. More than 90 percent of the food colorings now in use are coal-tar derivatives coming from petroleum. They are found in jams, jellies, fruit drinks, ice cream, pickles, processed meat, and fish. Caramel color and flavoring do not require certification, but must be labeled "artificially colored" or "flavored." The following list identifies seven of the most offensive colorings:

- FD&C Blue No. 1 is a coal-tar derivative used as a coloring in bottled soft drinks, desserts, gelatin, ice cream, ices, dry drink powders, candy, confections, bakery products, cereals, and puddings.
- FD&C Citrus Red No. 2 can damage internal organs and is a weak cancer-causing agent. This red dye colors the skin of some Florida oranges.
- FD&C Green No. 3 is a coloring used in mint-flavored jelly, frozen desserts, gelatin desserts, candy, confections, baking products, and cereals. It may cause allergic reactions.
- FD&C Red No. 3 is a coal-tar derivative used in canned fruit cocktail, fruit salad, cherry pie mix, maraschino cherries, gelatin desserts, ice cream, sherbets, candy, confectionery and bakery products, cereals, and puddings. It may interfere with the neurotransmitters in the brain.
- FD&C Yellow No. 5 (tartrazine) is a coal-tar derivative used as a coloring in prepared breakfast cereals, imitation strawberry jelly, bottled soft

drinks, gelatin desserts, ice cream, sherbets, drink powders, candy, confections, bakery products, spaghetti, and puddings. Food manufacturers add this yellow dye to almost every packaged food even though they are probably aware that about half of all aspirin-sensitive people, plus up to 100,000 other individuals, are sensitive to this dye. Life-threatening asthmatic symptoms are possible. This yellow dye is in about 60 percent of both over-the-counter and prescription drugs such as antihistamines, antibiotics, steroids, and sedatives. A product does not have to appear yellow to contain yellow dye. The average daily consumption of dyes is fifteen milligrams, of which 85 percent is Yellow No.5. Among children, consumption is usually higher. This dye can promote zinc deficiency and affects behavior in some children.

- FD&C Yellow No. 6 (sunset yellow) is a coal-tar dye used as coloring in carbonated drinks, gelatin desserts, dry drink powders, candy, and confectionery products that do not contain oils and fats. This dye is also in bakery products, cereals, puddings, and tablets.
- FD&C Lakes are pigments prepared by combining FD&C colors with a form of aluminum or calcium that makes the colors insoluble. Manufacturers use FD&C Lakes for dyeing egg shells and other products that are adversely affected by water. Confection and candy products commonly contain these pigments.

Avoid foods that list colors with numbers, by name, or simply state "artificial color." Colorings can be found in products you would never suspect. Red dye is used in white-colored items to make them look brighter. Yellow dyes are often used in baked goods and cake mixes so that buyers think they're getting a product made with eggs.

Are there natural colors that are acceptable? Annatto is a natural yellow color found in cheeses, butter and other products. Beta-carotene is also a yellow color used in some products. Carmine is a red color derived from a mealybug. Some manufacturers use spinach and beet powders to color pasta. Read the label of every food you buy.

ASPARTAME

The marketed names of aspartame are NutraSweet and Equal. Aspartame is an artificial sweetener about 200 times sweeter than sucrose. It intensifies the taste of other flavors and sweeteners. More than half of the people in this country currently consume aspartame—an easy thing to do since it is found in more than 4000 products. The FDA has recently approved aspartame for use in baked goods.

More than 80 percent of all complaints about foods and additives previously received by the FDA concerned aspartame products. About 6,000 consumers reported their health problems to this agency, including hundreds of instances of convulsions. Large amounts consumed over time can upset the amino acid and neurotransmitter balance in the body. A recent study found that memory loss attributed to diabetes was caused by aspartame. Another study found an increase in convulsions in people using aspartame-containing products.

BHA AND BHT

Butylated hydroxyanisole (BHA) is a preservative used in many products, including various drinks, chewing gum, ice cream, ices, candy, baked goods, gelatin desserts, soup bases, potatoes, potato flakes, dry breakfast cereals, dry yeast, dry mixes for desserts, lard, shortening, dry sausage, and shortenings. BHA affects liver and kidney function. Many people have allergic reactions to this product, and it has been associated with behavior problems in children.

Butylated hydroxytoluene (BHT) is chemically similar to BHA, but may be more toxic to the kidneys. Similar in use to BHA, BHT retards rancidity in frozen and fresh pork sausage, and freeze-dried meats. Food processors add it to potato and sweet potato flakes, enriched rice, and dry breakfast cereals. The base product used for chewing gum contains BHT. You can find it in shortenings and animal fats. Allergic reactions and enlargement of the liver have been the result of eating foods containing BHT. There is a link between hyperactivity and other behavior disturbances in children. England prohibits the use of this food additive.

CAFFEINE

Caffeine is a naturally occurring ingredient in coffee, cola, mate leaves, and tea. It is a flavor used in cola and root-beer drinks. Caffeine is a central nervous system, heart, and respiratory stimulant. It can cause nervousness, insomnia, irregular heartbeat, and noises in the ear. Caffeine can affect blood sugar release and uptake by the liver. The FDA asked for studies on the long-term effects of this additive to determine whether it causes other health problems. See the chapter "Caffeine" for more information

CARRAGEENAN

Carrageenan is an Irish moss derivative with a seaweed-like odor and salty taste. It acts as a stabilizer and emulsifier in chocolate products, chocolate-flavoring drinks, chocolate milk, pressure-dispensed whipped cream, syrups for frozen products, French dressing, confections, evaporated milk, cheese spreads and cheese foods, ice cream, and artificially sweetened jellies and jams. Some uncertainties now exist with this product requiring that additional studies be conducted. While these tests are being conducted, carrageenan is still being allowed in foods.

MSG

The most common flavor enhancer added to foods is monosodium glutamate (MSG). Flavor enhancers usually add no flavor of their own to foods, but heighten or modify existing flavor. More than 75 percent of the population may react to MSG. Snack foods, soups, canned tuna, and many of the prepared foods now found on grocery store shelves contain MSG.

An ingredient listed as "natural flavoring" can actually be MSG because the label doesn't have to call it MSG. There are several names being used on labels today including sodium caseinate, autolyzed yeast, hydrolyzed vegetable protein, or hydrolyzed yeast. Other names are calcium caseinate, textured protein, yeast food, hydrolyzed protein, yeast extract, natural chicken or turkey flavoring, natural flavoring, hydrolyzed yeast, and other spices. See the chapter "MSG" for more complete information.

NITRITES OR NITRATES

Nitrites will prevent the development of some bacteria and add a pink color to delicatessen meats. Nitrites and nitrates are common additives in processed meat and preserved poultry. Food manufacturers add nitrites to 60-65 percent of all pork products in the United States, as well as other meats, poultry, fish, and cheese. It is especially common in processed bacon, sausage, luncheon meats, and hot dogs.

ORRIS ROOT EXTRACT

Orris root extract causes frequent allergic reactions. It is used in chocolate, fruit, nuts, vanilla, drinks, ice cream, ices, candy, baked goods, gelatin desserts, and chewing gum.

PHOSPHATES

Phosphates prevent the physical and chemical changes that affect the color, flavor, texture, or appearance of food. There are phosphates in carbonated drinks, baked goods, cheese, canned meats, dry cereals, cola drinks, and powdered foods. Phosphates attract the trace minerals in foods and then continue to remove them from the body. Widespread use has led to dietary imbalances, especially calcium deficiencies.

SODIUM BENZOATE

Sodium benzoate is a flavoring and preservative in margarine, bottled soft drinks, maraschino cherries, dry drink mixes, dry soup mixes, salad dressings, condiments, snack foods, gum, and sauces. Ice used to preserve fish may contain sodium benzoate. It can cause intestinal upset.

SORBATE

Sorbate is a preservative and fungus preventive used in drinks, baked goods, chocolate syrups, soda-fountain syrups, fresh fruit cocktail, some deli salads, cake, cheesecake, pie fillings, and artificially sweetened jellies and preserves.

SULFITES

Sulfites appear on the labels of packages with names such as sulfur dioxide, sodium sulfite, sodium and potassium bisulfite, and sodium and potassium metabisulfite. They are preservatives and bleaching agents used in ale, wine, beer, and sliced fruit. Sulfites are commonly found in shellfish, soups, wine vinegar, packaged lemon juice, avocado dip, maraschino cherries, potatoes, salad dressings, sauces and gravies, corn syrup, and dehydrated potatoes. Fresh, peeled, frozen, canned, or dried vegetables may contain this preservative. They can be in jams, jellies, molasses, marmalades, stuffing, fruit juices, and tomato paste.

The primary use of sulfites is to prevent or reduce discoloration of light-colored fruits and vegetables such as dried apples and dehydrated potatoes. They allow vegetables and fruits to look fresh even when quite old and stale. Sulfites prevent rust and scale in the boiler water that comes in contact with food. Bottled lemon juice in your tea or splashed on your salad could be a source of sulfites. Fresh-squeezed lemon is okay, but bottled lemon juice often contains sodium bisulfite.

The FDA prohibits the use of sulfites in foods that are important sources of thiamine (vitamin B1), such as enriched flour, because sulfites destroy this nutrient. This additive also destroys vitamin A. Problems range from stomach aches, difficulty breathing, to hives. Some people had fatal allergic reactions to sulfites, especially asthmatics. Now, restaurants seldom add them to their food items. Sulfites may still be added at the manufacturing level.

Since 1985 hundreds of adverse reactions to sulfites have been reported to the FDA. More than one million asthmatics are allergic to this substance. The FDA plans to propose a ban on sulfites used on fresh, peeled potatoes, whether served in restaurants or sold unpackaged in stores. This ban will include French fries.

XANTHAN GUM

The fermentation of corn sugar by the bacterium *Xanthomonas campestris* produces xanthan gum. It thickens, suspends, emulsifies, and stabilizes water-based foods, like dairy products and salad dressings. It is an ingredient in packaged meat and poultry products. Gum takes away the thirst mechanism and sends a continuous signal to the stomach to produce acid.

Report Reactions

The only way the FDA can know about a problem with additives is through consumer and physician reports. Adverse reaction reporting is voluntary and the FDA encourages physicians to report patients' reactions. Most of the time the reaction is not medically treated because the individual doesn't go to the doctor, or the symptoms are not recognized as coming from an additive. The agency's Adverse Reaction Monitoring System collects and acts on complaints concerning all food ingredients including preservatives. If you experience an adverse reaction from eating a food that contains additives, describe the circumstances and your reaction to the FDA district office in your area (see local phone directory). It is important that you also send your report in writing to: Adverse Reaction Monitoring System (HFS-636), 200 C St., S.W., Washington, DC 20204.

Once you recognize your family's need to eliminate, or at least drastically reduce, the chemical food additives in the diet, you will accept the extra effort willingly. You may have to spend more preparation time with fresh, organic foods than you did with highly processed ones, but the effort is well worth it.

PHENOLICS

Phenolics are aromatic compounds found naturally in foods derived from plants, animals, and pollens. These compounds preserve, protect, color and flavor foods. They protect plants against pathogens and help attract flower pollinators. You can find these chemicals in practically every food you eat every day. They are a major underlying cause of allergic symptoms, as well as many learning disorders.

Foods containing phenolics such as salicylates, coumarin, and phenylalanine are frequently the cause of hyperactivity reactions. In one study, 57 percent of the people tested with phenolic compounds showed some sensitivity. The immune system of animals that were continuously exposed to the same phenols also became depressed. Even fetal hiccups suggest that phenolic compounds circulate in the blood to the fetus and possibly sensitize the child before birth.

The following phenolic compounds were found to most often cause reactions: acetyl salicylate, ethanol, dopamine, nor-epinephrine, histamine, coumarin, indole, malvin, ascorbic acid, gallic acid, phenylisothiocyanate, and phenylalanine,

Milk contains thirteen different phenolics, making it one of the most allergic foods in the diet. The main route for phenolics to leave a milk-producing animal is through its milk. Cows add a particularly reactive phenolic compound to their milk if they eat feed containing cottonseed. Gossypol, the phenolic compound found in cottonseed, is fat soluble, causing it to be concentrated in cream, ice cream, and other milk fat products. Foods at the top of the allergic list, besides dairy, are tomatoes with fourteen phenolics, and soy with nine. Phenolic compounds are also present in substances such as plastics, paper, and rubber.

Manufacturers select high-content phenolic plants for domestic food production because of their ability to resist disease and insects. The phenolics help to preserve, color, and flavor the plants. The same types of compounds are added artificially when food additives are used to preserve, color, and flavor foods. These common additives are yellow dye, BHA, BHT, and sodium benzoate.

It is conceivable that certain plant phenolics may be the allergic components of pollens, dust, or molds. Phenol, the standard preservative in conventional allergy injections, is itself a common allergen. Phenol has a special affinity for the brain and is known to suppress the immune system. Phenol is a major constituent of smoke, so anything smoked may cause a reaction in some people.

Allergies to a phenolic compound can cause a variety of symptoms. Some people begin crying for no apparent reason, some become depressed. Others experience abdominal pain, distention, and diarrhea, or other adverse reaction to foods. Smooth muscles may also be affected. This causes the constrictions often seen in respiratory problems such as asthma. Phenolic compounds appear more generally toxic if natural barriers, or the body's ability to detoxify, is not functioning properly. The more the body is overloaded with toxins and stress, the harder it is to defend itself from these chemicals. Various researchers have concluded that phenolics can also act as cardiac stimulants. This accounts for the accelerated pulse after eating certain foods. Many people react to tap water. It seems that chlorinated water normally contains hypochlorite, a molecule that combines with any phenolic compound to form an aromatic compound. This combining of chemicals can be very toxic to susceptible individuals and cause reactions in the body.

The thing to understand is that when an individual encounters a suspected phenol, the same allergic symptom, whatever it may be, occurs again and again. Learning disabilities, hyperactivity, the inability to concentrate, and other behaviors that are often diagnosed as attention deficit syndrome can be added to the long list of problems associated with these compounds. The many varieties of phenols may indicate why intolerances vary.

Complete avoidance of the offending food(s) or substance is a possible treatment of phenolic allergies, but many times it is very difficult, if not impossible. Another treatment is to neutralize the problem compound. When a neutralizing dose is given to stop an allergic reaction, the person starts smiling, laughing, joking, and the allergic symptoms disappear. A person can be desensitized to several foods all containing the same phenolic compound. Since phenolic compounds are often repeated throughout nature, desensitization to a few main chemicals could reduce most of the symptoms caused not only by foods, but also by pollens and environmental chemicals.

A treatment that neutralizes phenols has been successful with infants and children, especially with conditions such as autism, mental retardation, insomnia, bed wetting, dyslexia, hyperactivity, respiratory allergies, headaches, asthma, and abdominal pains. Investigate the possibility of phenolic sensitivity. Neutralizing doses can be obtained through physicians familiar with phenolic therapy. It may take a while to see the full results of your efforts, so have patience. Many people have overcome serious illness with the diagnosis and treatment of phenolic compounds.

CHAPTER 11

Salicylates and the Feingold Diet

SALICYLATES AND ALLERGIES

In the 1970s Dr. Ben Feingold, M.D., developed one of the first natural approaches to treating true hyperactivity. A pediatrician who taught at Northwestern University, Dr. Feingold was a pioneer in the fields of allergy and immunology. He was also Chief of Allergies at Kaiser Permanente Medical Center in San Francisco. According to Dr. Feingold, many children are sensitive to naturally occurring salicylates and phenolic compounds.

When Dr. Feingold introduced this program, he only had allergic and hyperactive children in mind, although the diet could be used on adults. He based this idea on over 1,200 cases where food additives seemed linked to learning and behavior disorders. In 1973, at a meeting of the American Medical Association, Dr. Feingold reported that he believed that salicylates, artificial colors, and artificial flavors in the diet were responsible for 40 to 50 percent of the hyperactive children he had seen in his practice. His statement set off an international furor. Even clinical ecologists were skeptical. How could such a small list of substances be such a frequent cause of symptoms?

Dr. Feingold proposed a diet management plan that adds nothing to the diet, but he recommended that artificial colors and flavors, BHT and BHA, and the flavor enhancer MSG be avoided. His plan included the removal of many processed foods, other additives, and most of the junk food available. These substances are the most common offenders of the central nervous system. The reason is they contain synthetic coloring and flavoring agents that are the causes of abnormal behavior. They can also cause symptoms of thought-to-be allergies. Any chemical compound—natural or synthetic—can induce neurological problems in an individual who is sensitive to that compound.

As far back as 1940 there were reports of sensitivities to dyes, especially to yellow dye no. 5 (tartrazine). Aspirin and other salicylate substances, naturally found in some fruits and vegetables, contain a chemical similar to this synthetic yellow dye. The chemical name for aspirin is acetyl salicylic acid. Aspirin is one of the primary offenders of the central nervous system; many other over-the-counter remedies, including artificially flavored vitamin pills, contain salicylates.

Other studies lend additional evidence to Dr. Feingold's claim that diet is a frequent cause of childhood symptoms. A study published in *Lancet* (1985) found that 82 percent of a relatively large group of hyperactive children responded to a hypoallergenic elimination diet. While on the diet, the behavior of many of the children became entirely normal. Most children don't react to only artificial colors and preservatives. This may explain why some previous double-blind studies that tested these substances alone had negative results.

An individual may need to make other diet changes if problems still remain after deleting some offending substances. A diet high in refined carbohydrates, especially refined sugar, is a common offender. Some children are more sensitive to additives when their compromised immune system is not capable of neutralizing toxic substances. Nonfood environmental allergens may cause undesired behavior, learning problems, or poor health.

THE FEINGOLD DIET

Dr. Feingold's diet starts with the elimination of two groups of foods. Group I contains a number of fruits and two vegetables. This group of foods has natural salicylates as part of their structure. You must omit them in all forms—fresh, frozen, canned, dried, juiced, or as an ingredient in other prepared foods.

When following the Group I diet, avoid any fruit or vegetable on the prohibited list. If you suspect a person has an intolerance to a food item that is not on the list, eliminate that food as well. In four to six weeks you will usually be able to introduce these foods back into the diet. The continued elimination of additives is usually beneficial to all members of the family.

Group I

FOODS TO AVOID

Fruits: almonds, apples, apricots, berries, cherries, currants, nectarines, oranges, peaches, plums and prunes, rose hips, grapes and raisins or any

product made from grapes such as wine, wine vinegar, jellies, etc.
Vegetables: tomatoes and all tomato products, cucumbers and pickles

If an individual shows a favorable response to this plan, the foods in this group may be slowly introduced back into the diet in four to six weeks. If either parent has a history of aspirin sensitivity, use caution in reintroducing the fruits and vegetables in group I. An aspirin sensitivity is usually related to an intolerance to salicylates. Try the foods one at a time for about three or four days. If the behavior seems normal, add another food item back into the diet. Follow this procedure until you test all the foods in group I. If these foods show no adverse reaction, you may allow them back in the diet.

Group II

If the symptoms continue even with the elimination of foods in group I, the next step is to avoid all foods that contain artificial color and artificial flavor. The Feingold plan specifically pinpoints the preservatives BHT and BHA. Do not use any foods that contain these substances. To be safe, even avoid any topical product that contains these additives including soaps, shampoos, and creams. Carefully read labels. Avoid non-permitted foods for five days if they contain the offending substances. You can have the permitted foods as long as they don't contain the offending products. When in doubt eat foods that are fresh, whole, and organic.

NON-PERMITTED FOODS (FOODS CONTAINING ADDITIVES)

- cereals with artificial colors or flavors
- manufactured bakery goods
- frozen baked goods
- luncheon meats
- turkey with prepared stuffing
- desserts with synthetic coloring/flavors
- beer
- instant-breakfast and quick-mix drinks
- tea (hot or cold)
- oleomargarine or colored butter
- mint-flavored items (toothpaste, etc.)
- commercial chocolate syrup or milk
- colored cheeses
- chili sauce, tabasco, tartar sauce
- instant-breakfast preparations
- cooking fats
- many packaged baking mixes
- all barbecued poultry
- frozen fish sticks
- manufactured candies
- soft drinks
- ice cream, yogurt, sherbet
- variety crackers
- mustard/catsup/mayonnaise
- soy sauce if flavored or colored
- barbecue-flavored chips
- distilled liquors, except vodka
- cloves

SOME PERMITTED FOODS

The following list contains some of the foods that an individual would be permitted to eat under the Feingold diet. These and any other basic foods are usually homemade or fresh and organically produced so that they contain no additives.

- milk
- all poultry, but not the organs
- grapefruit or pineapple juice
- homemade lemonade or limeade
- all cooking oils and fats
- mustard prepared at home

- distilled white vinegar
- all fresh fish
- pear or guava nectar
- homemade mayonnaise
- sweet butter
- jellies made from permitted fruits

Group III

If symptoms are still present after trying the above elimination diet, then you will need to avoid the following foods for an additional five days: avocado, banana, carob, carrot, cayenne, eggplant, grapefruit, green or red peppers, lemon, lime, melons, olives and olive oil, pineapple, pomegranate, potato, pumpkin, and squash.

General Guidelines for a Salicylate-Free Diet

- Keep a diet diary and write down everything the person being tested eats. Also note any symptoms that occur at the time. In the event an unfavorable behavioral pattern reoccurs, the diet record will show the pattern. Symptoms usually occur within two to four hours. If a change in behavior does occur, the food(s) that were eaten most recently are most suspect.
- Salicylates need to build up in the system before a reaction occurs. You may be able to tolerate a food on a four-day rotation diet, but find it causes problems when eaten daily.
- Carefully check all package and container labels. Manufacturers list the term "flavor" or "natural flavor" on the label without stating the actual ingredients. If you have doubts, do not use the product. It may contain MSG or other additives.
- To avoid artificial flavors and colors, you need to eliminate most baked goods—cakes, cookies, pies, pastries, and puddings. The most common dyes used in foods are FD&C Yellow no. 5 and no. 6, and FD & C Red no. 3. You can still eat these foods by baking them yourself at home, but without additives.
- Practically all candies on the market have artificial colors and flavors added. Make easily prepared candies at home.
- The greatest success comes when the entire family adheres to this diet.

The support of family members serves as an added incentive for the child. You can reduce temptation by not stocking the prohibited foods in the house.

- Adhere to this diet 100 percent or it can lead to failure. Remember, a single bite or a single drink of a non-permitted food can cause an undesired response that may persist for seventy-two hours or more. This will interfere with any desirable results. It can also keep a person in a persistent state of disturbed behavior throughout the week.

- When using medication, if it is contained in a colored capsule, only use the powder inside. A white pill is not necessarily a safe color to take either. Some white tablets have a small amount of red dye in them to make them look even whiter. Practically all pediatric medications and over-the-counter vitamins contain artificial colors and flavors. Consult your doctor and/or pharmacist to be sure. They can look up a medication to find out its contents.

- Check all toothpastes and toothpowders, mouthwashes, cough drops, throat lozenges, and perfumes. Health-conscious stores carry alternatives to additive-laden products.

- BHT is in some soaps, hand creams, and shampoos. Topical substances applied to the skin can absorb into the bloodstream and cause reactions. Remember that some people must avoid artificial colors and flavors throughout their lives.

Many individuals improve greatly after the elimination of salicylates in their diet, if this is the problem. The Feingold diet would be unsuitable for the management of non-salicylate foods related to behavior disturbances. While the Feingold diet is helpful for many hyperactive children, it is unusual that it relieves all of the symptoms. A large majority of children have to also stop all refined sugar and any other food(s) causing a reaction. This diet reduces behavior problems in enough individuals to warrant a trial for one to two months.

The Feingold Association researches foods to determine which brands are free of both obvious and hidden additives. This information, along with step-by-step guidance, is provided for members of the association. See the "Resource Guide" at the end of this book for more information.

CHAPTER 12

Non-Engineered & Organic Foods

The latest Frankenstein-like monster is in our food supply. Our foods may contain recombinant-based proteins and genetically engineered microorganisms adapted for and applied to the agricultural industry. All foods are targeted for this type of modification because it extends shelf life. In 1993 the United States government began approving patents for the manipulation of animal genes. The Food and Drug Administration (FDA) is now allowing gene splicing techniques to develop new plant varieties. This has the potential for adverse effects on the people eating these foods. Genetically engineered foods were not proven safe before marketing, but many of these new genetically altered food products are now on the grocery store shelves for sale. According to *Mother Jones* magazine, genetic engineering is popping up in fresh and processed foods all over.

Biotechnology creates genetically engineered food by splicing a gene from one organism or substance and placing it in another to get a desired trait. Favorite foods such as tomatoes are sold to consumers without advising them that the gene of a fish is embedded in the tomato. It makes the tomato look brighter and shiny and last for months without spoiling in the refrigerator. One of these altered tomatoes can sit on a store shelf for twelve weeks appearing fresh. Is this food still a tomato when it also has fish genes? Squash, melons, and corn are being made with virus genes; potatoes with chicken genes.

Over 27 different genetically engineered crops have been or are close to being approved for commercial production. Most of these products focus on virus-resistant, herbicide-resistant, or insect-tolerant plants to improve crop yields. At the moment most engineered foods are directed toward the animal feed business, rather than improving human nutrition. The protein, carbohydrate and oil composition of plants are open to genetic manipulation.

The Pure Food Campaign, a coalition boycotting genetically engineered foods and synthetic bovine growth hormone, has announced products to avoid and action to protect your family and community. The current products on the grocery store shelf to avoid are: Flavr Savr tomato by Monsanto/Calgene, Endless Summer tomato by DNAP and Zeneca, tomato paste by ICI/PetoSeed Corporation, Freedom II squash by Upjohn Corp/Asgrow Seed Co., Roundup Ready soybeans by Monsanto, Liberty Link corn by Hoechst/AgroEvo, and Bollguard cotton. Canola oil has also been modified and "enriched," yielding triglycerides with fatty acids of different chain length and different structures than from the original plant.

The FDA will not routinely test genetically engineered foods prior to marketing. They only require those biotech foods containing genetic material from common allergens to be labeled because the new food may also cause allergic reactions. These are foods containing peanuts, wheat, or soy.

The difficulty arises when these allergens may not be the common ones and therefore will not be labeled by the FDA, making it very hard to detect other food allergies and sensitivities. There are also ethical concerns with the genetic crossing of species. What about the insertion of human genes into farm animals, or animal genes into other animals and plants? All these issues are becoming a very real concern. A recent scientific survey found that 53 percent of the consuming public was morally opposed to animal genetic engineering and 85 percent wanted genetically engineered food to be labeled as such. There is also opposition because of religious dietary restrictions. How will you know if a food is Kosher or contains a pork gene? Will information be made available so that you can make an informed choice?

In 1992, the 62,000 member American Dietetic Association (ADA) took a stand in support of eating genetically altered food. They released a position paper stating "that the techniques of biotechnology are useful in enhancing quality, nutritional value and variety of food available for human consumption and in increasing the efficiency of food production, processing, distribution, and waste management." They approve the gene splicing that combines genes from dissimilar species. It appears that the future will bring thousands of genes from bacteria, viruses, animals, and plants into the food that all of us eat. These altered foods will then be served up by the dietitians who staff institutions such as schools and hospitals.

Once again, technology is entering new territory without concern for the effects on our health or the environment. They do not know the long-term effects. There are just too many unanswered questions to allow something like this to go on. Here's how to stop the distribution of genetically engineered foods:

• Contact Pure Food Campaign for more information at 1130 17th St. NW, Suite 300, Washington, D.C. 20036; or call (202) 775-1132.
• Contact and protest to your legislators with a phone call, fax, or letter. Encourage them to introduce legislation requiring mandatory labeling.
• Protest to the FDA, 5600 Fishers Lane, Rockville, Maryland 20857.
• Let your local grocery stores, restaurants, and school cafeterias know how you feel about genetically engineered foods. Tell them that you will not shop at any store or establishment that carries these foods.
• Request that the stores post signs stating whether they serve or sell these types of altered foods.
• Educate yourself on the dangers of the manufacturing and eating of genetically engineered food.

What About Irradiated Foods?

The reason manufacturers want to irradiate food is to kill pathogens. Information that is available on food irradiation from government agencies and international organizations gives assurances of safety and benefits, but none of the potential risks and drawbacks. Their assurances are not backed up by any credible testing because there isn't any adequate safety testing program. The safety studies are limited to animals, not humans, and they did not test for toxic or carcinogenic effects. The international studies were only for brief periods of time and did not adequately assure long-term safety.

Added or residual chemicals found in irradiated foods can result in the break down of more toxic compounds. There is some evidence that radiation can induce the decomposition of some pesticides and pollutants and form other dangerous compounds. Chlorinated pesticides in water can form free radicals forming new and dangerous chemical compounds in the food.

It is hard to find truthful information on the effects of food irradiation. One of the best sources is a book written by Karen M. Graham called *Food Irradiation, A Canadian Folly*. This information serves well for us and other countries where irradiation projects are being promoted. The book is definitive on the subject, including discussions of safety, nutritional impact, and the influence on the environment and its people.

It should also be noted that the killing of bacteria in our food does not remove the toxins made by that bacteria, such as aflatoxins. It also seems that the irradiation of food destroys up to 80 percent of vitamins A, B, C, D, and K, while vitamin E is almost completely destroyed. This doesn't include the losses of vitamins due to long-term storage and cooking. Fats may form more toxic and carcinogenic compounds because irradiation changes the composition of food at the molecular level.

The public should be aware that although radiation could reduce the number of some pathogens, it does not necessarily eliminate them. After treatment, the food can be re-contaminated. Radiation will only injure some organisms who can then repair themselves and grow in number again. Mild pathogens may be killed, but what about the more resistant ones? With the lack of competition after killing off the weaker ones, virulent pathogens could proliferate and possibly mutate. Radiation is not the solution. It would be a lot safer to improve food handling from the farm to the table.

The Quality of Our Food

In the past, the foods we ate were of higher quality. More plants were organically grown in soils rich in a wide range of important minerals. This was beneficial because plants use minerals just as we do to create necessary chemicals for their own biological function. We depend on plants to provide us with these essential chemicals and minerals.

According to the *American Journal of Natural Medicine*, 1996, a two year study compared the difference in the nutritional value of organic foods compared with commercial foods. Foods were bought at several stores in the Chicago area. Apples, pears, potatoes, and corn were selected, choosing specimens of similar variety and size. Results from element analysis showed that the organic foods were significantly lower in the heavy metals lead, mercury, cadmium, and aluminum, while the level of essential and trace minerals was roughly twice that of the supermarket varieties.

The additions of additives, preservatives, pasteurization, homogenization, hormones, steroids, and antibiotics are all good reasons to give up dairy products. It is routine to use Chloramphenicol, a dangerous antibiotic, to treat fevers in cows during their transport. Cattle are also frequently given steroids. All these toxins pass through the milk to you and your child. Unless you have information to the contrary, you need to assume that milk is contaminated and unfit for your child, and you. If you must use cow's milk, consider buying organic milk. It is free of pesticides, antibiotics, and hormones. Health food stores and co-ops usually carry it. And with all the publicity about mad cow disease, we now know that it is a common practice to add sheep parts to some animal feed, especially those fed to cows.

The best kind of diet would consist of 100 percent organically grown, unrefined foods, with absolutely no additives, colorings, preservatives, pesticides, or any other chemical adulterations. This includes avoiding sugar, canned foods, frozen foods, most commercially baked goods, and most restaurant foods. Be absolutely sure of the contents of every item consumed. Even a small amount of the offending chemicals can trigger symptoms lasting up to five days. If you only allowed one minor slip every three or four days, and it happened to be a primary irritant, the reaction would be continuous. Even after a lot of effort and hard work there would still be no improvement.

Shopping at the Average Supermarket

Putting together a chemically-free diet from the average supermarket is not an easy job. The following suggestions will help you find foods with lower chemical contamination.

- Buy lean red meat where the fat has been stripped.
- Buy frozen fish in large pieces or as whole fresh fish. Check for preservatives, especially if packaged. Shellfish is better if left in the shell.
- If you buy tuna be sure it is spring-water packed, but without MSG. Remember, MSG is called by many names such as "natural flavoring" or "hydrolyzed vegetable protein." See the chapter "MSG" for more information. Sardines packed in olive oil or spring water cause fewer problems than other canned fish.
- Razor clams, shrimp meat, and crab meat vacuum packed in cans from their local city water usually contain chlorine and maybe fluoride. It is best to buy fresh.
- Oysters in glass containers usually have no preservatives.
- Buy nuts in the shell only.
- Sometimes sprayed fresh vegetables are better tolerated if washed and peeled first. Use a food wash to remove as many toxins as possible.
- Eat potatoes peeled; do not bake in skins.

LABEL INFORMATION

The 1990 Nutrition Labeling and Education Act provided the FDA the opportunity to revise the regulations and impose a new structure on current labels. Nearly all labels display their contents and nutritional breakdown. Reference Daily Intakes (RDI) has replaced U.S. Recommended Daily Allowances (RDA). The RDI gives amounts per serving for proteins, carbohydrates, fats, cholesterol, along with some vitamins and minerals. The label focuses on the nutrients that the FDA believes are most important. It does not list all the vitamins and minerals as before.

You should know that the ingredients on a label are listed in descending order based on the quantity used in the product. Sometimes it's hard to be sure what some of the items are. Often, there are hidden ingredients such as sugar. The product may contain several types of sugars each called something different. Each sugar may be okay in small amounts, but when you add up all the different sugars listed in the product, the total amount is often unacceptable. Terms such as sugar, sucrose, fructose, maltose, lactose, honey, syrup, malt, corn syrup, high-fructose corn syrup, molasses, and fruit juice concentrate are used to describe sweeteners added to foods. If one of these terms appears first or second in the list of ingredients or if several of them appear, the food is likely to be high in added sugars. A wise shopper reads labels and avoids technical-sounding names that are obviously not natural foods.

It is important to note that a label that advertises "100%" of any substance such as "100% aloe vera gel," does not mean that the content in the container is 100 percent aloe vera. It means that the aloe vera used was the entire aloe vera plant, not just the juice or seeds. The product can still contain other substances such as petroleum products, artificial dyes or preservatives. Such advertising can be very deceiving.

There are various other ways in which labels can be very deceptive. Be aware that labeling on products that say "light" or "lite" does not necessarily mean fewer calories. It can mean that the oil used was lighter in color than the oil normally used. Also be careful to not be fooled by anything labeled "enriched." Manufacturers remove the original nutrients during processing and partly restore them afterwards. Another common practice is to state that a product has no added salt, but the product could already be naturally high in sodium.

In today's market it is also very common to see the word "natural" on a package. Do not be fooled. This does not mean the food is organic or additive-free because many additives are natural substances. It is possible to make a synthetic food from natural chemicals. "Natural" may refer to only one ingredient. It could also refer to the processing of the food and not to how it was grown. If you do not know a producer's practices, and if there is no certification label, it is anybody's guess how close the food really comes to being organic.

"Pure" is another misused word. It does not mean a product is additive-free. Unintentional additives such as pesticides and herbicides are sprayed on crops. The hormones and antibiotics given to animals are not on any label. Buy meats that are free of steroids and antibiotics and other toxic chemicals whenever possible. The newest fad is "low fat" items that usually contain large amounts of salt, sugar, MSG, or other taste-producing substances. The irony is that these items may be more harmful than the fat you are trying to avoid.

Manufacturers know that when specific claims are made on a food-product label most people believe them and buy the product. Maybe you shouldn't. Make reading labels a regular habit before you toss foods into your shopping cart. Though not all additives must be listed, most are on the package. Compare similar items and choose those that are prepared with the fewest or no additives, but don't overlook sugar and salt. They can also be detrimental to your health.

Why Eat Organic Foods?

There are various reasons why organic foods are worth the investment. A study done at Rutgers University almost 40 years ago, but buried in obscurity, found that organic foods are more nutritious than non-organic ones. They had a much higher mineral content than their non-organic counterparts: calcium was 2.6 times higher in organic snap beans, 3.4 times higher in organic cabbage, 4.4 times higher in organic lettuce, and five times higher in organic tomatoes. In 1993, another study found that organic produce contained more trace minerals and fewer toxic chemicals than any conventional produce tested.

Another reason organic foods are desirable is that they taste considerably better then non-organic ones. Organic farming starts with nourishing the soil. This leads to more vitamins, minerals, and other nutrients in the plant resulting in food that just tastes a whole lot better. You don't have to put sauces or cheese on your food to enhance the taste.

On the surface, organic foods may appear to be more expensive than conventional foods. What consumers need to realize is that because of the increased nutrition, our bodies will probably need to consume less on an organic food diet. There are also many hidden costs in conventional farming that are paid out by taxpayers. These include federal subsidies, pesticide regulation and testing, hazardous waste disposal and clean-up, and environmental damage.

It is interesting that many people are intent on paying as little as possible for their food, but will pick up a candy bar or other junk food without looking at the price. The real issue shouldn't be just expense, but value. You have to decide if you prefer your foods to be grown in healthier soils, contain fewer chemical residues, are picked riper, and arrive at the store quicker so they contain higher levels of vitamin and minerals, and taste better.

Those of us who buy organic foods are voting with our dollars. It sends a message that we support small-scale organic farmers who are attempting to achieve sufficient income to support a lifestyle in harmony with the earth instead of a large-scale production farm growing food in a conventional way that contains little nutrition and plenty of toxins. On an individual level we can make a new kind of agriculture possible. Where you spend your food dollars can directly promote an agricultural system that provides healthy food and improves environmental quality.

Diet plays a crucial role in the development and the treatment of allergies and sensitivities. As the saying goes, "We are what we eat." If a person does not eat healthy, there can be numerous repercussions. Awareness of the food we eat, the use of organic foods, and careful attention to food allergies and sensitivities can all help to change illnesses. With a varied and healthful diet, many adverse symptoms will often disappear.

Is the Food Really Organic?

"Organic" is the term used to describe plants grown without artificial fertilizers or pesticides. Farmers who use organic methods grow their crops in a way that enriches rather than depletes the environment. This also includes raising meat without growth hormones and without antibiotics. Unfortunately, "organic" is being tossed around carelessly by anyone wanting to make some money off this new trend.

In 1992, close to 700 new "organic" processed foods and drinks were introduced into the food market. Consumers have a right to be protected with federal regulations that define and govern the use of the term "organic." Meanwhile, numerous companies are incorporating "organic" into their advertising, implying that their product is somehow better than another. If organic or any of the following terms appear on packaged or processed foods there may be good reason not to trust their authenticity: pesticide-free, local organic, no spray, natural grown with pest management, all natural, and minimally processed with no artificial ingredients. These terms carry no guarantee that they are what we expect when we buy organic foods. In other words, the claim is meaningless.

At present, more than twenty-five states and many third-party organizations have established certain criteria and procedures for foods before they can carry the organic claim. The Federal Organic Foods Production Act defines "organic" and sets standards for the materials and practices used in the growing and processing of organic foods. The act also creates a national system of farm inspection and certification procedures. Only products labeled "certified organic" or "certified organically grown" by a state agency or a reputable third-party certifier are to be considered truly organic products. These products will carry the certifier's seal of approval or official endorsement.

When you purchase organic foods be sure to look for approval from certifying groups such as the following: California Certified Organic Farmers (CCOF), Farm Verified Organic, Maine Organic Farmers' and Gardeners' Association, Natural Organic Farmers' Association, Ohio Ecological Food and Farm Association, Organic Crop Improvement Association (OCIA), Organic Foods Production Association of North America (OFPANA),

Tilth (Oregon and Washington), and the Texas Department of Agriculture Organic Certification Program.

The natural products industry has gone a step further than the government and considers the term "organic certification of production" to guarantee that not only the ingredients, but also the manufacturing processes are certified to be free of contamination from toxic material. Certifying agencies have worked along with manufacturers to develop these standards. If a processed food carries a "certified organic" label, it means that each ingredient and every process qualifies it as organic and chemical-free.

Organic products generally contain a shorter list of ingredients than their conventional equivalents. By law, 95 percent of the ingredients of any product labeled "organic" must be certified organic. Typically, the 5 percent remaining represents minor ingredients such as herbs, spices and processing aids such as baking soda. Many products contain exclusively organic ingredients.

Consumers should read labels carefully. The placement of the word "organic" on the label identifies the amount of organic ingredients in the product. For example, "organic vegetable soup" must contain 95 percent or more certified organic ingredients. "Soup made with organic vegetables" can have no less than 50 percent organic vegetables. Vegetable soup containing less than 50 percent organic can choose to identify certified organic ingredients, but only on the ingredient panel.

You can usually find a store in your area that specializes in supplying organic foods. A farmer's market or vegetable stand may also supply you with fresh and organically grown foods. These toxin-free foods will improve the nutritional content of your diet.

The best way to replace the important nutrients lost in our current diet is to eat a greater variety of foods, shop for organically grown produce, and cook foods less and at lower temperatures. Consider adding an organic home garden to your yard, but a word of caution. Have your soil tested for heavy metals and other toxins before growing and eating foods from your yard. If organic food is not available in your area, there are many mail-order companies listed in the "Resource Guide."

CHAPTER 13

Yeast Infections and Diet

Yeasts do not really contribute anything to our well-being, but they are usually part of our non-pathogenic bowel flora. They are harmless when their growth is in balance with other organisms that live in the intestinal tract. If an imbalance occurs, then yeast organisms can become overabundant, leading to established colonies on the skin, and in the throat, ears, vagina, and colon. Candidiasis is the medical term for the condition that occurs when the levels of common yeast in the intestines are out of balance. Overgrowth of yeast in the intestinal tract is affecting at least one third of the people in this country, but standard lab tests often don't show anything wrong. *Candida albicans* is commonly the type of yeast that causes problems that can ultimately lead to allergies or sensitivities.

Understanding how yeast can affect us is important because many vague symptoms may be due to this organism. Yeast can interfere with the formation of fatty acid conversions. It can also overwhelm and damage the immune system, especially when antibiotics are used. There is an association that has been discovered between recurrent ear infections in infancy and attention deficit syndrome (ADD) that later develops.

Several studies have stated that many of the children being evaluated for school failure gave a history of more than ten ear infections. These children received repeated and prolonged courses of broad-spectrum antibiotic drugs. Drugs like these alter bowel flora, including the proliferation of yeast such as *Candida albicans*. As a result of these changes, there is an increase in the absorption of food antigens, putting the child at risk for food sensitivities. This may play a major role in causing hyperactivity, attention deficit syndrome, and related behavior and learning problems. Problems with yeast imbalance can present unique problems in children, resulting in symptoms and behavioral changes that are not usually seen in adults.

Symptoms of Yeast Infection

- digestive disturbances, including stomach aches, frequent diarrhea or constipation, distention and bloating, gas, irritable bowel, nausea, and cramps
- behavior and learning problems such as hyperactivity, learning disability, attention deficit disorders, poor memory, and aggressive or otherwise inappropriate behavior
- emotional problems, including rapid swings in mood, depression, irritability, anger, frustration, and unreasonable fears
- muscle problems, including muscle aches, cramps, muscle fatigue, and incoordination of muscle activity
- sugar cravings or a strong desire for sugar-containing foods
- allergic reactions, including asthma, hay fever, sinus infections, earaches, eczema, hives or skin rash, runny or stuffy nose, and known reactions to various foods, chemicals or other substances. Problems often begin after antibiotic use
- urinary problems, such as kidney and bladder infections, or vaginal or rectal itching or discharge
- a generalized set of symptoms that could include fatigue, cold hands and feet, sleep disturbance, blurred vision, itchy ears, and dizziness
- white patches in the mouth (oral thrush) or diaper rash

FOODS THAT ENCOURAGE YEAST GROWTH

The same foods that commonly upset the human body chemistry are the foods that keep the yeast fed: chocolate, most sweets, refined grains, fermented and aged dairy products, dried fruit and fruit juices, alcoholic beverages, pizza, and other refined carbohydrates. When these foods are commonly found in the diet it is easy for yeast to proliferate. Yeast organisms have hearty appetites and they create a craving for more of these foods. It is not unusual to lose the taste for vegetables and animal proteins when high levels of yeast are present, because these foods do not help the yeast thrive. An overabundance of yeast will produce cravings for fermented, pickled, smoked, or dried foods.

What you eat is important, but the way you eat may also be causing many problems. If you have poor digestion, the food becomes a welcome fuel source for the yeast in your lower digestive tract and colon. Along with diet, stress factors add an additional burden on the immune system and make a person more vulnerable to eating the wrong foods.

Causes of Yeast Infections

One of the worse offenders affecting bowel flora and the growth of *Candida albicans* is the repeated and prolonged use of broad-spectrum antibiotic drugs. Antibiotics kill bacteria, both beneficial and harmful ones, but they do not directly affect yeast or viruses. Of all the antibiotics used in the United States, 55 percent are routinely fed to livestock. Nearly all the animals raised for food in this country receive antibiotics sometime during their lifetimes. Eating in a restaurant once a week can increase the risk of yeast infections because of the antibiotics found in the animal fat and dairy products.

In 1994, antibiotic prescriptions for humans posted a record year of 281 million, or 15 percent of all prescriptions. Antibiotic overuse could be making chronic yeast infections into a classic example of physician-induced disease. By killing the bacteria that make up more than 95 percent of the normal bowel flora, the way is paved for yeast infections.

There are other factors that can upset the yeast balance and allow over-growth. A course of steroid therapy can give the yeast the foothold it needs and sugar in the diet keeps it fed. Poor nutrition, regardless of the reason, can lead to the increased growth of yeast.

Diagnosis of Candidiasis

Scientific proof that *Candida albicans* can cause problems like hyperactivity, learning disabilities, depression, anxiety, and various other psychiatric disorders is somewhat limited at the present time. One of the reasons is that there is not a reliable test for intestinal candida. A person's stool can be cultured for candida, but a high yield of the organism may or may not be diagnostic. It seems that the amount of yeast growing in the stool may have no relationship to the number of symptoms the person is experiencing.

Leo Galland, M.D., has found that individuals who have a positive candida culture are less likely to respond to antifungal drugs than those with a negative culture. Evidently, when candida is in the intestinal tract causing illness, the body responds by secreting a growth inhibitor into the bowel lumen, making the yeast more difficult to culture. People who are not being made ill by their intestinal yeast do not produce this inhibitor, so the yeast is easier to culture. Taking a yeast questionnaire, a good medical history, and a physical exam may be more helpful in determining risk to this organism. A therapeutic treatment trial may be the best way to see if symptoms will clear.

Effects of Candidiasis

- Yeast organisms can spread out from the lower bowel to colonize the entire digestive tract, including up through the stomach (especially in cases of low or no stomach acid) into the throat, mouth and nasal passages, and down into the lungs.

- Many people experience adverse food reactions because of abnormal bowel flora. There is a relationship between yeast overgrowth in the intestines and food sensitivities. The bowel wall itself is normally a very sturdy protective membrane that keeps the toxic products of digestion out of the bloodstream. In candida overgrowth, the yeast colonies dig deep into the wall with such a tenacious grasp that they damage the bowel wall itself. The lining becomes inflamed and less efficient in handling food. This can result in allergies and food sensitivities. This can also lead to a permeable intestinal lining. Another result is that the bowel walls become more permeable and start to allow large proteins through. In other words, they start to leak. This phenomenon leads to what is called the "leaky gut" syndrome. It is thought that incompletely digested proteins and toxic by-products of digestion leak into the blood where they cause different reactions at distant sites such as the joints, lungs, and especially the brain. Other results of a leaky gut may be chronic fatigue, food allergies, immune deficiency, autoimmune disease, inflammatory joint disease, and behavior disorders.

- There are almost eighty different toxins produced by yeast overgrowth. This is a tremendous load on the immune system and could contribute to an increase in other infections and allergies. These toxins make someone feel more sluggish, interrupt vitamin and mineral absorption and action, and cause other body processes to fail. They can affect body hormones and alter nerve transmission, resulting in incorrect signals being sent to the brain.

- Candida appears to attack the immune system. The immune system produces antibodies to everything at the slightest provocation. This may explain why people with candidiasis are allergic to so many different things. A person with *Candida albicans* has a hard time feeling well without treatment.

YEAST QUESTIONNAIRE

This questionnaire is designed for adults. It lists factors in a medical history that promote the growth of *Candida albicans* and symptoms commonly found when yeast are present in excessive amounts in the body. Filling out and scoring this questionnaire will help you and your physician evaluate how yeast may be contributing to your health problems. For each "yes" answer in Section A, circle the point score in that section. Total your score and add it to the other scores at the end of the questionnaire.

WOMEN'S SCORE

over 180 = yeast certainly present
over 120 = yeast probably present
less than 60 = the risk of yeast is low

MEN'S SCORE

over 140 = yeast certainly present
over 40 = yeast probably present
less than 40 = risk of yeast is low

Section A: History   POINT SCORE COLUMN

1. Have you ever taken tetracycline or other antibiotics for one month or longer?   25
2. Have you taken other broad-spectrum antibiotics for respiratory, urinary or other infections for more than two months at a time. Did you take several shorter courses of antibiotics within a one-year period?   20
3. Have you taken even a single course of broad-spectrum antibiotics?   6
4. Have you been bothered by persistent prostatitis, vaginitis, or other problems affecting your reproductive organs?   25
5. Have you been pregnant 2 or more times?   5
    1 time?   3
6. Have you taken birth control pills for more than 2 years?   15
    For 6 months to 2 years?   8
7. Have you taken prednisone or similar drug for more than 2 weeks?   15
    For less than 2 weeks?   6
8. Does exposure to perfumes, insecticides, fabric, shop odors, and other chemicals provoke symptoms moderate to severe symptoms?   20
    Mild symptoms?   5
9. Are your symptoms worse on humid days or in moldy places?   20
10. Have you had athlete's foot, ring worm, jock itch, or other chronic fungus infections of the skin or nails?
    Have these infections been severe or persistent?   20
    Have these infections been only mild or moderate?   10
11. Do you crave sugar?   10
12. Do you crave bread?   10
13. Do you crave alcoholic beverages?   10
14. Does tobacco smoke really bother you?   10

Score Section A _____

Section B: Major Symptoms

If a symptom is occasional or mild score 3 points.
If a symptom is frequent and/or moderately severe then score 6 points.
If a symptom is severe and/or disabling then score 9 points.

1. Fatigue or lethargy	_____	13. Bloating	_____
2. Feeling of being drained	_____	14. Troublesome vaginal discharge	_____
3. Poor memory	_____	15. Persistent vaginal	
4. Feeling spacey or unreal	_____	burning or itching	_____
5. Depression	_____	16. Prostatitis	_____
6. Numbness/burning/tingling	_____	17. Impotence	_____
7. Muscle aches	_____	18. Loss of sexual desire	_____
8. Muscle weakness/paralysis	_____	19. Endometriosis	_____
9. Pain/swelling in joints	_____	20. Cramps/menstrual	
10. Abdominal pain	_____	irregularities	_____
11. Constipation	_____	21. PMS	_____
12. Diarrhea	_____	22. Visual problems	_____
		Score Section B	_____

Section C: Other Symptoms

If a symptom is occasional or mild score 1 point.
If a symptom is frequent and/or moderately severe then score 2 points.
If a symptom is severe and/or disabling then score 3 points.

1. Drowsiness	_____	17. Dry mouth	_____
2. Irritability	_____	18. Rash or blisters in mouth	_____
3. Incoordination	_____	19. Bad breath	_____
4. Inability to concentrate	_____	20. Joint swelling or arthritis	_____
5. Frequent mood swings	_____	21. Postnasal drip	_____
6. Headache	_____	22. Sore or dry throat	_____
7. Dizziness/loss of balance	_____	23. Cough	_____
8. Pressure above ears	_____	24. Pain or tightness in chest	_____
9. Head swelling & tingling	_____	25. Wheezing/shortness of breath	_____
10. Itching	_____		
11. Other rashes	_____	26. Urgency/urinary frequency	_____
12. Heartburn	_____	27. Burning on urination	_____
13. Indigestion	_____	28. Failing vision	_____
14. Belching/intestinal gas	_____	29. Eyes burning or tearing	_____
15. Mucus in the stools	_____	30. Recurrent infections	_____
16. Hemorrhoids	_____	31. Ear pain or deafness	_____
		Score Section C	_____
		TOTAL SCORE	_____

THE DIET AND CANDIDIASIS

The following food plan will essentially starve out yeast. It may help detect food sensitivities as well. On a yeast-free food diet, prepare all foods plainly. They can be fresh, frozen or canned, without added sweetener. You can bake, roast, steam, broil, or boil the food. Look for antibiotic-free meat and eggs. You will usually pay more for these products, but it is certainly worth it.

Allowed Foods

MEATS

• all meats (fresh or frozen) without hormones or antibiotics
• all seafood
• poultry
• red meat
• game meat
• eggs

GRAINS, STARCHES, AND LEGUMES

• all grains except corn
• sweet potato or yams
• winter squash
• non-yeast breads and crackers
• all fresh, dried, or cooked beans and peas
• tapioca

DAIRY

• no dairy, but rice milk, soy milk, and other grain or nut milks are allowed

VEGETABLES

• all fresh, raw, or lightly steamed vegetables, properly washed and peeled (because the surfaces may contain mold)

FRUITS

• all fruits, fresh or frozen (without sugar), but limit the intake of fruit. It's best to eat fruit alone and not combine it with other types of food. Limit yourself to two servings a day, but avoid fruit juice and dried fruit
• melons if washed carefully before cutting open; eat melon by itself
• scrub or peel fruit because the surfaces may contain mold

NUTS AND SEEDS

• most kinds, especially if fresh and raw

OILS

• all oils, but cold-pressed organic oils are preferred

MISCELLANEOUS

• most seasonings without sugar
• most thickeners

SWEETENERS

• none (preferably)

DRINKS (UNSWEETENED)

• herbal teas
• water, especially if purified

SALAD DRESSINGS/CONDIMENTS

• if made with lemon or lime juice instead of vinegar

Foods to be Avoided

MEATS

• barbecue and cheese sauces and marinades
• meats if they contain antibiotics and hormones
• processed, aged, cured, and smoke meats and fish; includes bacon, sausages, hot
  dogs, corned beef, pastrami, salami, etc.

GRAINS, STARCHES AND LEGUMES

• malt and malted products
• corn is high in natural sugar; try to decrease it's use
• Avoid yeast-containing products. The following substances may be derived from
  yeast and should be avoided: multiple vitamins, and capsules or tablets containing B vitamins. Check all vitamin products and supplements to be sure that
  they are yeast-free. Many products that contain vitamin B12 also contain yeast.

DAIRY

• All products made from cow's milk including cultured or aged milk products
  such as cheese, buttermilk, sour cream, or sour milk products. Milk products
  are high in lactose and usually contain antibiotics. Both of these factors promote the overgrowth of candida.

VEGETABLES
• none have to be avoided

FRUITS
•dried fruit and fruit juice

NUTS AND SEEDS
• peanuts and pistachios because of the high mold content

OILS & MISCELLANEOUS PRODUCTS
• vinegar
• soy sauce
• edible fungi (mushrooms)

SWEETENERS
• all types of sugars and sugar-rich foods (see the chapter "Sugar")

DRINKS
• alcoholic beverages
• cider
• fermented drinks (root beer, wine, whiskey, brandy, etc.)
• soft drinks in general
• regular or instant coffee
• all concentrated natural sweeteners
• extracts, tinctures, cough syrups and other medications that are not yeast, mold, and sugar-free

SALAD DRESSINGS & CONDIMENTS
• vinegar or vinegar-containing foods like mustard, catsup, mayonnaise, pickles, and commercially prepared salad dressings
• worcestershire sauce, steak sauce, tartar sauce
• accent, miso and tamari

Additional Treatments for Yeast Infections

• The use of an herbal yeast killer containing undecenoic acid is part of the preferred method of treatment. It is very effective with minimal side effects. This herb combines well with caprylic acid to kill the different stages of yeast over-growth. Sorbic and propionic acids selectively inhibit the pathogenic form of *Candida albicans*. There are very effective homeopathic and herbal remedies that help the body regain a healthy balance. All products must be free of sugar, alcohol, and yeast.
• Digestive enzymes containing proteases are often needed to keep the

small intestine free from yeast. Pancreatic enzymes appear to help rid the body of yeast cells, too. Full-strength pancreatin products are preferred because lower potency products are often diluted with salt, lactose, or galactose to achieve the desired strength.

- Nystatin is a drug that kills yeast, but often has side effects of gastrointestinal upset. This is easily remedied by taking the dose with meals rather than between meals, or by lowering the dosage. Sometimes it is best to increase the dosage gradually because as the yeast is killed, toxins are released causing symptoms to become worse for awhile. Vitamin C helps neutralize these reactions. The maintenance dose is extremely variable between individuals. The duration of treatment is equally variable from person to person. Using undecenoic acid is just as effective without the side effects.

- Supportive treatment includes beneficial bacteria. Buy products containing *Lactobacillus acidophilus, Lactobacillus bifidus,* and *Lactobacillus bulgaricus.* These are friendly bacteria that exist in the intestine, but are killed by antibiotics. They are important in rebalancing the intestinal tract. The acidophilus found in milk and yogurt does not adequately replenish the intestinal flora, because most of the organisms are killed during the digestive process. Take the Lactobacillus on an empty stomach only accompanied by water.

- Garlic has demonstrated significant antifungal activity. It is as potent as nystatin and other reputed antifungal agents, but without the side effects. The use of commercial preparations are designed to offer the benefits of garlic without the odor. Raw garlic can antidote homeopathic remedies.

- Enteric-coated volatile oils made from oregano, thyme, peppermint, and rosemary are powerful antifungal agents. Tests have indicated that oregano oil is more than 100 times more potent than caprylic acid. These volatile oils are quickly absorbed, but have been known to cause heartburn in some individuals unless prepared with enteric-coating to ensure delivery to the small and large intestine.

- Other herbal medications may be helpful in the treatment of *Candida albicans.* The herbs that have been found the most effective are: berberine-containing plants including goldenseal (*Hydrastic canadensis*), barberry (*Berberis vulgaris*), Oregon grape (*Berberis aquifolium*), and goldthread (*Coptis chinesis*). Uva ursi (*Arctostaphylos uva ursi*)has also been used successfully.

- It is helpful to use some type of herbal cleanse to detoxify the intestinal system, move the bowels more regularly, and provide an environment for the desired intestinal flora to flourish.

- Vitamin A helps to restore intestinal wall integrity and the immune system. Do not take high doses of vitamin A without being monitored by a physician.
- Support the immune system by decreasing stress, avoiding allergens, providing a proper diet, and getting adequate rest and sleep. It is also important to support thymus gland function.
- Remove strong odors and toxic household cleansers from the home because they place an additional toxic burden on the body. People with candida are usually unable to tolerate chemical smells, household cleansers, perfume, etc. Avoid processed foods contaminated with industrial solvents, artificial flavorings, colorings, and preservatives.
- Avoid antibiotics and immune suppressant drugs such as prednisone and cortisone. If an antibiotic is necessary because of illness, then supplement with a high-count *L. acidophilus* and *L. bifidus* for at least a month after you discontinue the drug. Products are available that contain several other types of intestinal flora helpful to the intestinal tract. It is important not to feed the yeast during this time with refined carbohydrates. Treatment of *Candida albicans* requires aggressive action.

Most people view *Candida albicans* as a sort of parasite. They see themselves as the innocent victim of a malicious, opportunistic organism that invades and attacks their body. In reality, we are not necessarily the innocent victims of disease, but often have control over our health. If we pay attention to our body, we will realize that every symptom is a signal—an important message that something in our life needs to change. When we have made the proper changes, our self-healing mechanisms will be free to perform. Our body gives us signals when drugs, foods, and other forms of distress have weakened our defenses. It's our smoke detector, our burglar alarm, our seat-belt buzzer. The signal may be annoying, but the early warning enables us to seek change for better health.

CHAPTER 14

The Immune System, Liver and Adrenals

The immune system closely interacts with the nervous and endocrine systems to maintain stability of the body. The allergic state is triggered or worsened by a combination of things such as infections, metabolism errors, nutritional deficiencies, digestive disorders, environmental stress, and blood sugar abnormalities. When a person is stressed they release a chemical called adrenalin from the adrenal glands. This chemical causes an increase in blood flow to the muscles and brain and increases the sugar delivery to body cells. When chronic stress exists the digestive system begins to get less blood, oxygen, and nutrition, and so does the immune system. This results in impaired nutrition and leads to an increased risk of infection and illness. Excessive stress can cause common conditions such as:

Hypothyroidism	Hypoglycemia	Pre-diabetes
Food sensitivities	Airborne allergies	Yeast infections
Indigestion	Irritable bowel syndrome	Malabsorption
Depression	Anemia	Low hydrochloric acid
Alcoholism	Insomnia	Ulcers
PMS	Behavior problems	Chronic viral infections

DIET AND THE IMMUNE SYSTEM

- The consistent eating of intolerant foods impairs the immune system and increases the stress response.
- Sugar and other refined and simple carbohydrates such as sucrose, fructose, honey, and concentrated fruit juice all reduce white blood cell production by 50 percent within thirty minutes of ingestion. This impaired immunity can last for over five hours. Most Americans consume daily 150 grams of sucrose, including other refined simple sugars, and may be suffering from a chronic weakened immune system as a result.

- Overconsumption of caffeine reduces levels of immunoglobulins in the serum. These globulins are a necessary part of the immune response.
- Having high cholesterol or triglycerides impairs the immune system.
- Excessive use of alcohol increases the risk of infections, hypoglycemia (low blood sugar), and depression. This reduces the body's ability to manage stress effectively.
- The development of intestinal toxins weakens the immune response, impairs digestion, and increases the stress response. To help minimize this problem take a regular supply of acidophilus plus other "good" organisms of the intestines. Include a cleansing diet.
- Malabsorption, a result of diarrhea, irritable bowel syndrome, intestinal food allergies, intestinal infection, or bacterial flora imbalances, impairs the immune system and increases stress.
- A lack of adequate calories or protein intake will dramatically decrease the body's ability to cope with stress. This type of malnutrition impairs immunity.

Dietary Recommendations for a Healthy Immune System

- It is better to eat five smaller meals each day then three big meals. Eating breakfast is important. If you think you are hypoglycemic then add adequate healthy snacks.
- Restrict saturated animal fats, as well as other high cholesterol foods such as shellfish. This includes fatty beef, chicken with skin, dairy products that are not fat-free.
- Eat a high-fiber diet with plenty of grains, vegetables, and fresh fruit.
- Test for existing food allergies and sensitivities.
- Enjoy your food and meal planning so that your new diet never becomes a burden or an obsessive-compulsive neurosis. Allow yourself to be flexible when you need to be. A perfect diet is not helpful if you can't do it. It is better to indulge yourself 10-20 percent of the time if you are usually eating well.
- Chew your food well. Eat consciously and slowly.
- Try to drink away from mealtime to prevent your digestive juices from becoming diluted. If you feel a need to drink with your meals, minimize the amount.

EXERCISE

Stretching exercises in combination with deep breathing are extremely effective as a method of stress reduction. Aerobic exercise at your target heart rate for twenty minutes every other day further reduces stress as well as your risk for heart disease and other chronic illnesses. Muscle building and strengthening exercises are beneficial when combined with aerobic and stretching exercises.

REST

Sleeping eight hours daily is essential for most working adults. Daily therapeutic relaxation is also an essential component. Allow yourself to re-experience inner peace and poise daily with meditation, prayer, chanting, listening to peaceful music without distraction or interruptions, or having a quiet bath by candlelight.

SUPPLEMENTS

The improvement of immune function with specific nutrients has begun to appear more frequently in medical literature. In the early stages of stress the adrenal glands become hyperactive to meet the demand. As the stressors continue in an unregulated manner, the adrenal glands can become exhausted. Continued unmanaged stress increases the need and utilization of several vitamins, minerals, and other supplements. It becomes important to consume the essential nutrients that help feed, support, and aid the adrenal glands to meet the demands of stress.

CHANGES IN MENTAL ATTITUDE DECREASES STRESS

The ability to manage stress is profoundly affected and controlled by a person's mental attitude. Negative and pessimistic thinking creates stress while positive changes in attitude reduces stress.

• Be more spontaneous and live fully in the moment.
• Embrace joy and enthusiasm in everyday life.
• Learn to ask for what you need. Meet your needs while being sensitive to others.
• Be more open-hearted, willing and able to love, and be loved.
• Let go of fear.
• Let go of control.
• Surrender your self-guilt, self-pity, grudges, and depression.
• Let go of the past.
• Live life from the inside out, rather than from the outside in.
• Love yourself.

YEAST AND THE IMMUNE SYSTEM

Immune dysfunction can come from many different causes, yet the most perplexing is the involvement of *Candida albicans*. This organism probably lives within most people and remains entirely compatible for an individual's lifetime. At any time it can establish itself in the tissues and release its byproducts into the bloodstream. This yeast has an affect on the immune, endocrine, and nervous systems. It also appears to be a complicating factor in many allergic symptoms, as well as other immune dysfunctions.

EATING HABITS

To really help your immune system you must change eating habits and emphasize healthy, live food. It is important not to mix too many foods at one meal and to properly combine foods. What is put into your body must be easily digested and assimilated and not adding additional stress to the digestive system. Dealing with stress, whether it comes from emotional, psychological, or biological causes requires enzyme-rich balanced meals. The most harmful foods that you can eat are the wrong fats, dairy products, white flour, sugar and sugar substitutes, and meat injected with hormones, steroids, and antibiotics. Foods become even more dangerous when treated with pesticides. This all affects the immune system and can ultimately cause allergic reactions or less-evident sensitivities.

INTERNAL BODY CLEAN-UP PROCEDURES

The body is constantly being given products that contain additives, preservatives, and other toxins, as well as toxic substances occurring naturally through food metabolism. To maintain a healthy environment for cell growth and body maintenance the body must eliminate these toxins. The five organs responsible for eliminating the body's waste products and toxins are: the skin, lungs, kidney, liver, and intestines. A health program, diet, or supplements only work if your organs of elimination and excretion are fully functioning.

A wide variety of health conditions can play a part in digestive disease due to toxic conditions. Lack of exercise, poor air quality, and emotional stress increase toxic waste in the body. Devitalized foods, drugs, and chemicals add to the toxic build-up in the body. This allows poor health habits to continue and even become worse. The following outline the different systems and organs the body employs to dispose of wastes.

- *The skin* eliminates water, salts, and urea. Keep it clean of dry dead skin cells so it will function properly. Use a loofah sponge when bathing because soap tends to block the pores. Dry brush the skin with a vegetable bristle brush, but always brush toward the heart.

- *The lungs* eliminate carbon dioxide and water. They function better with exercise. Develop a habit of doing 2 or 3 deep breaths before each meal, but avoid doing this in a smoky environment. A brisk daily walk is very beneficial.

- *The kidneys* eliminate salts, urea, uric acid, creatinine, metabolized hormones, and water. Thirst is usually the determining factor for the intake of water. Juices are often acceptable, but filtered water is best. You could use distilled water that is free of all chemicals and minerals. A lack of potassium can cause damage to renal tubules. Foods high in potassium are oranges, tomatoes, figs, apricots, bananas, dates, kelp, sunflower seeds, wheat germ, almonds, raisins, parsley, and sesame seeds.

- *The liver* eliminates bile salts, pigment, and bilirubin. It is also the primary storage organ for nutrients and some toxins. To detoxify the liver and gall bladder use herbs and homeopathic medications. Periodically cleanse the liver by drinking the juice of a fresh lemon in a cup of very warm water. This should be done first thing in the morning when the stomach is empty.

- *The intestines* eliminate roughage, water, salts, and dead cells. If the small intestines are building up excessive amounts of mucus, absorption will be reduced, slowing down all nutrient utilization. The cleaner the small intestines, the faster any course of action will show results. Eating foods that don't produce additional mucus will gradually improve absorption. Your diet should avoid foods such as salt, sugar, and milk. Fifty percent of your diet, or more, should be raw foods. To further reduce mucus make sure that 50 percent of your diet is from alkaline forming foods.

YOUR ADRENAL GLANDS AND ALLERGIES

The body has two almond-size adrenal glands—one gland sits directly on top of each kidney. One of their jobs is to direct the chemical defenses against allergies. Mold, house dust, pollens, foods, and all the other allergy-producing substances are invaders that can attack our immune system. When the adrenal glands fail to direct our chemical defenders, then the attacking invaders get in and cause damage. This results in symptoms such as sneezing, a runny nose, hives, rashes, and skin eruptions. It also sets up the body for the chronic repetition of the same occurrence.

Often, the difference between the non-allergic person and the allergic one is the difference between strong, responsive adrenal glands that can direct the body's defenses quickly, and weak, sluggish glands that do not have the capacity to do the necessary work. Allergic people, including asthmatics, usually have poorly functioning adrenal glands. When these glands work properly, allergic symptoms decrease. The identity of the sensitizing agent is not always as important as knowing how to treat the glands that direct the body's defenses, the adrenals.

The adrenal glands see a typical case of hay fever as an emergency. Foreign substances that enter the body break down and convert chemicals to things that the body can use, but there are many foreign substances that the body can't handle. Then a process begins that leads to inflammation and swelling of the mucous membranes as more of the allergens get in. The body's alarm system goes off and contacts the core of the adrenal glands, the medulla. The adrenal glands then secrete a chemical that is carried to the other parts of the body and back to another part of the adrenal gland called the cortex.

The medulla's hormone stimulates the lungs into providing more oxygen, a faster blood flow in the heart, and the secretion of hormones by the adrenal cortex that neutralize the invading allergens. This process happens very quickly. If the defensive attack is successful, the body does not have an allergic response. This process takes place anywhere the attack occurs, whether it is in the bronchial passages, the stomach lining, or in the skin. If this defense system fails in the bronchial passages it results in asthma; in the stomach lining it is a food sensitivity or allergy; in the skin the results could be a rash, hives, and itching.

It is in the lymph nodes that cells called lymphocytes are manufactured to collect the newly formed antibodies and carry them to where the invading antigens are. Antibodies will not form and lymphocytes will not release their antibodies without the assistance of chemicals from the adrenal cortex. If the adrenal cortex is unable to function adequately for whatever reason, there are going to be allergies and infections.

When the adrenal cortex is functioning at its best, it secretes more than 32 hormones. The body cannot function without these hormones and the ones produced by the adrenal medulla. The adrenal hormones prepare the body to withstand stress. They also regulate the chemical conversion of food into the fuel and building material our body needs. The adrenal glands then regulate the transport of this fuel throughout the body and transport the building material for the repair and replacement of old cells and tissues.

What if the adrenal glands are exhausted because of poor nutrition, genetically weak organs, or insufficient amounts of hormones? How much reserve strength do they have? If the time comes that even the reserves are exhausted, the whole body is going to suffer. This may be one of the reasons some people have many allergies and infections while others never seem to get sick. The adrenal glands have recuperative powers if given a chance. The first place to start is by eating a proper diet and getting the nutrition that your body needs in order to be healthy.

YOUR LIVER AND ALLERGIES

The liver is the principal organ that treats toxic substances and prepares them for elimination from the body. It also stores and distributes nourishment for the entire body. Food particles are delivered to the liver from the portal blood system and over several hours the liver selects, removes, synthesizes and detoxifies the final products of digestion. Besides storing glycogen and all the vitamins (except vitamin C), the liver manufactures enzymes, cholesterol, amino acids, and proteins. It also produces the bile that emulsifies fat.

Liver congestion due to an improper diet may be a factor in allergies. Undigested foods usually stimulate the immune system to increase histamine. The body's liver produces the most effective antihistamines available to neutralize the allergic or sensitivity reaction, but if it is compromised and not functioning efficiently, histamines build up and trigger symptoms. Under normal circumstances an individual never notices a problem, but a liver that is "plugged up" with toxins and fatty tissue cannot neutralize the allergic reaction. The excessive use of over-the-counter antihistamines may cause more liver damage, allowing the liver to handle histamines less and less.

Toxins may be produced by the body or enter the body from the environment, drugs, foods, or drinks. Today we are exposed to an increasingly higher level of toxins from gasoline exhaust, paint fumes, carpet cleaning agents, and commonly prescribed drugs. It is important to have a healthy liver in order to cope more efficiently with these toxic substances. The liver normally removes toxic chemicals from the blood and stores them in its own cells until it is able to dump them into the lymph system or into the bile for removal from the body. The liver's ability to detoxify itself is dependent on two conditions: the number of toxins needing to be eliminated and a healthy functioning detoxification system. If chemical exposure is too great, the liver may stop dumping the toxins for removal and begin reabsorbing them back into the circulation. The liver will then try to hold on to the toxins so that the level of circulating poisons do not increase.

Symptoms of a Poorly Functioning Liver

There are usually vague symptoms including headaches, low energy, digestive problems with bloating and constipation, or allergies and sensitivities to a variety of substances. Pain may come from under the right rib cage or there is a yellow color to the skin or whites of the eyes. A poorly functioning liver affects the entire body, including the emotions. Anger, irritability, and lethargy are often associated with a sluggish liver. The liver needs to be healthy and functioning well to perform its many tasks and destroy harmful substances such as histamine, drugs, poisons, chemicals, and toxins from bacterial infections. A liver cleansing program should incorporate various steps.

- It is best to eat a diet low in fat, high in fiber, and with plenty of vegetables, both raw and cooked. Green leafy vegetables such as watercress and romaine should be a large part of the diet. Lunch might be a green salad with olive oil, lemon and garlic dressing. For dinner include lightly steamed vegetables that are warm, not hot.
- Do not eat fried foods.
- Avoid white flour products and nuts, nut butters, avocado, mayonnaise, meat, coffee, poultry, and dairy products. Instead of nuts, substitute seeds. Instead of animal protein, use tofu, beans, legumes or white meat fish.
- Hot lemon water or herbal teas may be substituted for coffee and caffeinated teas.
- Take an acidophilus culture with live bacteria to cleanse, detoxify and implant beneficial intestinal flora. Take on an empty stomach 1/2 hour before food and beverages, except for water.
- If you take a glandular product that has desiccated liver, find sources that are non-chemically derived. You may need to substitute liver glandulars with herbs if you also have a sensitivity to animal products. There are herbs that stimulate the liver to produce and dump bile. Herbs can heal most toxin-induced liver damage.
- People recommended for a liver detoxification program are usually overweight, drink excessive alcohol, use prescription or recreational drugs, consume excessive junk food, suffer from chronic fatigue, have allergies and sensitivities, or have a history of liver problems.

Illnesses Resulting from a Toxic Liver

In one reported case, a man was poisoned with a lawn insecticide that resulted in severe debilitating neurological problems. He was hypersensitive to the insecticide because he was taking an anti-ulcer medication called Tagamet. It blocked his major liver detoxifying enzyme system. As a consequence, the numerous doctors who evaluated him believed that the medication caused the poison to accumulate throughout his body and become very potent in its attack on his nervous system. This happens because the body becomes very toxic if the accumulation of toxins is greater than the liver's ability to detoxify them.

People with Parkinson's whose liver detoxification systems were evaluated, found out that they were unable to detoxify and excrete controlled doses of various drugs. Research suggests that they may be unusually susceptible to toxins. This might allow many individuals to suffer from brain chemical disturbances because they have a poorly functioning detoxication system. People with conditions such as chronic fatigue syndrome and those with a history of chronic illness were found to have a higher correlation between depressed liver detoxication ability and the severity of their symptoms.

The ability to test and therapeutically treat the liver to correct this inability to detoxify may also be the needed treatment for such illnesses as blood sugar irregularities, yeast infections, environmental allergies and sensitivities. The excessive burden of toxic substances placed on the liver causes it to not function properly resulting in symptoms. A sensible liver detoxification diet and supplement program may be necessary if you experience any of these problems.

Help the Liver Detoxify

The liver is a key detoxifying organ. It cleans house for us by filtering the toxins, bacteria, and chemicals out of the body. The liver is known to have at least 650 different functions, one of which is to produce natural anti-histamines to keep allergies low. Help keep it clean and it will serve you well during the allergy season. Clean it at least twice a year, in the early spring and fall. At this time, it is best to avoid red meats, sugars, refined starches, dairy products, alcohol, and caffeine. Drink adequate amounts of pure water.

There are several homeopathic remedies that protect, support, and help to detoxify the liver. They also help to reduce the histamine level in the liver thus reducing allergy symptoms, especially hay fever. One formulation combines the homeopathic potencies of: *Beta vulgaris, Carduus marianies, Chelidonium majus, Hydrastis canadensis, Lycopodium clavatum, Raphanus sativus, Natrum sulphuricum, Picrorrhiza kurroa, and Ptelea trifoliata,* as well as homeopathic liver and gallbladder glandulars.

Broccoli possesses several compounds that activate liver detoxication enzymes. Prepare broccoli lightly steamed or raw in order to preserve the active compounds. Pure apple juice helps to cleanse the liver and is beneficial in all liver conditions. Drink freely. Carrot juice is an excellent liver cleanser stimulating the system to eliminate waste. Other juices to drink are cherry, cranberry or mixes of these fruits, but without added sugar. The following are other recommendations to help the liver detoxify.

• Stop putting toxic chemicals into your body.
• Constitutional hydrotherapy, a form of water therapy, helps the liver detoxify.
• There are natural forms of chelation therapy that bind many of the toxic chemicals and heavy metals and pulls them out of the body.
• Exercise increases blood flow and initiates fat mobilization throughout the body. This helps the liver detoxify.
• Good elimination from the intestinal tract is vital so that the detoxification pathway is not blocked. Avoid being constipated.
• If you are exposed to emotional and stressful situations that are unresolved, your liver may not detoxify efficiently and could store toxins.

HERBS THAT HELP THE LIVER DETOXIFY ARE:

• *Artium lappa* (Burdock): Burdock has been used historically as a blood purifier. It is a strong liver purifying and is valuable for skin problems and all blood cleansing and detoxification problems.
• Berberine-Containing Plants: Herbs that contain berberine have been used for centuries to treat the liver. They increase the secretion of bile, eliminating the stress on the liver because of impure blood. Berberine has the ability to reduce inflammatory conditions induced by allergies or infections. It is used for the treatment of gallbladder inflammation and to correct metabolic abnormalities in liver diseases. Berberine is found in the herbs goldenseal (*Hydrastic canadensis*), Oregon grape root (*Berberis aquifolium*), and barberry (*Berberis vulgaris*). Goldenseal root effectively supports the lymphatic system during a detoxification program, but only take it for a limited time.
• *Beta vulgaris* (Beet roots): Drink one cup raw beet juice first thing in the morning to stimulate and help cleanse the liver. Sip slowly and do not repeat for several days. Beet leaves also have liver cleansing properties.
• *Chelidonium majus* (Chelidonium): This plant is good for sluggish, toxic, or congested livers. The symptoms include localized pain radiating to the right shoulder blade and light-colored stools. Chelidonium increases bile production and flow. It is best to take in the morning, but only use for a limited time.
• *Panax ginseng* (Ginseng): Also referred to as Korean or Chinese ginseng, this plant aids the liver in detoxification by helping it to remove toxins and debris from the circulation and protects the liver from chemical

damage. Ginseng's liver actions are quite broad and support the many functions of this organ.

- *Picrorrhiza kurroa* (Picrorrhiza): Picrorrhiza is an important herb in the Indian system of Ayurvedic medicine. It is used for the treatment of liver ailments and immune disorders. In many tests it was comparable or superior to silymarin, the active ingredient in milk thistle.
- *Rubus idaeus* (Raspberry Leaves): The leaves of this plant help to clear liver congestion. Use one ounce of the leaves in 1/2 pint boiling water. Simmer for twenty minutes and drink cold. Take two to three cups throughout the day. Continue treatment for three to five days.
- *Rumex crispus* (Yellow Dock): Yellow dock is an excellent blood cleanser, tonic, and immune builder. It increases the ability of the liver and related organs to strain and purify the blood and lymph system. It is used to treat skin diseases, liver disorders, and nourish the spleen. It is also good for skin itch.
- *Silybum marianum* (Milk Thistle): This is often the herb of choice to help detoxify and heal the liver. It is a well-known herb used for many years with the unique ability to detoxify, protect, and regenerate the liver. The active medicinal ingredient in milk thistle is silymarin. The desired potency is 70 percent. The best symptom to indicate the use of this herb is pain extending up under the left shoulder blade.
- *Taraxacum officinale* (Dandelion): The use of dandelion not only helps to detoxify the liver, but the entire system. This herb is best known for its ability to induce the flow of bile from the liver and improve digestion. European and Indian herbalist have used dandelion for centuries to treat liver diseases.

Section 3

COMMON ALLERGY-CAUSING FOODS

CHAPTER 15

Dairy-Containing Foods

As far back as the 1950s there were reports that cow's milk was the leading offender of symptoms in children. William Crook, M.D., reported these findings to the American Academy of Pediatrics in Chicago and published his observations in *Pediatrics* on fifty children in 1961. For 40 years he has been writing and talking about sensitivities to milk and other foods, but most doctors haven't been interested in his findings. Why? One reason is that the advertising campaigns from the dairy association has been very effective. Another reason is that most sensitivities to milk are probably not IgE mediated. This means that it is not detected by the usual allergy tests. It also takes a lot of time to explain how to do an elimination-challenge diet and the subsequent rotation diet. Doctors are not likely to spend that amount of time working with you.

Traces of milk solids occur in a wide variety of foods, but most people tolerate the limited amount found in bakery products if they avoid other dairy items. Milk is usually an important item in the diet of the average child, but can be harmful to anyone hypersensitive to it. Use a calcium supplement if milk elimination continues for long periods of time. If you want to confirm a milk sensitivity try the following method:

- Allow only foods that are dairy-free for at least two full weeks. It often takes that long to clear dairy from the body's intestinal system. Notice if any symptoms have decreased or been eliminated. You may need to avoid dairy for at least thirty days before symptoms disappear. Of course, if other foods are also part of the cause then all symptoms may not disappear.
- Use the elimination-then-challenge method before adding dairy back into the diet.

Foods to Eliminate

- There are four parts to whole milk: casein, whey, lactose, and lactalbumin (milk protein). They should all be avoided when found in products unless there is not a sensitivity to a particular part.

- Whey is found in imitation milk products and other dairy substitutes, cream soups, soup mixes, most margarines, and store bought pastries and cookies. Whey is added to many processed foods to improve its nutritional content. It is a by-product of the cheese making process and should be avoided by all people allergic to milk.
- Avoid lactalbumin or lactalbumin phosphate since it contains concentrated milk protein. This causes a strong reactions to those sensitive to milk.
- Avoid all liquid milk, cream, or half and half including evaporated and dried milk.
- Look for on labels words such as buttermilk solids, milk derivatives, milk solids, and sour milk solids. Avoid these products.
- Avoid cottage cheese and all other cheeses. Most soy and almond cheeses contain casein, a dairy product. Processed cheese foods and spreads contain dairy.
- Avoid ice cream; sherbet contains milk solids.
- Avoid creamed or milk soups, sauces, gravies, and milk puddings.
- Avoid pancakes and waffles made with cow's milk. Many mixes contain dried milk.
- Avoid chocolate milk, candy, pie, cakes and beverages that contain milk products.
- "Non-dairy" substitutes often contain caseinate. These are products such as Coffee-mate, Cereal Blend, Preem, Cool Whip, etc. Caseinate is a milk product.
- Read the labels of baby food carefully. They often contain milk products.
- Avoid products containing sodium caseinate.
- Avoid products containing acidophilus or labeled "lactose reduced."

Allowed Foods

- Any foods that are not specifically eliminated in the above list are allowed. This includes meats, fruits, and vegetables.
- If a label says Pareve or Parve, it is milk-free in order to conform to Jewish food laws. Kosher milk-free foods are available at any Jewish delicatessen or the kosher food section in a large supermarket.
- Instead of cow's cheese, try tofu, soy cheese or almond cheese.
- A good substitute for mayonnaise is tofu sour cream, soy yogurt, nut butters, or avocado.
- Substitute rice, soy, nut and seed milk for cow's milk in the diet. Some of the brand names are Rice Dream, Amasake (rice milk nectar), West Soy and White Wave Silk. There are recipe books available on how to prepare different kinds of non-cow's milk such as nut milks.

- Many people enjoy peach or pear juice or apricot nectar on their dry cereal. Fresh fruit can be added to dry cereal if it does not cause any digestion problems. Mixing fruit with other foods may not be the best food combination, but it may be a better choice than using dairy products.
- Fruit ices that do not contain milk are available at some stores or ask to have them carried. Keep a supply on hand in your freezer of fruit ices, popsicles, Rice Dream frozen desserts, juice ice cubes, frozen fruit smoothies, or Ice Bean made from soy. There are also delicious ice cream-type products made from soy and rice.
- You can use raw potato water instead of milk in any recipe. Dice the potato into a blender, add 1/2 cup warm water, and then blend.
- Fruit and vegetables juices/purees are great substitutes to be used in recipes.
- Many people who are sensitive to cow's milk can tolerate goat's milk.
- The following foods have traces of milk solids, but often are tolerated if eaten in very small amounts: bakery products including bread and rolls, butter and margarine. Of course it would be best to buy products without any dairy ingredients included.

Butter is mostly milk fat and can often be tolerated by people with milk allergies. Butter can be "clarified" so that all milk residue is removed. Melt the butter over low heat and continue to heat until the foam disappears and there is a light-brown sediment in the bottom of the pan. Pour off the clear butter and leave any sediment in the pan.

At a restaurant inquire whether the food you are ordering contains dairy products. Put your question in this way, "Do you use butter, margarine, cream, cheese of any kind, fresh milk, buttermilk, dried milk, powdered milk, condensed milk, evaporated milk, or yogurt in this food?"

Other Reasons Not to Drink Milk

1. Milk is high in lactose, but two-thirds of the world's population cannot tolerate milk lactose. This includes 80 percent of the black population, almost all Asians, American Indians, South Americans, and 24 percent of Caucasians.
2. Pasteurized and raw cow's milk contains antibodies of grass pollen, house dust mites, Aspergillus mold, and wheat proteins. There are enough allergens present to cause an allergic reaction in someone sensitive to these substances. The presence of these antibodies is probably because the cow is being exposed to the allergens in the feed: pollen and mold from grain, wheat protein from feed grain, and mites from barns or pastures. Sometimes, it even affects people who are not truly allergic to pollen, dust, mold, or wheat.

3. Lactalbumin is the protein found in cow's milk. These proteins can be absorbed in the intestinal tract of a human and result in an allergic reaction. A recent report said that several patients had allergic reactions to milk protein after eating processed meats. There was no labeling on the product saying it contained milk. The companies responded by stating that the United States Department of Agriculture (U.S.D.A.) allows the listing of milk protein hydrolysate to be called 'flavoring' on the label. Because it is important to know what is in your food, it is best to buy your food in the whole form, unrefined, fresh, or without packaging.

4. Highly concentrated protein foods are too concentrated and can cause difficulty for most diabetic and hypoglycemic patients.

5. Homogenized milk is worse than just pasteurized milk because it contains xanthine oxidase, a damaging enzyme that is absorbed from homogenized milk. It is thought that xanthine oxidase damages arteries and causes heart disease.

6. Exposure to cow's milk in the first three months of life increases the risk of diabetes (IDDM) by almost two times. This includes infant feeding formulas based on cow's milk. It is best not to feed infants anything but human milk for at least the first six months of their lives. Apparently, proteins in cow's milk cause the human body to make antibodies. These antibodies attack the protein and destroy pancreatic cells that produce insulin. A study published in the *American Journal of Clinical Nutrition*, 1990, found a significant correlation between the consumption of unfermented milk protein and diabetes in 13 countries. Japan had the lowest incidence and the lowest consumption of milk protein per capita. The Scandinavian countries had the highest.

7. Remember, pasteurization (cooking milk) is for the purposed of keeping bad milk in a saleable condition and for no other purpose. Pasteurized milk products lack the necessary enzymes, vitamins and minerals to maintain good health. Any farmer knows that if you feed only pasteurized milk to a baby calf, it will die in 6 weeks from malnutrition. Pasteurization may destroy pathological bacteria, but it also destroys the friendly bacteria and the casein. Casein then changes to calcium caseinate. This makes the milk virtually indigestible. Most nutritional experts agree that unpasteurized, unhomogenized, raw dairy products are more healthy to consume. However, this is not the form most food markets carry. Pasteurization and homogenization of dairy products destroy much of their nutritive value.

8. Recent studies on the addition of vitamin D to milk suggest that this action may contribute to the development of hardening of the arteries (atherosclerosis) and the formation of kidney stones.

9. Many people have a hard time digesting milk in the gastrointestinal tract, leading to bloating, gas, cramps, diarrhea, or constipation. This may be due to allergies, a lactose intolerance, enzyme deficiencies, chemical additives, and toxic substances given to the cow.

10. Milk drinkers are always full of mucus. They tend to have more coughs, headaches, ear infections, post-nasal drip, colds and flu than nonmilk drinkers. Beside the other negative results of drinking milk or eating dairy products, it causes all kinds of allergies, intolerances, and sensitivities.

11. Recurrent ear infection is strongly associated with early bottle feeding of cow's milk, whereas breast feeding (minimum of 4 months) has a protective effect. This may be due to the protective effect of human milk against infections, nursing reduces the development of allergies, or a combination of both. Most studies show that about 85 to 90 percent of children drinking cow's milk also have allergies: 16 percent to inhalants, 14 percent to food, and 70 percent to both. Breast feeding often prevents food allergies and sensitivities, especially if the mother avoids the foods that she is sensitive to during pregnancy and lactation. If she also avoids the most common allergic foods of children (wheat, dairy, eggs, sugar, and caffeine) then the child has a good chance of not being a victim of repeated ear infection and other childhood problems.

12. Mother's breast milk is high in phosphorous (a brain food) and cow's milk is high in calcium (for bone structure). The human baby develops its brain first while the calf develops its bone structure first. It's absurd to feed a human baby milk from a cow. It is also very interesting that cow's milk is 300 times more potent in casein than human breast milk. Casein increases bone structure. A human develops twice its weight in 7 months while a calf develops twice its weight in 7 weeks. It appears that cow's milk is for cows and human milk is for human infants.

13. Heavy dairy-product consumption is correlated with magnesium deficiency because the calcium to magnesium ratio in dairy products is very high. This can create a relative magnesium deficiency leading to insomnia, constipation, anxiety, irritability, muscle spasms and cramps, and irregularities of the heart beat.

14. It is unknown at this time how much bovine growth hormone (BGH) gets into the current milk supply. It may not be the amount of BGH getting into the milk that is as important as what is happening to the cows. The udder infections that result because of this added hormone have more consequences to our health. It may increase the amount of milk production, but it also makes the cows sick causing an 80 percent incidence of udder infections, as well as other health problems. This increas-

es the use of antibiotics to treat the infected cows. It is likely that anyone consuming the milk will be getting more antibiotics.

Bovine growth hormone causes an increase in growth factor in cow's milk that results in the regulation of cell growth, division, and differentiation, particularly in infants. Pasteurization and digestion do not destroy BGH, and it absorbs easily in the gut. Synthetic BGH caused significant increases in body and liver weights and bone length in just two weeks when tested on mature rats by the manufacturer, Monsanto. Neither Monsanto nor the FDA tested the long-term effects of this hormone on infants of any species, and certainly not in humans.

Consumer awareness of the problems with BGH is growing. More information is surfacing that clearly indicates this hormone may cause long-term damage to consumers who use milk with the added BGH. BGH increases levels of Insulin Growth Factor I in supplemented cows and this may increase the incidence of high blood pressure, breast cancer, and glucose intolerance in milk consumers. Currently, there is no test available to determine if BGH is added to the milk.

The FDA has issued restrictive guidelines to prevent manufacturers from labeling dairy products "bovine growth hormone-free." Monsanto, the drug's manufacturer, has taken aggressive legal action to prevent any perception that the resulting dairy products are somehow dangerous or inferior.

The FDA says that milk produced with man-made bovine growth hormone is virtually the same as naturally occurring growth hormone found in milk. The FDA also says that dairy product labels cannot claim BGH-free because the hormone also occurs naturally in milk. Small dairy companies that buy directly from the farmer have more control over this addition than large companies who use milk from thousands of herds. The approval of this growth hormone drug is legal for cows, but is not being used in goat's milk.

15. In the book *Diet for a New America,* John Robbins discusses the toxic contents of the various food groups. It seems only wise to eat or drink foods with the least amount of toxins that are also the easiest to digest. Animal products (meats) and dairy products (milk, cheese, yogurt) contain a high level of toxins unless you buy organic or chemical-free products. There are traces of many different drugs and chemicals in the cow's milk sold in supermarkets in North America. Antibiotics and chlorine are just two of these substances.

16. Vegetarian diets, even with the inclusion of dairy products, are usually low in iron. Eating dairy products increases the dietary need for more calcium and this competes with iron for uptake inside the body.

Calcium-rich foods may decrease iron absorption by up to 50 percent. Vegetarians who live on wheat and dairy products, with little or no fruit or vegetables, are likely to be deficient in iron and zinc. Children may exhibit behavioral problems as a result.

17. The American Academy of Pediatrics recommends against giving infants under one year whole cow's milk because it can cause blood loss from the intestinal tract.

18. Until the age of 6 months the infant's gut wall is relatively "leaky." It is possible that proteins from the cow's milk may gain entry into the bloodstream and compromise the immune system.

19. Pasteurizing milk reduces its vitamin, mineral, and enzyme content, making an already imperfect food less adequate. It also destroys milk's natural antibodies against bacteria.

20. Kurt A. Oster, M.D., former Chief of Cardiology at Park City Hospital, Bridgeport, Conneticut, contends that xanthine oxidase, an enzyme found in milk fat, initiates over 50 percent of all heart disease. Homogenization breaks milk fat into tiny globules and allows this enzyme to be absorbed through the intestinal wall and into the circulatory system.

Forms of Dairy That Can Be Tolerated

Lactalbumin becomes insoluble in heated milk and forms a scum on the surface. Since high temperatures render most of the lactalbumin out of the milk, some milk-sensitive people can tolerate an evaporated milk formula. In the making of cheese, they separate the proteins into curds and whey. Lactalbumin primarily remains in the whey. Because of the removal of the lactalbumin, many milk-sensitive people can tolerate hard cheeses. Some milk-sensitive people can also tolerate yogurt. Goat's milk and cheese are usually more digestible then milk from a cow. Others can tolerate fermented dairy products or skim milk. Non-dairy foods such as soy, rice, or oat milk could be used as a replacement. A variety of nuts can also be made into nut milk.

CHAPTER 16

High-Calcium Non-Dairy Foods

A number of health problems are the result of calcium-related imbalances including premenstrual syndrome, arthritis, and osteoporosis. The typical diet in this country relies on dairy products for 72 percent of its calcium, but dairy is a common allergen. All or some of these milk parts (lactalbumin, lactose, whey, and casein) may be added to many prepared foods. It is better to select from other available foods to derive sufficient calcium from the diet. Research shows that children with a dairy sensitivity have changes in the permeability of their intestinal tract that increases after eating the offending food. Also, products made from cow's milk are not readily digestible.

Enhance Calcium Absorption and Utilization

A variety of vitamins and minerals help calcium absorption, but improper methods of food preparation can cause a loss. Minerals are more stable than vitamins, but usually lost in commercial processing or in the left over cooking liquid. The assimilation of calcium depends on vitamin D, vitamin C, zinc, boron, magnesium, folic acid, manganese, vitamin B6, copper, and strontium. Usually the ingestion of a good multi-vitamin and mineral preparation will supply the factors needed to help the body assimilate calcium. Most of the foods that are high in calcium are also high in the synergistic nutrients that help to assimilate calcium.

If you decide to supplement with calcium, bedtime is the best time. During sleep you are not taking in other food stuffs that can interfere with the absorption of calcium. Some people can't take calcium on an empty stomach; then have it with a small snack.

When cooking dried beans or leafy greens, add an acid such as vinegar, lemon, lime, or ascorbic acid (vitamin C) to increase calcium availability. When making soup stock from bones, add one or two tablespoons vinegar during the boiling process. The acid in the vinegar will dissolve the calcium out of the bone providing a soup stock unusually rich in calcium. Sea vegetables (kelp, kombu, nori) add substantial amounts of calcium to the diet.

Factors That Affect Calcium Metabolism

- Avoid fast foods or items that are over-processed.
- Avoid cigarette smoking.
- Physical inactivity decreases bone density.
- The pasteurization of cow's milk may interfere with calcium absorption.
- The lack of stomach acid (hydrochloric acid) or a sufficient decrease may affect calcium metabolism. Many people with allergies are low in hydrochloric acid.
- Commonly prescribed drugs such as tetracycline, heparin, corticosteroids, or diuretics interfere with calcium absorption.
- The excess meat protein found in the typical American diet may drive down calcium levels. A heavy daily consumption of meat can lead to a relative calcium deficiency. Excessive calcium loss from bone can be deposited in soft tissues (hair, joints, arteries, kidneys) as well as lost in the urine in high amounts.
- Foods high in something called oxalates can bind the available calcium, making it unavailable for use by the body. Foods high in oxalates are spinach, rhubarb, beets, and beet greens, almonds, cashews, cocoa, and chocolate. Do not consume large quantities of these foods, especially at the same time you take calcium.
- Excessive phosphorus may drive down calcium levels. A major source is the various carbonated cola drinks.
- Caffeine found in coffee, tea, cola, and many other drinks may be involved in decreased calcium metabolism.
- A diet high in sugar and salt decreases calcium absorption. Excessive sugar causes calcium to be leached out of the bones.
- Don't take fiber simultaneously with your calcium supplements. It can bind the calcium and make it unavailable to the body. Dietary phytates adversely affect the uptake and utilization of many minerals, including calcium. Foods high in phytates are grains, beans, and nuts.
- If you drink alcohol every day, your calcium intake won't do you much good. Alcohol interferes with the body's absorption of calcium and may block the benefit of this nutrient.
- How much calcium you digest and absorb is even more important that adding calcium-rich foods to your diet or taking calcium supplements. Many people do not absorb calcium because the diet doesn't contain enough magnesium.

Recent studies do not agree that a high calcium intake has a positive affect on continued bone health. The more calcium one ingests at any given time, the smaller the percentage of absorbed calcium. Eating dairy products increases the dietary need for more calcium. When the body adapts to a low-calcium diet, it actually excretes less calcium in the urine and increases absorption.

Excessive calcium in the body could result in soft tissue calcification or arthritis. One possible beneficial nutrient to help counteract this effect is magnesium. In recent studies there was an increase in bone density in post menopausal women who took more magnesium and less than the recommended calcium.

Magnesium helps move calcium into our bones, preventing osteoarthritis and osteoporosis. A magnesium deficiency, however, will prevent this chemical action. Taking more calcium is not the solution. While magnesium helps the body absorb and utilize calcium, excessive calcium prevents the absorption of magnesium. What amount is adequate for one woman may be insufficient for another. Magnesium helps the body utilize B-vitamins, as well as inactivate excessive estrogen, and decreases PMS symptoms.

Studies indicate that it is magnesium, not calcium, that forms the hard enamel that resists tooth decay. Milk, poor in magnesium, not only interferes with magnesium metabolism, but also interferes with the mineral responsible for the prevention of tooth decay. Milk is also the greatest producer of lactic acid than any other food. Lactic acid dissolves calcium in the protective layer of the tooth. Remember, a high calcium level in the diet increases the magnesium requirement. Since there is usually a deficiency of magnesium in the population, drinking large quantities of milk could be one of the causes of dental caries.

Exercise is the best way, short of potent medication, to significantly increase bone mass after growth has stopped. People who exercise for one hour, three times a week, actually gain bone mass. A comparison group of sedentary women lost bone mass. The best kind of exercise for healthy bones is weight-bearing exercise. Over-exercising can be a distress on the body and lead to bone loss. It is best not to exercise until exhaustion. Exercise will not be enough to prevent osteoporosis if your body chemistry is not in balance.

Sources of Calcium

The actual milligrams of calcium are different from milligrams of a compound containing calcium. There is about 91 milligrams calcium in 1000 milligrams calcium gluconate, so read the labels! Take calcium along with its complementary mineral, magnesium. The ratio is usually 2:1 calcium to magnesium. Some sources say a 1:1 ratio is better.

The following are the different types of calcium supplements and their advantages and disadvantages. They are listed in order from best to worse type of calcium for the body:

1. Calcium microcrystalline hydroxyapatite is 25 percent calcium, very well absorbed, can reduce bone loss, absorbed by some malabsorbers, and a complete bone food.
2. Calcium citrate is 24 percent calcium, very well absorbed, absorbed by those with poor digestion, but not a complete bone food.
3. Calcium aspartate is 20 percent calcium, well absorbed, but not a complete bone food.
4. Calcium ascorbate is 10 percent calcium, well absorbed, non-acidic vitamin C, but not a complete bone food.
5. Calcium lactate is 15 percent calcium, well absorbed, may contain milk and/or yeast by-products, and not a complete bone food.
6. Calcium carbonate is 40 percent calcium, the cheapest source of calcium, not a complete bone food, may be malabsorbed by those with poor stomach digestion, and can cause gas. Calcium carbonate acts as an antacid and decreases stomach acid. With the decrease of stomach acid calcium absorption may also decrease. This form of calcium is not a good source, at least in theory, not to mention altering your stomach acid levels every time you take it. Calcium derived from oyster or egg shell is mostly calcium carbonate.
7. Bone meal is 39 percent calcium, contains multiple minerals needed for bone, but may contain high levels of lead, arsenic, cadmium, etc. Organic constituents are destroyed leading to reduced effectiveness. Bone meal is derived from beef and can cause problems if there is a beef sensitivity.
8. Calcium gluconate is 91 percent gluconate, not calcium.
9. Calcium phosphate absorbs poorly.

Food Sources of Calcium

The following list of calcium foods will help you find additional sources of calcium from your diet that is not dependent on cow's milk. The RDA for calcium is 800-1000 milligrams a day. This high amount of calcium is based on a calcium that has a low absorption rate. The list contains foods rich in calcium as well as low-calcium foods. Compare these foods to one cup of cow's milk that contains about 300 milligrams of calcium. The approximate calcium content of the foods in the list below is the number of milligrams per 8 ounces or 1 cup, unless stated otherwise.

Wakame	3500 mg.	Broccoli (1 stalk)	160 mg.
Komnu	2100	Navy beans	140
Nori	1200	Figs	126
Agar-agar	1000	Tortillas (2)	120
Sesame seeds	2100	Corn, canned	100
Sardines with bones	1000	Pinto beans	100
Green peas, dried	1000	Quinoa, cooked	80
Almonds	750	Black beans	60
Mackerel with bones	680	Eggs, hard cooked (2)	60
Banana, dried	620	Lima beans	60
Chestnuts	600	Raisins, raw (3.5 oz.)	60
Salmon with bones	490	Corn meal	50
Soybeans, cooked	450	Squash, boiled	50
Hazel nuts (filberts)	450	Soy sprouts, raw	50
Turnip greens, cooked	450	Sweet potato (1 small)	50
Blackstrap molasses	410	Whole wheat flour	50
Tofu	400	Olive, green (12)	48
Garbanzo beans, cooked	340	Banana, raw	40
Goat's milk	320	Oats	40
Orange juice (calcium fortified)	320	Romaine lettuce leaf	40
Collard greens, cooked	302	Rye flour, dark	40
Shrimp	300	Cashews, raw (50)	36
Tapioca, dried	300	Mung beans	35
Mustard greens, cooked	280	Alfalfa sprouts	25
Walnuts	280	Peanuts (1/4 cup)	25
Sunflower seeds, hulled	260	Rice	25
Spinach, cooked	250	Rye flour, light	20
Oysters, raw	240	Grapefruit, raw	16
Rhubarb, cooked	210	Tomato, raw (1)	15
Kale, cooked	200	Head lettuce	10

CHAPTER 17

Corn-Containing Foods

C orn is one of the most hidden allergens found in foods. Many processed food products contain sugar derived from corn. Commercial medications made into tablets, wafers, and capsules often contain corn, as well as vitamin and nutritional supplements. If there is any doubt about a product's content, write the manufacturer for up-to-date information. Check labels for corn-free products or make food dishes corn-free at home.

Different Forms of Corn

- Green corn (from fresh): baby corn, canned, frozen, roasting ear, fritters, succotash, tamales
- Dried corn: corn flour, cornmeal, cornstarch, hominy grits, parched corn, popcorn
- Refined forms of corn: corn flakes, corn oil, corn sugar, corn syrup, glucose, dextrose, high fructose corn syrup, and artificial sweeteners; most commercial fructose is derived from corn, not fruit

Types of Exposure to Corn

- Inhalant exposure: fumes from cooking corn, ironing starched clothes (corn starch), and body or bath powders, talcum
- Contact exposure: starched clothing and corn-containing adhesives (envelopes, stamps, stickers, etc.), soaps, toothpaste, paper cartons or containers and cups
- Food exposure: corn products and foods containing corn products. Restaurants may use an oil that contains corn such as when cooking French fries.

Avoiding Corn

Cook corn-free by using only fresh, non-packaged fruits, vegetables, meats, or home-canned foods. Use corn-free oils derived from soy or olive oil, pure safflower oil, sunflower or canola oil. Water-packed foods are usually corn-free. Substitute arrowroot in recipes calling for cornstarch. Many cardboard containers are powdered with cornstarch including many milk cartons.

If you suspect a corn sensitivity, an elimination or rotation diet will be necessary. Manufacturers can add small amounts of corn to a product without stating it on the label. Unfortunately, items such as nectars with "cane sugar" on the label permit up to 25 percent corn syrup without appearing on the label. Since the syrup used in canned fruits is usually corn syrup, use only syrup-free products. Avoid foods that you suspect contain corn until they are thoroughly checked out. The best label is one that states the product is corn-free.

Sugars That May Be Derived From Corn

1. Corn dextrin is a white or yellow powder obtained by enzymatic action of barley malt on corn flours. Milk and milk products often contain corn dextrin as a modifier or thickening agent.
2. Corn syrups are the result of using enzymes or acids on cornstarch to make it sweeter. They can be in maple, nut, and root-beer flavorings, and in ice cream, candy, and baked goods. Glue has corn syrup added to it and applied to envelopes, stamps, and sticker tapes. It may be in ale, aspirin, bacon, baking mixes, beer, bourbon, breads, breakfast cereals, pastries, candy, catsup, cheeses, chop suey, chow mein, fish products, ginger ale, hams, jellies, processed meats, peanut butter, canned peas, plastic food wraps, whiskey, and American wines.
3. Dextrose (corn sugar) is often sold blended with white sugar. Many artificial sweeteners contain dextrose. If you are sensitive to corn you will need to read the ingredients carefully of so-called "artificial" sweeteners. Dextrose is usually the first ingredient on the label. It is an ingredient in intravenous solutions commonly used in hospitals. Many people have "surgical complications" due to an allergic reaction after receiving intravenous dextrose. Dextrose may be derived from other noncorn sources, but it is getting harder to know the actual source of many sugar products.
4. Fructose (or Levulose) is often derived from fruit sugar. The fructose commonly found in stores comes from corn, cane or beet sugar, not from fruits. It is sometimes very difficult to identify the source of the fructose in a food item, because of the confusion between fructose derived from fruit or fructose made from high-fructose corn syrup.
5. Glucose is a commercially processed sugar derived from cornstarch. The main problem with glucose is its low sweetness level. You could eat a

large quantity without being aware of its presence in a food. Glucose is a flavor found in ground-meat dishes, luncheon meats, and in maple syrup. Confectioners generally use glucose in candy making because it gives the hard-boiled candies a clear appearance.

6. Honey farmed in the United States usually ends up in supermarkets as a refined sweet liquid with all its nutritional properties strained out. It is not uncommon to find honey adulterated with corn syrup or other sugars.

7. Maltodextrins are less sweet than dextrose. They are processed from corn or maize and used to convert liquid flavors into dry powders. They are also used as texturizers and flavor enhancers in candies, particularly chocolate. Maltodextrins are in many dehydrated products such as soup and gravy mixes, spice blends, seasonings, salad dressing mixes, instant coffee, doughnuts, frozen desserts, infant foods, jelly beans, peanut butter, sausages, and cookies.

8. NutraSweet contains dextrose and aspartame. Dextrose is a refined sugar made from corn.

9. Sorbitol is a nonglucose carbohydrate called a sugar alcohol. Sorbitol occurs naturally in fruits, seaweed, and algae, but is commercially produced from such sources as dextrose (a corn derivative).

10. Xylitol is also a nonglucose carbohydrate called a sugar alcohol. It can come from birch trees, corn cobs, peanut shells, wheat straw, cotton seed hulls, and coconut shells. It has the same sweetness as sucrose (table sugar) and leaves a pleasant, cool taste in the mouth. It is still being used in some chewing gums.

CHAPTER 18

Pork-Containing Foods

If you need to be on a pork-free diet, avoid foods and products that could contain pork.

FRESH PORK PRODUCTS

Pork roast	Pork brains	Pork liver
Pork chops	Pork kidneys	Souse (head cheese)
Pork sausage	Cracklings or chitterlings	

CURED PORK

Pickled pig's feet	Sausage	Bacon or bacon drippings
Ham	Rinds (pork rinds)	Salt Pork

PROCESSED PORK

Wieners	Mincemeat	Liverwurst
Vienna sausage	Spam	Luncheon meats
Canned meats such as "potted" meats		

FOODS/PRODUCTS THAT MAY CONTAIN DERIVATIVES OF PORK

Lard	Prepared cake and pancake mixes	Bakery products
Bacon drippings	Pre-breaded frozen foods	Ice cream
Shortening	Frozen seafood and fish	Potato chips, fritos
Margarine	Fried foods in restaurants	Gelatin, Jell-O
Mashed potatoes	Soaps	Candy bars
Mayonnaise	Vegetables seasoned with salt pork	Puddings
Mexican food	Glue in milk cartons	Salad dressing
Nondairy cream	Instant foods	Cosmetics

DRUGS THAT MAY CONTAIN PORK

Calcium and magnesium stearates	ACTH
Thyroid tablets	Capsules,pills for anemia
Intrinsic factor (from hog stomach)	Glycerin capsules

CHAPTER 19

Potatoes and Potato-Containing Foods

If you know you suffer from a sensitivity or allergy to potatoes, the following list will help you select potato-free products:

- Most yeast such as baking yeast, beer yeast, and baking powder contain potato. Yeast and nutritional yeast are usually grown on potato products. Instead use Red Star yeast. It is potato free.
- Beers that are potato-free are: Henry Weinhard, Tuborg, Corona, and Olympia.
- Some people who are sensitive to potatoes are also sensitive to part or the entire nightshade family. This includes potato, tomato, eggplant, peppers (red and green), chili peppers, paprika, pimiento, tobacco, and cayenne.
- Some inexpensive yogurts, baby foods, and egg replacers contain potato.
- Spray starch used on clothing may be derived from potato.
- Dextrose may be made from potato sugar.

The following products are derived from potato or may contain potato:

many prepared soups, noodles, and sauces	potato starch
modified starch	iodized salt
potato flour	vitamin A palmitate
baby foods	beef stew or hash
some breads or biscuits	clam chowder
potato chips	meatloaf or meat pies
taco sauce	doughnuts (some)
gravies (some)	meatballs

CHAPTER 20

Foods and Products Containing Soybeans

A sian countries have grown and eaten soybeans for centuries, especially China, whereas American farmers have grown and fed soybeans for years to their livestock or plowed it under for fertilizer. Lately, many uses for this bean have been discovered proving to be a treasure and a bonanza in this country. If you know you are sensitive to soybean products, the following list will be helpful in identifying items containing soybeans:

- Bakery goods: Many bakers use soybean flour in their dough mixtures for breads, rolls, cakes, and pastries. This keeps their goods moist and saleable several days longer. K-Biscuits and several crisp crackers have soybean flour in them.
- Sauces: La Choy, Lea & Perrin's, and Heinz's Worcestershire sauce contain soy.
- Cereals: Sunlets and Cellu Soy flakes are soy cereals. Look for soy as an added ingredient in other cereals.
- Salad Dressings: Many dressings and mayonnaise contain soy oil. Sometimes the only hint on the label is that the product says vegetable oil, and it doesn't say soy-free. Soy oil is now being added to many brands of oil previously free of soybean. If the contents are in question, contact the company for more information.
- Meats: Pork-link sausage and luncheon meats may contain soybeans. The allergic individual should buy only pure meat products.
- Candies: Hard candy, nut candy, and caramels often contain soy flour. Lecithin is usually derived from soybean and is used in candy to prevent drying and to emulsify the fats.
- Milk Substitutes: Due to rising cost, many pizza parlors are using cheese made from soybeans. If you are having reactions after eating pizza, ask the restaurant to let you read the label from the cheeses they use. Many

varieties and flavors of soy milk are available such as Sobec and Mull-Soy. Some bakeries use soy milk instead of cow's milk in their products. If in doubt, ask!

- Ice Cream: There are several varieties of soy ice cream available. Soy may also be an ingredient in ice cream made from cow's milk.
- Soups: Soy is frequently an ingredient found in prepared soup.
- Vegetables: Chinese dishes often use fresh soy sprouts as a vegetable. They also include soy in many dishes in the form of tofu, soy sauce and other sauces.
- Nuts: Soybeans are roasted, salted, and used instead of peanuts.
- Shortenings, Fats, and Oils: Crisco, Spry, and other shortenings may contain soy oil. Margarine and butter substitutes often contain soy products.
- Noodles: Soybeans made into macaroni and spaghetti noodles are available.
- Miscellaneous: Tofu, Natto, and Miso are soy products. Soy cheese is available, and it usually contains casein (derived from cow's milk).

Other Common Soy Products

blankets	glycerin	adhesives
varnish	grease	lubricating oil
candles	linoleum	soap
celluloid	massage creams	paints
nitroglycerin	fertilizer	coffee substitute
cloth	printing ink	custards
paper finishes/sizing		

New Contacts with Soy Products

Expect many new contacts with soybean products. Commercial lecithin previously came from eggs, but now most of the lecithin used in food processing is from soybean oil and is added to many foods. Because lecithin is so highly refined, and since very little is used in food preparation, it is unlikely to cause a problem for soy-sensitive people, at least that is what the FDA says. It would probably be best to have any product containing lecithin tested for individual sensitivity. Soy is also being added to many cosmetics.

Researchers in New Zealand found that soybeans can adversely affect hormonal development in infants and recommends caution using infant soy formula. Another study associated the development of autoimmune thyroid disease with soy formula. All legumes are rich in substances that act similar to estrogen in the body. When soy is combined with a diet that also contains a variety of whole foods and prepared by soaking and cooked slowly, there doesn't seem to be a problem. When soy protein is used in concentrated amounts such as in most modern soy products and supplements, deficiencies in several minerals and vitamins can also occur. In Asian countries, soy is consumed as a condiment, not as a replacement for animal foods, so fewer health problems are seen using soy.

CHAPTER 21

Wheat In The Diet

Food sensitivities have become commonplace. Wheat is one of the most common food allergens and gut intolerant foods, besides dairy. Eating the same food day after day contributes to food problems. The staff of life, for some people, is not bread made from wheat. It can cause bloating, headaches, constipation, fatigue, and other digestive symptoms.

Some people tolerate certain forms of wheat such as white bread, but not whole wheat. Other individuals can eat pasta, but not bread. Still others cannot eat any form of wheat because of the gluten content (see the chapter "About Gluten"). Those who cannot tolerate wheat fiber often have stomachs and intestinal linings that are delicate. and cannot handle raw vegetables or fiber-rich foods. Many sensitive people react to the yeast used to make bread. They can eat yeast-free crackers and pasta, or yeast-free bread, but not products using yeast to make the dough rise. An intolerance to wheat can be difficult to manage because of the prevalence of this grain in the American diet.

It is best to eat in a way that simplifies digestion through proper food combination and food rotation. For some individuals a digestive aid helps to reduce digestive symptoms because it helps to break down the food. In the beginning even a small amount of the offending food can cause problems, but it is possible to resolve a sensitivity to foods over time. This treatment may have to include desensitization to some of the particularly intolerant foods. The best way to detect wheat in your diet is to read labels.

The following are common names of wheat products: gluten, semolina, durham, couscous, triticale, kamut, white flour, graham flour, all-purpose flours. Wheat is often mixed with other flours such as rye or legume flour. Whiskey, vodka, gin, beer, and other alcoholic beverages that contain grains usually contain wheat. Wheat is often included with other grains in products such as multi-grain cereals or breads. It is usually the grain of choice in battered and breaded products, meat mixes, pastas, and pastries. Many seasonings and condiments contain wheat. It is used as a thickener in corn starch, ice cream, and commercially made sauces and mustards.

Tamari and soy sauce contain wheat unless you buy the wheat-free variety. You can find wheat in foods containing malt; commercially prepared casseroles, souffles, and creamed soups; and vinegar derived from wheat grains. MSG can be prepared from wheat.

Alternatives to Eating Wheat

Some people who are sensitive to wheat are also intolerant to gluten. Other grains besides wheat contain gluten. If you are gluten intolerant, then some of these foods may be a problem and cause reactions. See the chapters "About Gluten" and "Grains" for more information.

Other foods you can use to replace wheat include: spelt, quinoa, rice, millet, rye, oats, barley, corn, soy, amaranth, buckwheat, potato. Many of these foods are available as flours, breads, cereals, and pastas. Check cookbooks for wheat-free baking. When making sauces or gravies, use potato or soy flour, arrowroot, kudzu, agar-agar, spelt flour, corn starch, or tapioca.

CHAPTER 22

About Gluten

WHAT IS GLUTEN?

Gluten is a mixture of proteins present in some cereal grains, especially wheat. It consists almost entirely of two proteins, gliadin and glutelin. The exact proportions depend upon the variety of grain. However, gluten does not agree with everyone. Some digestive problems are associated with a gluten intolerance such as celiac's disease. Gluten is a syrupy substance that binds the dough and is responsible for making bread springy. Gliadin is also the protein in rye flour and in a wheat-and-rye blend called triticale.

What is a Gluten Intolerance?

A digestive tract that cannot tolerate gluten is characterized by malabsorption due to damage to the small intestine. When a gluten intolerance becomes an extreme condition, it is called celiac's disease, non-tropical sprue, or gluten-sensitive enteropathy. Symptoms may include weight loss, greasy and foul-smelling stools, and diarrhea. There is often multiple vitamin and nutrient deficiencies and an eczema-like skin conditions usually occurs.

One of the hallmark signs of celiac's disease is iron-deficiency anemia and extreme fatigue, not corrected by iron supplements. Also present are low serum calcium levels. Breast-fed children, along with the delayed introduction of cereals and cow's milk, can provide a protective effect that greatly reduces the risk of developing a gluten intolerance. Most children diagnosed with celiac's disease experience relief soon after starting a gluten-free diet.

Dermatitis, herpetiformis, psoriasis, irritable bowel syndrome, and inflammatory bowel disease may also be the results of a gluten intolerance. It is a common problem for food-sensitive individuals and can trigger more symptoms such as fatigue, joint pains, and headaches. There has recently been an association between gluten intolerance and lichen planus.

A blood test is now available for diagnosing gluten intolerance. Testers use the alpha gliadin antibody level to identify individuals who are likely to respond to a gluten-free diet. People with recurrent oral ulcerations, but who had normal small intestinal biopsies, were studied. People with a gluten intolerance had raised levels of antibodies to alpha gliadin. In three out of these four people the ulceration disappeared on a gluten-free diet and relapsed after again having gluten. Among the people who did not have raised alpha gliadin antibody levels, none responded to a gluten-free diet.

AM I SENSITIVE TO WHEAT BECAUSE IT CONTAINS GLUTEN?

You can be sensitive to wheat, but not because it contains gluten. Other factors to consider are the many molds that grow on wheat and the use of pesticides. When introducing wheat back into the diet, try organic wheat first.

WHAT OTHER FOODS BESIDES WHEAT CONTAIN GLUTEN?

Oat, rye, most beers, Postum, products containing cereals, barley, and anything containing barely malt, triticale, kamut, quinoa, millet, spelt, and possibly buckwheat and teff. Products derived from cereal grains are likely to contain gluten. People who are not able to eat other gluten-containing grains can often tolerate spelt and millet since they are some of the easiest grains to digest. Check with your health-food store for availability.

Millet has small amounts of gluten, but virtually no gliadin. Malt comes from sprouted barley and from the hydrolyzed starch of other grains. Barley contains hordein, a protein with similar properties to gliadin. Hordein is so similar to gliadin that it should be avoided by people intolerant to gluten.

WHAT GLUTEN-CONTAINING FLOURS SHOULD BE AVOIDED?

Barley, buckwheat (kasha), oat, rye, spelt, triticale, quinoa, millet, and wheat (white, semolina, durum, kamut, couscous, bulgur, whole wheat).

WHAT GLUTEN-CONTAINING PASTAS SHOULD I AVOID?

Artichoke, buckwheat, durum, semolina, secale, spelt, quinoa, wheat. If you are in doubt about the contents of a flour product, write or call the company that makes the product before using it. Read labels!

WHAT ARE SOME SUBSTITUTES FOR GLUTEN-CONTAINING GRAINS?

Gluten-free foods are corn, rice, wild rice, amaranth, soybean, and potatoes. Although not a grain, soy products are free of gluten and often used as a grain substitute.

WHAT ARE SOME GLUTEN-FREE FLOURS?

They are arrowroot, kudzu, amaranth, rice, garbanzo (chick pea), corn, potato, soybean and other bean flours, and all nuts and seeds. Make sure these flours are wheat-free. It is common to find wheat added to many other types of flours.

What About Other Food Intolerances?

People who cannot tolerate wheat fiber or gluten often have delicate stomachs or intestinal linings creating a sensitivity to many foods. They may experience difficulty tolerating raw vegetables and other fiber-rich foods.

ALLOWED	AVOID
Beverages	
carbonated beverages, milk, buttermilk, skim milk, tea, vodka, wine, and coffee that is not made from cereal grains	coffee substitutes chocolate, malted milk, Postum, Ovaltine, ale, beer, and brandy and other alcoholic beverages, instant coffee
Breads	
bread products made from arrowroot, corn, gluten-free starch flours, rice, or soybean	all bread products made from wheat, rye, oats, or barley, all commercial products and mixes, flour mixes, and bread crumbs
Cereal	
hot cereals made from corn meal and rice, all other ready-to-eat cereals made from corn and rice products with allowed ingredients	many commercial cereals contain gluten
Condiments	
salt, pepper, sugar, herbs, and spices	none
Desserts	
homemade custard, gelatin, cornstarch, or tapioca puddings; ice cream and sherbet without gluten stabilizers; desserts prepared with allowed flours and starches	desserts prepared from wheat, rye, oats, or barley; all commercial desserts and mixes; ice cream and sherbet

Fats

butter, cream, margarine, fats, real mayonnaise; commercial salad dressings without gluten stabilizers, shortenings, vegetable oil, and lard

commercial salad dressings with gluten stabilizers

Fruit and Fruit Juices

all

Meats and Substitutes

beef, fish, lamb, pork, poultry, veal, and liver; pure all-meat cold cuts, frankfurters, and sausage; cheese, eggs, and peanut butter; all prepared meats without the addition of wheat, rye, oats, or barley

commercially prepared entrees; processed cheese and cheese products containing gluten stabilizers, meat with fillers; meat alternatives or protein substitutes that have gluten stabilizers

Potato and Substitutes

white and sweet potatoes; grits, rice, hominy, and any non-gluten products

barley, macaroni, noodles, and spahetti made from wheat; any prepared with wheat, rye, or oats

Soups

clear broth, homemade cream soups thickened with allowed flours, and allowed vegetable soups

any containing wheat, rye, oats, or barley; canned soups containing prohibited ingredients

Sweets

pure candies, honey, jams, jellies, marshmallows, sugars, syrups, molasses, and corn syrup

any containing wheat, rye, oats, or barley

Vegetables and Vegetable Juices

all

any with wheat, rye, oat, or barley such as cream sauces and bread crumbs

Miscellaneous

baking powder, baking soda, chocolate, cocoa, coconut, gravies made with allowed flours and starches, nuts, olives, vinegar, mustard, catsup, pickles

any containing wheat, rye, oats, or barley

CHAPTER 23

Egg Substitutes

WHAT TO LOOK FOR ON LABELS

Eggs may be listed on food labels as egg, egg white, albumin, ovalbumin, egg protein, globulin, powdered egg, ovomucin, ovovitellin, ovomucoid, ovalbumin, or vitellin. The following items may contain eggs. If they do, avoid them when on an egg-free diet:

whole eggs	baked goods (except most breads)
batter-fried foods	creamy fillings, puddings, custards
breakfast cereals	bouillon
cake flours	prepared frostings
French toast, waffles, etc.	hollandaise sauce
ice cream	malted cocoa drinks
egg noodles and macaroni	meat loaf and meat balls
marshmallow	mayonnaise
meringues	omelets
baking mixes of all kinds	salad dressings
sausages	sherbet
souffles	spaghetti
soups	wines (cleared with egg white)
bread or breaded foods	fritters
glazed rolls	macaroons
icings	Caesar's salads
sausages	sauces, tartar sauce

There are several ways to make up for a lack of eggs in cooking. Do not try to replace more than two eggs at a time or there will not be enough leavening. The following list suggests a variety of ways to substitute eggs:

1 Egg= 2 tablespoons flour +
1/2 teaspoon cold-pressed oil +
1/2 teaspoon (egg-free) baking powder +
2 tablespoons liquid

1 Egg =	2 tablespoons liquid + 1 tablespoon oil + 2 tablespoon baking powder
1 Egg =	1 tablespoon ground flax or psyllium seed + 3 tablespoons water. This is a good binder.
1 Egg =	2 tablespoons water + 2 teaspoons baking powder
Egg white =	1 tablespoon plain unflavored gelatin. (Dissolve gelatin in one tablespoon water. Place in freezer until thickened and beat until frothy. Chill and whip again.
1 Egg, large =	2 ounces of firm tofu for each large egg in most recipes.

You can get a good commercial egg replacer, available from Ener-G Foods, Box 24724, Seattle, Washington, 98124. It is also found in most health-food stores and contains potato starch.

ADDITIONAL HINTS

- Use Jolly Joan Egg Replacer; this contains no egg derivatives.
- Add 1 extra tablespoon of egg-free baking powder for each egg missing.
- You can use 1 package of Knox gelatin as a binder or use agar-agar.
- In baked goods use shortening instead of oil. You can beat air into it better.
- Use one mashed banana as a binder in place of one egg.
- Beat one minute extra for each egg needed. This incorporates more air to substitute for the leavening.
- Add one teaspoon vinegar (if tolerated) as leavening for each egg in a cake recipe.
- To give body and stickiness, use pureed, cooked starchy vegetables, apple or other fruit sauce, or nut butter.

CHAPTER 24

Magnesium

A long with potassium, magnesium is the major intracellular element in the cells of the body, and is required for hundreds of critical enzymatic functions within the cell. A deficiency of magnesium at the cellular membrane level can interfere with the cell's ability to take up all other nutrients. Energy production depends directly upon the availability of adequate magnesium and is essential for normal heart function. It is also a sedative and may be helpful in hyperactivity and insomnia. Magnesium is intimately associated with calcium metabolism and helps to prevent the formation of kidney stones and the development of arterial plaque, along with vitamin B6. For many women, getting sufficient magnesium is the missing link to reducing the risks of osteoporosis and arthritis and reducing the symptoms of PMS.

HOW MUCH MAGNESIUM DOES YOUR BODY NEED?

The RDA only recommends 350 milligrams per day for women of all ages. It is more likely to be about 200 milligrams more than what is in the average diet. Older adults who eat a good diet need to take between 700 and 800 milligrams of magnesium each day. Post-menopausal women may need up to 1000 milligrams of magnesium a day to strengthen their bones. If you've been taking mineral supplements that are higher in calcium than magnesium, you may want to reverse the proportions and take more magnesium than calcium.

CAN YOU TAKE TOO MUCH MAGNESIUM?

It seems unlikely that you can take too much magnesium. There have been no known cases of magnesium toxicity from taking supplements, but excessive amounts can cause chemical imbalances in the body such as inhibiting insulin release from the pancreas resulting in fatigue and depression. When tissue magnesium levels become very high, bio-unavailability occurs. This can create a peculiar combination of symptoms of both magnesium deficiency and excess.

How did this trend in magnesium deficiencies begin?

We have assumed that high quantities of nonfat dairy products such as milk and yogurt were both safe and beneficial, but it has upset the body's balance of calcium and magnesium. Dairy products contain nine times as much calcium as magnesium. The high protein content of dairy, especially when combined with other animal products, can pull calcium from the bones where it is needed. If you have been eating many dairy products, along with few or no grains and beans (that are rich in magnesium), you have probably upset your calcium and magnesium ratio even further.

The processing of grains such as whole wheat or brown rice, reduced down to bleached white flour and bleached white rice, loses most of the magnesium. The average American diet provides only 40 percent of the recommended daily amount of this mineral. If you add sugar to this depleted diet, phosphates that are high in processed foods and soft drinks, alcohol, stress, caffeine in coffee and black tea, chocolate, and a high-fat diet, then magnesium levels are reduced even more. This also includes the lowering of B-complex vitamins and essential minerals. Leading authorities estimate that 80 percent of the population is deficient in magnesium.

What are good sources of magnesium?

An increase in whole grains such as brown rice, millet, buckwheat (kasha), whole wheat, millet, triticale, quinoa, rye, and all varieties of beans will provide a magnesium-rich diet. Eat plenty of fresh green vegetables, too. Fresh produce will provide your body with calcium and magnesium as well as other important nutrients. Feature greater amounts of tofu (soybean curd) and seafoods, because these foods contain high levels of magnesium. Reduce refined sugar and alcohol in the diet to prevent excessive magnesium from being excreted in the urine.

What symptoms are common with a magnesium deficiency?

A cardiologist may consider it of little importance that his patient with arrhythmia also sees an orthopedist for chronic lumbosacral pain. No attention is paid to the patient's history of irritable bowel syndrome, depression, and fatigue. All of these are common magnesium deficiency symptoms. Making connections between symptoms that cross specialty lines is important. For example, you can have eye-muscle twitches or leg cramps, chronic back problems, cardiac arrhythmia or palpitations, and chemical sensitivities because of a single magnesium deficiency. There is more evidence that a magnesium deficiency is a frequent cause of cardiac arrhythmias resulting in arterial spasms, hypertension, and heart attacks.

An American diet does not provide the daily requirement for magnesium. The *Journal of the American Medical Association* showed that in over one thousand patients hospitalized for heart problems, 90 percent of the doctors did not think of checking for a magnesium deficiency. Eighty percent of doctors are now telling men over 40 to take aspirin to keep from having a heart attack, but no mention is made of how increasing magnesium intake could reduce heart attack deaths.

A child that is ticklish, sensitive, impulsive, and excitable can be low in calcium and magnesium, especially magnesium. Rhythmical activities like thumb sucking, bed rocking, hair twisting, and foot jiggling usually indicate low levels of calcium and magnesium. More stress increases these activities. These children are restless, squirmy, disturb others, and fail to finish tasks. They tend to be more restless in a crowd or the classroom, but less trouble on a one-to-one basis.

What Does Chocolate Do to the Body?

The metabolizing of chocolate in the body creates the neurotransmitter phenylalanine. This can lead to mood problems such as depression, lethargy, and anxiety. As a result of this neurochemical imbalance, there can be strong cravings for chocolate. Chocolate cravings may also be an indication that there is a calcium or magnesium imbalance. Cocoa powder contains more magnesium than any other food. This means that a person can be a "chocoholic" because the body needs more magnesium. Don't rush out and stock up on candy bars and other chocolate-containing foods to get more magnesium, because this will only create more imbalance.

Chocolate contains an excessive amount of sugar, which leeches calcium out of the bones, ultimately leading to a greater imablance of calcium and magnesium. The solution may be to take a calcium and magnesium supplement that is two parts calcium to one part magnesium. If this doesn't work, then try a different combination. There may be a need to further increase the magnesium and decrease the calcium. When you find the correct balance between these two minerals, chocolate cravings usually disappear.

Sensitivity to chocolate is very common. It is necessary to eliminate any food or drink containing chocolate or cocoa for at least two weeks. Then return chocolate to the diet and eat it several times to see if the symptoms appear. If any form of chocolate causes symptoms, eliminate it from the diet again for at least two months, then introduce it back into the diet only occasionally.

Carob is a good substitute for chocolate and is available at most health-food stores. It comes from the fruit pod of a Middle Eastern locust tree. Carob contains no caffeine, is naturally sweet, is available in powdered form, and can substitute for cocoa. Watch out for carob chips because they may contain sugar or some other ingredient you are trying to avoid.

Carob has less than half the calories, one-hundredth the amount of fat, and two and one-half times the amount of calcium as contained in chocolate. It does not interfere with the assimilation of calcium as does chocolate and cocoa. You might notice a slight raw taste that will disappear by mixing it with hot water or when heated briefly in a double-boiler. It dissolves better in oil then in water. The following list contains foods that commonly contain chocolate or cocoa:

- Candy, cake, cookies, pie, and ice cream
- Hershey's and other chocolate flavorings
- Chocolate-covered nuts
- All "cola" drinks, including low-calorie colas, often contain chocolate derivatives
- Chocolate that is colored-coated
- Doritos taco chips have cocoa added

CHAPTER 25

Fruits, Meats, Salt, and Hard-to-Digest Foods

Some of the following foods may need to be avoided if you are found sensitive to them or they cause digestion problems. It may be important to know what indicates fruit, meat, salt, and foods that are hard to digest.

FRUITS

Apple	Citric acid	Grapes/raisins	Papaya
Apricot	Citrus fruit (all)	Kiwi	Peach
Avocado	Coconut	Mango	Pears
Banana	Cranberries	Olives	Pineapple
Berries (all)	Dates	Palm oil	Tomato
Cherry			

Also consider products made from fruit such as wine, wine vinegar, apple cider vinegar, fruit liquors, and all oils, barks, and peels from these foods. This includes any food cooked with or flavored with fruit or fruit extracts. Almost all canned tomato products contain citric acid, derived from fruit. Read labels. You can find products without citric acid, or make your own. The following foods are not classified as fruits, but as melons:

Cantaloupe	Crenshaw	Honeydew	Rhubarb
Casaba	Ground cherry	Muskmelon	Watermelon

MEATS

Meats include beef, pork, mutton, chicken, and turkey. They include meat products and by-products including lard, some solid shortenings and margarines, soups made from meat stock, gravies, gelatin, Jell-O, gelatin capsules, marshmallows, some ice creams, and soups with meat stock or bouillon. Fish and other seafoods are not classified as meat.

SALT

Ordinary table salt is inorganic mined salt and nearly all prepared foods contain it. Many people do not tolerate mined salt well. Ocean salt or sea salt is an organic compound and does not share the same intolerance characteristics. Buy products containing sea salt at your health-food store and carry your own salt shaker when you eat out. It is best to get pure, unprocessed sea salt. It is gray or pink in color and contains a multitude of valuable minerals and trace elements. Read labels and use only products that specify sea salt. If you must buy products with ordinary table salt, try to reduce the amount when possible. It is usually better to reduce your intake of salt, no matter what kind it is.

Hard-To-Digest Foods

Chocolate, oatmeal, bananas, nuts, peanut butter, pork, lunch meats, oils, fats, salmon, halibut, hard-cooked eggs, oysters, shrimp, lobster, crab, shellfish, organ meats, processed cheese, little white navy beans, corn on the cob, canned corn, turnips, parsnips, onions, cooked cabbage, cucumbers, head lettuce, radishes, cherries, out-of-season melons, pickles, and strong spices. Rhubarb and tomatoes often aggravate symptoms. The body has a difficult time digesting fried, barbecued, pasteurized, dried, and other over-processed and over-cooked foods that you find in cake mixes, dried milk, dried eggs, pizza mixes, dairy products and other boxed and processed foods.

CHAPTER 26

Mucus-Forming Foods

Excess mucus production can affect many areas of the body. Any factor that irritates or inflames the mucous membranes will stimulate excess mucus secretion. An imbalance in the digestive system is a common cause for such excess. When digestive organs become irritated or inflamed, proper digestion is impossible and a mucus condition will develop. Some conditions that result are headaches, postnasal drip, sinusitis, digestive disorders, ear infections, gallbladder disease, and recurrent colds.

Sugar is especially good at making excessive mucus in the body. As a test, take a spoonful of sugar at bedtime and note how you have a full throat of phlegm in the morning. Salt and dairy products are also a major cause of mucus. A lack of exercise and poor circulation will further contribute to the body's congestion, leading to more irritation and more mucus formation.

There are other causes of excess mucus. The most frequently seen problem is an extremely unbalanced diet. The excessive consumption of even the best unrefined whole-wheat bread will produce too much mucus. The situation will be worse if you add refined white flour and sugar. Not eating an abundance of vegetables can also create a mucus-forming and acidic condition, or if the diet consists mostly of starches. Toxic chemicals, pesticides, and hormones add to the burden.

MUCUS PRODUCERS

Refined foods	Lack of exercise
Very hot or very cold foods	Alcohol, black tea, coffee
Very spicy foods	Additives
Sweets	Dairy products
Oily foods	Excess salt
Known allergy-causing foods	Excess saturated fats
Fried foods	Green vegetable deficiency
Poor food combinations	Poor elimination
Excess acidic foods	Digestive enzyme deficiency
Inhalant irritants(fumes, cleaners, etc.)	

Any allergy or food sensitivity can result in excess mucus production. The most common food allergens are wheat, dairy products, sugar, and eggs, but any food may present a problem. It would be wise to eliminate the foods most frequently associated with excess mucus production. Also exclude from the diet all refined carbohydrates such as sugar, alcohol, coffee, tea (except herbal without caffeine), pepper, strong spices, junk foods, and tobacco. It is best to keep dietary fats to a minimum.

To avoid excess mucus, it is necessary to increase vegetables and fruit in the diet. Citrus fruit juices such as grapefruit and lemon are useful in some mucus conditions if they are not too concentrated. They help to break up congestion. In some conditions, such as bladder infections or acute stomach problems, citrus can be very irritating. Apple juice seems to be more gentle on the stomach and usually does not cause any problems. Vegetable juice, onions, and odorless garlic capsules are very useful mucus solvents, as well as strawberries, blackberries, raspberries, cranberries, and all other berries. Pineapple, if not excessively sweet, is a good mucus solvent and so are whole oranges, grapefruits, lemons, cherries, and tomatoes. Avoid vegetable fats such as coconuts or avocados and increase consumption of raw vegetables, kelp, and brown rice.

There have never been such large quantities of polyunsaturated fats in the diet. There have also never been such high incidents of mucus-laden conditions such as asthma, inner ear infections, postnasal drip, sinusitis, etc. The two trends may be linked by more than coincidence. A research team from the University of California at Davis claims that high levels of commonly consumed vegetable oils might increase the severity of asthma. One consequence of eating a diet high in certain polyunsaturated oils, (found in corn oil, mayonnaise, and many packaged foods), may be the increased production of compounds that make mucus secretion worse. Not all oils pose the same danger. Those of the omega-3 fatty acid variety found in fatty fish and flax oil may reduce the risk. At least with asthmatics, it may be best to increase the monounsaturates such as those found in olive and canola oils, as well as fish intake, especially salmon, mackerel, and cod.

An improvement in mucus production results if there is an avoidance of mucus-forming foods such as dairy, wheat, and sugar products for at least two months. There also needs to be a diet free of food sensitivities, the increase of foods and liquids that decrease mucus in the body, and a balance of acid and alkaline foods in the diet. Other considerations are using exercise, nutritional supplements, and botanical remedies to further increase the general health of the individual. It is also important to establish and maintain proper bowel function.

CHAPTER 27

The Harmful Effects of Caffeine

Caffeine has become a common component of the Western diet and has substantial and harmful effects. What does coffee do for you? It's a "pick-me-up." In response to the caffeine, the liver will increase the secretion of glucose or blood sugar. This gives you energy and increased alertness, shortens reaction time, and increases capacity for attention-requiring tasks. However, within one hour the drug absorbs into the digestive tract and reaches its peak levels. It then passes to the central nervous system and various tissues. With increasing doses of caffeine, the mental effects become negative. Nervousness, restlessness and insomnia commonly occur. Even in relatively small doses, sensitive individuals will experience these negative symptoms.

The most commonly consumed caffeine beverages outside the home are soft drinks and coffee. It is difficult today to get away from coffee with all the coffee shops, coffee breaks, and coffee advertising that surrounds us. Most people know how many alcoholic drinks they have each day, but coffee drinkers usually don't keep track. Coffee contains caffeine, but so does cola, decafs, black tea, chocolate, cocoa, and many prescriptions and non-prescription drugs. Several so-called "weight loss" medications contain high levels of caffeine.

Too many people are not even aware of the effect coffee has on them. It is a powerful stimulant that temporarily provides a feeling of energy and alertness, but at a cost to your health. It stimulates the adrenal glands and keeps the body in a perpetual state of arousal. Common side effects of this over stimulation include anxiety, insomnia and nervousness. It also depletes the body of the essential nutrients: potassium, magnesium, calcium, and the B-complex vitamins. With caffeine you are also depleting the body of the nutrients that maintain a stable mood and good energy levels.

The medical profession uses caffeine as a stimulant and diuretic. A therapeutic dosage is 250 milligrams. That is the equivalent of two cups of coffee or four cola drinks. Medication such as antacids, cold remedies, and pain relievers often contain caffeine. It can act as a stimulant for the central nervous system or heart, and as a relaxant for bronchial muscles. Twelve or more cups a day can lead to "caffeinism." Habitual drinkers can exhibit withdrawal symptoms such as fatigue, headaches, and irritability.

Roasted and ground coffee contains about 85-150 milligrams of caffeine in a five-ounce cup. Instant coffee has about 60 milligrams and some decaffeinated coffees contain 15 milligrams per cup. By comparison there are 30-70 milligrams in a cup of tea, cocoa can have as many as 42 milligrams, cola drinks 35-70 milligrams in a twelve-ounce can or bottle, and a regular chocolate bar has 20-25 milligrams. Other products high in caffeine are two tablets of No-Doz with 200 milligrams and two tablets of Excedrin at 130 milligrams. Espresso doesn't contain less caffeine than other types of coffee. A five-ounce cup of espresso could contain a whopping 200 to 250 milligrams.

The method of preparation of your coffee also matters. Percolated coffee (including espresso) generally has a little less caffeine than drip coffee. A two-ounce cup of espresso and a five-ounce cup of regular percolated coffee contain about 80 to 100 milligrams of caffeine. A five-ounce drip cup contains 100 to 150 milligrams. Decaffeinated is not the same as caffeine-free. Brewed decaffeinated coffee usually contains one to five milligrams of caffeine per cup. Even this much can keep some people going.

Coffee may seem to increase energy, but it probably works best if you're bored or experiencing fatigue. It increases alertness and enhances performance on various tasks, but it helps performance levels that are already low. Different personalities have different experiences with coffee. It seems to help extroverts stay attentive more than it helps introverts with the same tasks. Caffeine can also cause the following problems:

1. Caffeine stimulates acid secretion in the stomach. Two small cups of coffee provoke an increase in hydrochloric acid. This effect can last for more than an hour. If there is a digestive ulcer present, then the effect can be greater and last for more than two hours. Caffeine can add to the cause of an ulcer, irritate any existing ulcer, and interfere with healing.
2. Caffeols, the volatile oils that give coffee its characteristic flavor and aroma, irritate the lining of the stomach and digestive tract. It is possible to induce digestive problems by having caffeols.
3. More than five cups of coffee a day increases the risk of stomach cancer.
4. It hasn't been decided if caffeine is addictive or not. It does fit several standards of drug addiction such as compulsion to continue use, and symptoms when the substance is withdrawn. Coffee drinkers, deprived

of their favorite beverage, usually suffer from irritability, in........, work well, restlessness, fatigue, headaches, sluggishness, and depression until the caffeine withdrawal passes.

5. Psychological problems are beginning to surface called "caffeinism." Several mental hospitals, including Walter Reed Medical Center, have noted psychiatric symptoms such as anxiety neurosis. This can include insomnia, headaches, agitation, and restlessness. The symptoms resolve with the elimination of caffeine.

6. Studies have proven that caffeine will interfere with the repair of DNA, the building blocks of the body.

7. Caffeine crosses the placenta and affects unborn children. A newborn infant does not have developed enzymes for the detoxification of caffeine. This could cause injury to the baby.

8. There is an increase risk of bladder cancer with four or more cups of coffee per day.

9. It raises blood pressure, increases heart rate, and can cause cardiac arrhythmia.

10. Caffeine increases blood coagulation thus increasing the risk of blood clots. It lowers the levels of a special enzyme (tissue lipase) that removes fats from the blood.

11. Caffeine impairs motor coordination, but increases mental speed. The improved mental efficiency will drop to below normal from one to three hours after drinking coffee.

12. Caffeine aggravates hypoglycemia (low blood sugar) and diabetes. Just two cups of coffee significantly raise blood sugar. There are more people with unstable blood sugars among coffee drinkers, because even very small quantities of caffeine improperly stimulate the pancreas. A study suggested that after the ingestion of caffeine individuals experienced a higher incident of hypoglycemic symptoms, such as trembling, sweating, and palpitations. Many people experience blood-sugar symptoms, but still have normal glucose tolerance tests. When they discontinue refined sugar, caffeine, and alcohol, their symptoms improve. This is why glucose tolerance tests are not necessarily reliable for diagnosing "reactive hypoglycemia."

13. Caffeine aggravates coronary heart disease by interfering with fatty acid and glucose balance in the blood. Heart attack risk is 60 percent higher with one to five cups of coffee daily than if you drink none. With six or more cups each day the risk is even 20 percent higher.

14. With the addition of caffeine to the diet, experimental animals voluntarily drank two to four times more alcohol than those who did not drink coffee.

15. Caffeine is a stimulant to the central nervous system. It prolongs the electrical messages transmitted by nerve cells and stimulates the higher center of the brain. The amount of caffeine in a cup of coffee will make a person seem to feel more alert. According to scientific experiments a person also experiences more confusion and nervousness. Excessive caffeine can also cause irritability and irregular heart beats. Chocolate and cocoa contain theobromine, which can cause a strong cardiac stimulation and an increased flow of urine.

16. Boiled coffee elevates blood cholesterol levels. When researchers prepare coffee by the drip method, using double filter paper, it did not cause a cholesterol elevation. This suggests that the villain is not caffeine in this case, but some other substance that is filtered out of the coffee. Other ingredients in coffee are trigonelline, chlorogenic acid, tannin, caffeic acid, and quinic acid. There are also volatile acids such as acetoin, ketones, furfural and acidic carbonyl compounds present.

17. Caffeine can deplete the body of a number of essential minerals, including calcium and potassium. It seems that moderate amounts of caffeine (400 milligrams per day) had no significant affect on these minerals, but produced a slight change in bone remodeling and rebuilding. Women who drink a cup or more of coffee a day did have lower bone density after they reached menopause according to researchers at the University of California, San Diego. A study from Tufts University found that consumption of caffeine in amounts equal or greater than two to three servings of brewed coffee per day appear to accelerate bone loss from the spine and the total body in women with low calcium intakes. A moderate intake of caffeine can increase the excretion of potassium resulting in a deficiency, especially if the individual does not consume adequate dietary potassium.

18. The more caffeine a woman consumes the greater her risk of having fibrocystic breast disease. This problem is higher in women who drink four or more cups of coffee a day or the caffeine equivalent.

19. Increasing the intake of caffeine during pregnancy can increase the risk of spontaneous abortion. For each 100 milligrams of caffeine ingested daily, the risk increased by approximately 22 percent. The National Institutes of Health announced in 1993 that miscarriage was strongly linked to a woman's caffeine intake during pregnancy. This study reported that even the caffeine in a cup and a half of coffee could double the risk of miscarriage in the first trimester. It could also increase the risk of gestational diabetes, pregnancy hypertension, leg cramps, and other common pregnancy complications.

The Food and Drug Administration (FDA) and the Center for Science in the Public Interest stands by their long-time recommendation that pregnant women avoid or greatly limit their intake of caffeine. It does pass through the placenta to the fetus. Caffeine is structurally similar to DNA and can produce chromosomal aberrations in mammals. In addition, there is evidence that caffeine interferes with fetal growth.

20. Actual studies on high-intensity performance activities indicate that caffeine has little or no effect, but does seem to enhance endurance performance.

21. Women who drink caffeinated beverages (coffee, tea, cola) took significantly longer to conceive, as reported in a recent study published in the British medical journal, *Lancet.* Women drinking more than one cup of coffee a day are half as likely to conceive during each cycle as those who drink less than one cup a day.

22. There is a clear link between moderate intake of caffeine and PMS.

23. The effects of black tea are similar to coffee. It contains caffeine, caffeols, tannic acid, and theophylline. A strong brew of tannic acid retards the digestion process. Theophylline is often worse than caffeine in releasing fats and sugar into the bloodstream.

24. Both black tea and coffee seem to interfere with the absorption of "non-heme" iron.

25. Caffeine acts as both a diuretic and a laxative.

26. Do not rely on caffeine as a diet aid. It does speed up the metabolism, but only for a short time.

27. Methylene chloride is the chemical solvent used in the process by which coffee is decaffeinated. Supposedly, methylene chloride is safe in the small amounts left in a cup of decaf. It has been said that there is no more methylene chloride in decaf than the equivalent found in the air of many large cities. That is really a comforting thought! The process used to make water process decaf may strip most of the flavoring compounds out of the coffee, but at least it contains no methylene chloride. No matter how safe it appears to be, it may be better not to take the chance.

28. The most commonly used coffee filters contain chlorine. It would be better to use brown unbleached paper filters, oxygen bleached white filters, unbleached cotton filters, or a reusable gold-plated mesh basket. Devices exist that do not even use filters.

29. The cheaper the coffee the more caffeine it may contain. Truck-stop-style coffee can have up to 25 percent more caffeine than a similar cup of designer coffee. The cheaper robusta beans contain more caffeine than the more expensive Arabica beans sold at specialty stores.

30. Coffee may antidote homeopathic medicines.
31. The caffeine habit is hard to kick. Habitual drinkers can exhibit withdrawal symptoms such as fatigue, headaches, and irritability, and a case of the blahs bad enough to look like depression. Caffeine withdrawal is a real problem and may be one thing that insures its intake. It is best to eliminate caffeine gradually over a period of a few days. Withdrawal is no fun, but after a couple of days your symptoms will disappear.

What does all this mean for sufferers of allergies? As you can tell, caffeine can affect the body in a myriad of ways, including the manifestations of allergic-type symptoms. Caffeine ranks in the top ten of allergy-causing substances.

CHAPTER 28

Sugar

It used to be only the rich who could afford the luxury of sugar, but by 1840 the sugar pushers were handing out free samples. Today, the American sugar industry has the largest advertising in the world, essentially making us a land of "sugarholics." The most common sugar, sucrose, is the white sugar used at the table. The average American consumes more than 25 percent of their calories as sugars, with an annual consumption of over 113 pounds per person. This only refers to the consumption of refined cane and beet sugar. It does not reflect the increasing impact of a variety of other sweeteners, especially high fructose corn syrup.

The beverage industry—producers of beer, wine, and soft drinks—uses more sugar than anyone, including the candy industry. These companies consume over 26 percent of refined cane and beet-derived sucrose and about 40 percent of corn syrups used in the food industry. The bakery and cereal industries use about 13 percent of the sugar produced for food purposes.

Is Sugar Addictive?

Sugar is one of the most destructive and punishing food items in our diet. It acts very similar to a drug when eaten in large amounts or consumed daily. Sugar can easily cause allergic responses and decrease the ability of the immune system to function properly. If you need a sweetener, it is healthier to use molasses, pure maple syrup, rice syrup, honey, sucanat, date sugar, sorghum, or stevia.

Those who attempt to quit the sugar habit find they have quite a struggle on their hands. Sugar, like alcohol, is intoxicating. It creates an imbalance of neurotransmitters in the brain. Going off sugar invites withdrawal symptoms with the most common ones being headaches, chills, and body aches. Sugar-addicted individuals often have a family history of alcoholism, diabetes, or both.

Sugar and Behavior

Studies have shown that destructive, aggressive, and restless behavior significantly increases with the amount of sugar consumed. Refined carbohydrates also appear to be the major factor in promoting unstable blood sugars. If every person experiencing hyperactivity, attention deficit disorder, or related behavior and learning problems tried a food elimination diet, the health of most of them would greatly improve.

Researchers at the New York Institute of Child Development suspected that sugar might be a complication in the treatment of hyperactivity in children. They studied the blood sugar metabolism of 265 children and found that 74 percent did not have the ability to properly digest and assimilate sugar and other refined carbohydrates. When these children were put on a corrective diet that promoted a more stable blood sugar, after only two to three weeks they were no longer hyperactive.

Sugar may not be the only culprit of hyperactivity. Also involved may be the carbohydrate to protein ratio. By increasing the protein intake, the needed amino acids produce neurotransmitters like serotonin, which ultimately has a calming effect. Hyperactive children usually have lower than normal levels of serotonin in the blood.

Too Much Sugar—Detrimental to Good Health

When you eat a candy bar, a piece of cake, cookies, or anything containing highly refined sugar, there is a rush of energy as the sugar enters the bloodstream. This energy is short-lived; in twenty minutes or so, you will probably feel sluggish, tired, cranky, or even mildly depressed. Candy bar ads promise quick energy, and energy is precisely what sugar provides— pure, unadulterated calories. But it doesn't provide vitamins, minerals, or fiber. Empty sugar calories can easily crowd out nutritious foods. If you sip sodas and eat candy but skip on meals, you are opening the door to poor health. Blood sugar imbalances and diabetes often appear after years of sugar abuse. Side effects resulting from sugar consumption may include:

- malabsorption of protein, calcium, and other minerals
- retarded growth of valuable intestinal bacteria
- injury to the pancreas so that it does not provide the proper digestive juices and insulin to the body
- a decrease in the ability to concentrate and an increase in mood swings
- unstable blood sugar levels
- a decrease in the immune system function

Symptoms of Sugar Sensitivity

Many children are highly sensitive to sugar and most of the sweets in their diet. This is because most children are fast metabolizers. They burn their foods at a faster than normal adult rate. When there is the combination of a fast metabolism and excessive sugar intake, the result can be behavior that is bizarre, antisocial, or even destructive. A high-sugar diet can aggravate other problems, including hyperactivity, anxiety, poor concentration, nervousness, and irritability. If children get aggressive just before lunch, three to four hours after a breakfast of sweet rolls and juice, there may be a blood sugar problem. Some children get headaches after this type of breakfast, others get stomachaches, and still others become hyperactive.

Where Does Sugar Hide?

Many foods contain hidden sugar largely as the result of industrial practices that are unfamiliar to the public. A common practice is to feed sugar to animals before slaughter to improve the color and flavor of the meat. The preparation of meat in packing houses and restaurants often involves the addition of sugar. This added sugar is not required to be listed on any label.

Products advertised as "reduced fat," "low fat," or "fat free" usually have increased sugar in them. When food processors reduce the amount of fat, the taste and texture are also reduced. Hamburger meat may have corn syrup added to reduce shrinkage and improve color, flavor, and juiciness. French fries usually have a sugar coating that turns brown when immersed in hot grease. The batters on fried foods contain some sugar, often sucrose or corn sweeteners. Manufacturers hide sugar in hot dogs and salad dressings, nondairy creamers, frozen pizzas, and peanut butter. There are hundreds of these "standardized" type foods that may contain sugar without any declaration on the label. These also include canned vegetables, vanilla extract, baby foods, and even iodized salt. Some foods are even required to have sugar in them by the FDA. For instance, catsup cannot be called catsup if it does not contain sugar.

The first ingredient on a food label is the most plentiful ingredient in the product, the second item listed is second most plentiful, and so on. When food processors found out that consumers were becoming aware of the dangers from sugar, they substituted three or four different types of other sugars so that the word "sugar" would not appear on the label, or would not appear as the first ingredient. For example, a breakfast cereal now contains oats, brown sugar, corn syrup, malted barley, malt syrup, honey, and dextrose. Count it up—that is six different kinds of sugar. Add them together and they would easily be the most plentiful ingredient in that box of cereal.

It is important to read labels because so much sugar is hidden in products such as ketchup, salad dressings, canned soups, peanut butter, luncheon meats and canned and frozen vegetables. It comes in many names and in many forms. Avoid foods containing corn syrup and any ingredients that ends in "ose." Even fructose is usually not derived from fruit, but from corn syrup. Fructose that is derived from fruit still puts a strain on the liver and elevates the bad cholesterol.

Over 50 percent of the sugar the average American consumes every year is from hidden sources. Partly as a result of this, junk food junkies develop large appetites for salt and sugar and then crave and eat more salt and sugar. The best way to avoid problems and cravings associated with sugar is to eat foods that are fresh and not packaged, canned, bottled, treated, or sweetened.

Is One Type Of Sugar Better than Another?

Don't let yourself be fooled by sugar or its many aliases. Sugar, whether cane sugar, beet sugar, or corn sugar, is completely refined and has no nutritional value except for providing empty calories. Sugar in any form is readily absorbed into the bloodstream and provides quick energy to the cells. Sucrose, fructose, dextrose—the body just converts them all to glucose. Glucose circulates in the bloodstream as fuel or is stored in the liver and muscles or elsewhere as fat.

Fruit juices are not necessary healthy for the diet—even the unsweetened juices. They are often high in natural concentrated sugar, and can have the same harmful effects as candy or other sweets. "Sweetened with fruit juice" sounds like a good thing, but what it really means is that the product is sweetened with juice that is refined down to practically pure sugar. Diets high in juice intake can contribute to a large part of a child's daily calories. The juice replaces other more nutritious foods and leads to a reduction in healthy protein, fat, vitamins and minerals.

How Does Sugar Affect the Body?

To digest simple carbohydrates such as sugar, the body requires additional vitamins and minerals, especially the B vitamins and minerals, but eating refined sugar depletes these nutrient reserves. Without B vitamins, carbohydrate consumption cannot take place. When sugar and other carbohydrates do not break down properly, they ferment in the body adding more of a toxic burden to the body. The body has to rob its reserves to obtain needed nutrients. As the reserves continue to be depleted, it is harder for the body to fend off disease.

Diets that are high in sugar increase urinary chromium losses as much as 300 percent. A lack of necessary chromium will manifest itself in a sugar craving. This mineral is necessary to maintain a healthy blood sugar level and contributes to the proper use of carbohydrates and fats. The more sugar eaten, the more chromium the body loses, which makes the body crave more sugar, and so on.

A deficiency of protein may also contribute to sweet cravings. It is critical to consume adequate protein, oils and fats. Otherwise, there will be hunger and more sweet cravings. Children deprived of foods such as eggs, avocado, nuts, seeds, and protein-rich foods often crave and eat more sugar, leading to sugar addiction.

Pediatric researchers at Yale University School of Medicine found that sugar causes a noticeable physiological reaction in normal healthy children. Twenty-five children and twenty-three young adults were given the sugar equivalent of two twelve-ounce cans of cola on an empty stomach while resting in bed. The blood sugar levels fell significantly further in the children than in the adults. The children's adrenaline levels rose twice as high as the adults and remained elevated during the five hours of scientific observation. The body releases adrenaline to counteract the effect of too much insulin and the resulting low blood sugar. The children's brain waves also showed that the ability to pay attention was affected ("Kids Really Do Get a Sugar Buzz," by Jane Brody, *The Seattle Post-Intelligencer,* March 15, 1995).

Complex carbohydrate-based sweeteners, such as organic brown rice syrup and barley malt, are less stimulating than refined sugar. Natural sweeteners, such as real maple syrup and molasses, don't seem to cause the overwhelming cravings that white refined sugar produces. Two herbal sweeteners that really work well are stevia and licorice. Natural sweeteners also tend to be much less sweet than refined sugars, reducing the likelihood of a sweet-habit developing. Even natural sweets are best consumed sparingly. Remember that any sweet is a concentrated source of sugar. Control your food instead of letting it control you. For more information on the effects of sugar and their relationship to blood sugar levels, complex carbohydrates and overall digestion/health, see the chapter on hypoglycemia.

Types of Sugars

Below is a list of other commonly used sugars. They are names you are likely to discover on the labels of processed supermarket foods.

• Aspartame is found in both the products NutraSweet and Equal. It is one of the most successful synthetic chemicals ever produced. The dominant producer is the NutraSweet Corporation, a subsidiary of Monsanto. Recently published estimates suggested that world sales amounted to approximately $1 billion in 1995. This chemical contains phenylalanine (50 percent), aspartic acid (40 percent), and methyl alcohol (10 percent).

Aspartame was originally synthesized as a possible antigastrin drug for treating peptic ulcers. Today, it is found in more than 4000 products. It is an artificial sweetener about 200 times sweeter than sucrose (table sugar) and intensifies the taste of other flavors and sweeteners. Large amounts consumed over time can upset the amino acid and neurotransmitter balance in the body. It also disturbs hormonal homeostasis.

In February of 1994, the U.S. Department of Health and Human Services released the listing of adverse reactions reported to the FDA with aspartame accounting for more than 75 percent of all adverse reactions reported. Many reactions were very serious including seizures. Other reactions reported included: headaches and migraines, nausea, dizziness, disorientation, severe anxiety, hyperactivity, personality changes, sleepiness, insomnia, numbness, atypical facial pain, breathing difficulties, tinnitus, vertigo, irritability, vision loss, severe depression, slurred speech, convulsions, memory loss, confusion, and other neurological disorders.

These adverse reaction reports detail well over 10,000 complains of 92 different symptoms, and most of them central nervous system related. Many other people may have had reactions, but did not report them to anyone. In a study that appeared in the *Journal of Applied Nutrition*, 1988, people who reported reactions to aspartame were surveyed. The following is an additional list of adverse health effects that were found: decreased vision and/or other eye problems, decreased tears, trouble with contact lens, blindness, hearing loss, unsteady gait, tremors, restless legs, chest pains, abdominal pain, pain on swallowing, severe itching, hives, thinning or loss of hair, frequency of urination, excessive thirst, joint pains, bloating and fluid retention.

Many people with low blood sugar are adversely affected by these sugar-free products. There have been cases of severe reactive hypoglycemia (low blood sugar), particularly during the night. Aspartame can make hypoglycemia worse, especially because of the severe caloric restriction and the increased release of insulin. With the use of NutraSweet, some diabetic patients had increased symptoms of memory loss, confusion and severe vision loss. When NutraSweet was eliminated from their diet, vision and memory returned, and blood sugar levels were controlled. According to researchers and physicians studying the adverse effects of aspartame, the following list contains a selection of chronic illnesses that may be triggered or worsened by ingesting aspartame: brain tumors, multiple sclerosis, epilepsy, chronic fatigue syndrome, Parkinson's disease, Alzheimer's, mental retardation, birth deficits, fibromyalgia, and diabetes.

The U.S. Air Force's magazine, *Flying Safety*, and the U.S. Navy's magazine, *Navy Physiology*, published articles warning about the many dangers of aspartame, including the cumulative adverse effects. The articles noted that the ingestion of aspartame may make pilots more susceptible to seizures and vertigo. Nearly 1,000 pilots reported symptoms including some who reported suffering grand mal seizures in the cockpit due to aspartame. The dangers of tunnel vision, blurred vision, seizures, vertigo and other serious adverse reactions are so great that articles and letters warning about aspartame have appeared in many aviation-related journals including *The Aviation Consumer* (1988), *Aviation Medical Bulletin* (1988), *Pacific Flyer* (1988) *National Business Aircraft Association Digest* (1993), and *Plane & Pilot* (1995).

In 1996, Mary Nash Stoddard, founder of the Aspartame Consumer Safety Network, gave a press conference about the connection between aspartame and brain tumors. The *Journal of Neuropathology and Experimental Neurology* (1996) reveals a study by Dr. John Olney about the association of increasing brain tumor rates and the link to aspartame. Dr. Russell Blaylock, professor of Neurosurgery at the Medical University of Mississippi, has researched the damage that is caused by the ingestion of excessive aspartic acid (aspartame) in the food supply causing serious chronic neurological disorders and other acute symptoms.

Aspartame also affects people with hypothyroidism because they often cannot metabolize chemicals and drugs. Since abnormal thyroid function is often unrecognized, symptoms due to aspartame may also go unrecognized. There has also been an increase in Graves' disease (hyperthyroidism) while consuming aspartame products. The factors leading up to this condition are usually a voluntary severe caloric restriction, increased energy demands relating to excessive exercise and other physical activity, and metabolic derangements caused by aspartame and its metabolites. Symptoms usually improve within weeks after avoiding aspartame.

Often the people and associations that give us information on aspartame are funded by the companies that produce aspartame. It is like putting the fox in charge of the hen house. The American Dietetics and American Diabetic Association get funding from NutraSweet. These organizations tell physicians how safe it is, so doctors are often unaware of the dangers.

• Acesulfame potassium (Sweet & Safe) is a sugar-free, low calorie sweetener without a chemical after taste. There have been over 90 clinical studies to support the safety of this product and it has been approved by the FDA. This product does not contain either aspartame (NutraSweet) or saccharin. It is based on a stable potassium compound that has been used successfully in Europe as a sweetener for over ten years without any side effects reported. The diet soft drinks, candy, and sugar-free chewing gum in Europe currently utilize this ingredient.

• Brown sugar is the result of processed molasses. Brown sugar is mostly sucrose and is often more refined than white sugar.

• Corn dextrin is a white or yellow powder obtained by enzymatic action of barley malt or corn flour. Milk and milk products often contain corn dextrin as a modifier or thickening agent.

• Corn sweeteners include various forms of corn, such as high fructose, dextrose, corn syrups, sorbitol, and mannitol (usually made from dextrose). The use of corn sweeteners is increasing—an average individual will eat more than eighteen pounds per year. More than half the cornstarch processed in this country is used to produce corn sweeteners. Corn-derived sugars are very common allergic substances.

• Corn syrups are highly allergic foods and addictive to many people. They can be in maple, nut, and root beer flavorings, and are found in ice cream, candy, and baked goods. Envelope, stamp, and sticker glues contain corn syrup. It is also found in ale, aspirin, bacon, baking mixes, beer, breads, breakfast cereals, catsup, cheeses, chop suey, chow mein, fish products, ginger ale, ham, jellies, processed meats, peanut butter, canned peas, and plastic food wrap.

• Dextrose (corn sugar) is often blended with white sugar. Many artificial sweeteners contain dextrose.

• Fructose occurs naturally in many fruits, vegetables, berries, and honey. It is considerably sweeter than sucrose (table sugar). The fructose commonly found in grocery store foods usually comes from cane or beet sugar, not from fruits. It can be very difficult to identify the source of fructose in a food item because of the confusion between fructose derived from fruit, or fructose made from high-fructose corn syrups. Fructose does not seem to cause the changes in blood sugar that other types of sugars do. Remember, fructose derived from fruit sugar is still a highly processed sugar, and it does contain calories.

- Glucose is a commercially processed sugar derived from cornstarch. There may be confusion with this name because the body's blood sugar is also referred to as glucose. The main problem with glucose is its low sweetness level. You could eat a large quantity without being aware of its presence in a food. Ground-meat dishes and luncheon meats often contain glucose, as well as some maple syrups. Confectioners generally use glucose in candy making for several reasons. It gives the hard-boiled candies a clear appearance and costs only half the price of cane sugar.

- Honey is commonly adulterated with corn syrup or other sugars. To get any nutrition out of refined honey you would have to eat an enormous quantity. There may be contaminants in honey, such as traces of sulfa drugs and antibiotics used to control bee diseases. Labels citing the source of the honey may not be accurate since bees often visit other plants in the area besides the ones listed on the bottle. A bottle of honey may contain several different blended honeys. Only unrefined raw honey is a nutritive food. This type of honey is getting harder and harder to find. Health-food stores are the best sources for finding this unrefined liquid gold rich with suspended bee pollen.

- Malt is sprouted grain, usually derived from barley, or from the hydrolyzed starch of other grains. It forms a thick sweet syrup that is added to foods to improve taste. Barley contains a protein similar in properties to gluten and should be avoided by gluten intolerant individuals. Malt is a major ingredient of malt beverages and non-alcoholic drinks. It can be dried into malt extract and added to an array of foods and beverages. Most dry breakfast cereals contain malt or malt extract. It is a common ingredient in all-purpose and enriched flour, barbecue sauces, canned and dried soup mixes, condiments, salad dressing, milk shakes, maltodextrin, meat sauces, pre-cooked meats, soups, unbleached flour, caramel flavoring and coloring, cola sodas of all kinds that contain caramel coloring. Caramel color and flavoring are considered natural and do not require certification, but must be labeled "artificially colored or flavored." Malt is used in most baked goods and deli meats. The sweet taste in carob candies may come from the addition of malt.

- Mannitol is one of the nonglucose carbohydrates called sugar alcohols. They absorb poorly because the body does not have the proper enzymes to process them. Mannitol is a constituent of many plants, but is usually derived from seaweed. It digests poorly in the body often causing diarrhea, and can induce or worsen kidney disease. Because it leaves a cool sweet taste in the mouth, antacid tablets, breath fresheners, chewing gum, children's aspirin tablets, and sugarless candies may contain mannitol.

- Raw sugar is cane sugar contaminated with so many insecticides, bacteria, fibers, dirt, lice, mold, and yeast that the government classifies it as unfit for sale. All other brown sugars, including ones called "raw," are simply refined sugars darkened with a small amount of molasses or some other coloring agent.
- Sorbitol is another nonglucose carbohydrate. Sorbitol can affect the body's ability to absorb and use nutrients such as the B vitamins. It is also hard to digest resulting in fermentation in the colon. The fermentation produced by the sorbitol can last as much as six hours. This can lead to increased pathogenic (bad) bacteria and reduced colonies of good bacteria. It can cause diarrhea if consumed in large amounts. Sorbitol occurs naturally in fruits, seaweed, and algae, but is commercially produced from such sources as dextrose.
- Stevia (*Stevia rebaudiana*) tastes sweet, but will not stimulate the body's metabolism. This herb's origin is in South America, where it has been used to sweeten foods and beverages for centuries. Its leaves have thirty times the sweetening power of sugar and only one calorie per ten leaves, a combination that makes it desirable in food production. While it tastes sweeter than honey, it is about as fattening as water. It is a harmless herb with some beneficial effects. One compound in stevia shows antibacterial activity against the bacteria that fosters tooth decay making it a good ingredient to add to toothpaste.

The FDA has tried to prevent the importation and sale of stevia into this country. The American Herbal Products Association (AHPA) has recently submitted a petition to the FDA requesting that stevia be granted "generally recognized as safe" (GRAS) status, allowing it to be used freely in various products for consumption. The AHPA submitted a petition to the FDA listing more than 900 articles documenting that the herb has been used safely for "hundreds of years" by millions of people. The FDA still wants more proof. Other companies wanting to use stevia in food products have meet the same resistance from the FDA.

The FDA launched a particularly aggressive search-and-seizure campaign that was followed in 1991 by a virtual blockade of stevia through the issuance of an "import alert." In the fall of 1994, the FDA was forced to modify the alert after Congress passed the Dietary Supplement Health and Education Act, because it allows the herb to be sold if it is formulated and labeled strictly for use as a dietary supplement. The agency still restricts stevia's use in teas and other food products and does not permit any mention of the herb's sweetening ability. Countries such as South Korea, Israel, Japan, China, and countries in Central and South America already permit stevia in their foods and consider it very safe.

The probable reason that stevia is having a hard time becoming a legal sweetener is not because of any health hazards, but because there is a big investment by U.S. manufacturers to keep products such as aspartame and sugar in our food products. They are not likely to invest money in getting FDA approval for a nonpatentable substance such as stevia. It seems that one of the companies that has a lot to gain from stevia staying illegal is Monsanto, the manufacturer of NutraSweet.

Japan has used stevia since the 1970s and has subjected stevia extract to extensive testing and found it without health risk. They now include it in candies, ice cream, pickles and soft drinks. In 1988, stevia extract commanded a 41 percent share of Japan's multimillion-dollar market for high-intensity sweeteners, outselling the American-made chemical compound NutraSweet. Coca Cola uses stevia as a sweetener when it exports their drink to other countries such as Japan.

Once you buy stevia as a dietary supplement, you can use it however you like. Add a pinch of dried leaves to your favorite tea. The liquid extracts and powders can be used in cooking and as tabletop sweeteners. Because of its intense sweetness, the powdered extract is often mixed with water and used by the drop. The liquid form is easier to use in cooking. To use stevia leaf, simply make a tea (1/2 teaspoon to a cup of water and let steep for fifteen minutes) and add 1/8 cup to a small amount of barley malt or brown rice syrup to enhance the sweet flavor. This combination helps mask stevia's slightly bitter flavor. For stevia suppliers see the section "Resources."

- Sucrose (table sugar) comes from sugar cane and beets. Table sugar is refined raw sugar after the molasses has been removed. It is just empty calories, providing no vitamins, minerals, enzymes, fiber, protein, or anything of nutritional value. Sucrose is also a highly allergic and addictive substance. A hidden source of sucrose is the coating of medication tablets.
- Sucanat is the registered name for an organically grown granulated cane sugar juice with the water removed. It is unrefined and used in products such as cough drops, candies, hot cocoa, ice cream, and in food preparation.
- Total invert sugar is a liquid sweetener more sweet than white table sugar. Manufacturers take sucrose and split it chemically and enzymatically to form glucose and fructose. This process is called inversion.
- Turbinado sugar is a raw sugar that has gone through a refining process to remove the molasses and impurities. It needs to meet only the minimum sanitary level set by the government. Molasses is the part of sugar that contains most of the nutrients found in unrefined cane and raw

sugar. This leaves turbinado sugar with fewer nutrients and more "empty" calories.

- Xylitol is a sugar alcohol, just like Mannitol and Sorbitol. It comes from birch trees, corn cobs, peanut shells, wheat straw, cotton-seed hulls, and coconut shells. It has the same sweetness as sucrose (table sugar) and leaves a pleasant, cool taste in the mouth. In high doses it can cause diarrhea. It is still being used in some chewing gums.

CHAPTER 29

MSG and Its Many Names

Glutamic acid is an amino acid most commonly found in its salt form, glutamate. It comes in two forms; one bound to protein and one free of protein. Free glutamate is used as a flavoring even though it does not have any flavor itself. What it does is affect the way the brain senses flavors. When a product contains 99 percent free glutamic acid it is called monosodium glutamate (MSG) and labeled this way. If a product consists of less than 99 percent free glutamic acid, then a variety of other names are commonly used. Usually, the amount of free glutamic acid in these products ranges between 8 and 40 percent.

Free glutamate is used in one form or another in almost all processed or manufactured food as a flavor enhancer. The food manufacturer can use a reduced amount of a food product and some cheap glutamate while getting a big taste and saving a lot of money. Unfortunately, about 30 percent of the population will experience some adverse reaction when they use this substance at the dosages available in food products.

There has been no long-term evaluation of free glutamate in humans. Manufacturers can currently produce "reaction flavors" without regulation or supervision. The FDA still has not proven that the ingestion of glutamate, in any form, is safe. Free glutamate, the active ingredient in MSG, is a naturally occurring substance and the FDA has defined "naturally occurring" as anything that comes initially from nature. Manufacturers advertise their products as "natural" or "all natural," but this does not mean they are good for you and it does not let you know if free glutamate has been added to the food.

Free glutamate works by stimulating your taste buds and changing your perception of how the food taste, but it has no nutritional value. It also increases flavor and odor appeal by suppressing bitterness and sourness. Because of its flavor enhancing qualities, free glutamate stretches the flavor of ingredients used in process foods and enhances their natural flavor while cutting production cost. Glutamic acid is an excitotoxic amino acid because it is known to excite and even kill brain cells in laboratory animals.

According to the *L.A. Time-Washington Post* news service, a new labeling rule proposed by the Food and Drug Administration (FDA) would require food producers to disclose whether their products contain free glutamate. Presently, it must be disclosed only if it is added to food in its pure ingredient form, MSG, but free glutamate is also present in many ingredients. Current labeling allows for free glutamate to be hidden in processed food with more than 40 different names. Because free glutamate is not clearly identified on product labels it is extremely difficult to confirm if this substance is causing reactions. Glutamate-sensitive individuals need to know what products contain this substance and the FDA should require the labeling of all free glutamate in processed foods.

The proposed labeling rule would cause manufacturers of prepared foods to disclose the presence of free glutamate on the label and not advertise themselves as MSG-free. There are critics for and against this ruling. Those against the use of glutamate say that it can trigger reactions ranging from dizziness and shortness of breath to headaches and drowsiness. However, the Glutamate Association, the Institute of Food Technologists, the Meat Institute and other food industry groups, say these claims are unfounded. They say that the levels of these ingredients used in the food supply probably do not cause adverse reactions in the general population. They also say that glutamate labeling would unfairly stigmatize products many consumers have been eating for a long time. The Atlanta-based Glutamate Association supports the use of MSG. Could it be because most of the organization's fifteen members are the nation's top food processors?

According to the Truth in Labeling Campaign, (TLC) a not-for-profit consumer group, the FDA has built its case for the safety of MSG and free glutamate on misleading studies sponsored by the glutamate industry. The FDA dismisses much of the research that clearly demonstrates that free glutamate poses certain risks. The FDA's announcement that this substance is essentially safe and only causes mild adverse reactions in a small percentage of people is an inaccurate reflection of the actual report. The Truth in Labeling Campaign says that MSG and free glutamate adversely affect the health of millions of Americans and its presence in food should be disclosed.

Some food products advertise that they contain "No MSG" or "No added MSG," but actually contain large amounts of free glutamate. The FDA acknowledges that these processed foods are misbranded and therefore illegal. It wishes to redefine the conditions under which such label claims can be made. One suggestion offered by the FDA would allow the use of these terms if the product contains less than .2 grams of free glutamic acid per serving, provided that MSG is not the result of a manufacturing process. Unfortunately, this cannot be determined by lab analysis.

In its lawsuit against the FDA, the Truth in Labeling Campaign has asked the court to order the agency to require that all processed food be measured for free glutamic acid following completion of processing. These food labels would refer to free glutamic acid as "MSG" with the amount given in grams. If the label says "No MSG" it should mean no MSG. Consumers should know what they are buying. The Truth in Labeling Campaign can be reached at P.O. Box 2532, Darien, Illinois 60561 or call them at (312) 642-9333 for more information.

OTHER COMMON NAMES OF FREE GLUTAMATE

Monosodium glutamate (MSG)
Calcium caseinate
Sodium caseinate
Textured protein
Natural flavoring
Yeast food
Autolyzed yeast
Hydrolyzed protein
Hydrolyzed vegetable protein
Yeast extract
Hydrolyzed yeast
Natural chicken or turkey flavoring
And other spices
Modified food starch

Glutamate can be found in anything protein-fortified, enzyme-modified, or fermented. It can appear where consumers least expect it, such as in the new chicken pox vaccine. Most canned tuna packed in water contains free glutamate as hydrolyzed protein. Sesame Street Pasta Shapes with Mini Meatballs in Tomato Sauce falsely advertises "No MSG" on its label. Restaurants are being supplied with soup labeled "No MSG Added" when there is free glutamate in it. The substance is even in Gerber's "Graduates" toddler food.

The most obvious products have ingredients called "hydrolyzed protein." These are not required to be listed as containing free glutamate. Since there is no restriction to this type of labeling, any new name could appear containing this substance. Various products may make no mention that an ingredient is glutamate derived. Manufacturers call it "flavoring," "natural chicken flavoring," "natural turkey flavoring," etc. Be cautious of any ingredient list containing the word "flavoring" or "natural flavoring."

The list of food products containing glutamate is growing. It is found in most salad dressing, processed meat, snack foods, soups, and prepared foods on the grocery store shelves. It is common in crackers, bread, frozen entrees, ice cream and frozen yogurt, and low-fat foods. Be careful of the "light" foods with reduced fat. They usually replace the lost flavor with flavor enhancing free glutamate. Restaurants often add it during preparation. Drinks, chewing gum, and candies are also potential sources. Food is not the only source. Soaps, shampoos, hair conditioners, and cosmetics can contain free glutamate, as well as binders for medication, nutrients, and supplements.

Symptoms of MSG and Free Glutamate

It is unclear why some people react to glutamic acid, but it may only become a problem when it becomes unbound in the manufacturing process forming free glutamate. When it occurs naturally in vegetables, glutamic acid doesn't seem to be harmful. Some people eat a food containing MSG and react immediately. Others do not react for at least 48 hours. Some reactions are dose related; the more you eat the more reaction you will have. Some highly sensitive individuals will react when a very small amount is present in their food. Usually, the reaction will be the same and within the same period of time.

There has been an enormous amount of evidence that the ingestion of free glutamate can bring on serious health problems. It can extend far beyond the so-called "Chinese restaurant syndrome." The reactions usually involve different body systems, especially the brain. Many people are experiencing adverse reactions to free glutamate and do not know the cause. In sufficient quantities, free glutamate is toxic to everyone. To those who cannot metabolize it effectively, even smaller doses can act like a poison.

Larger amounts of glutamate can cause mild states of intoxication. Its use can also result in a state of uneasiness with a flushed face and a clouded mind. High levels of MSG can affect young children. Studies have indicated that the damage done at the time of initial exposure may not produce any obvious outward effects. Later in a child's development there may be signs of learning disability or emotional instability. Symptoms from MSG are often called "Chinese restaurant syndrome" even though MSG is commonly used in most restaurants. To avoid this risk, eliminate all food and drinks that contain this substance.

Women who ingest MSG while pregnant increase the risk of the developing fetus having a smaller pituitary, thyroid, ovary, or testes. This results in reproductive dysfunction in both females and males. MSG also increases the allergic load, putting someone at risk of developing sensitivities to numerous chemicals and other substances. It can make consumers more sensitive to products containing aspartame (NutraSweet).

There is also the issue of whether the widespread promotion of MSG may contribute to the dramatic increase of Alzheimer's disease, ALS (Lou Gehrig's disease), and Parkinson's disease. The blood-brain barrier, once thought to protect the brain from the unregulated flow of MSG, is damaged by conditions such as trauma to the head, stroke, diabetes, hypoglycemia, and aging, allowing the MSG to pass through.

The symptoms of free glutamate toxicity are many and varied. So many symptoms can occur that it is often difficult to believe that it is the free glutamate causing them. How could a single substance cause such diverse reactions? One of the reasons is that it acts like a neurotropic drug, a substance that affects the nervous system. This substance can affect insulin metabolism and diabetes, resulting in both excessive insulin secretion and insulin resistance. If you experience any of these symptoms, you must be aware that there could be other reasons for experiencing these types of symptoms besides consuming some form of free glutamate. It would be wise to seek medical advice. Common symptoms due to free glutamate are:

Anxiety attacks	Attention deficit disorder	Asthmas
Bloating	Burning sensations	Carpel tunnel
Chest pains	Depression	Diarrhea
Disorientation/confusion	Dizziness	Drowsiness
Fatigue	Flushing	Gastric distress
Headaches and migraines	Hyperactivity	Infertility
Insomnia	Irregular or rapid heart beat	Joint pain
Mood swings	Mouth lesions	Nausea
Numbness (i.e., fingertips)	Shortness of breath	Seizures
Simple skin rash	Skin rash	Slurred speech
Stomach aches	Stunted growth	Tremors
Vomiting	Endocrine problems	Weakness

CHAPTER 30

Fats & Oils

D uring the past century or so, the amount of total fat in the American diet has nearly doubled due to the inclusion of margarine and highly processed vegetable oils. These oils did not exist before 1800. Manufacturers now want products that last indefinitely on the shelves of grocery stores. They have introduced oils that contain unnatural and unhealthy acids, as well as fats and oils that are deficient in essential substances.

WHAT ARE ESSENTIAL FATTY ACIDS (EFAS)?

While most fats are recognized as being bad for health, there are some fats that are necessary. These are the essential fatty acids (EFAs). They function as building blocks in the membranes of every cell in the body. About twenty specific fatty acids are required by the human body to maintain normal function. The body can make all of them but two—Omega-3 (linolenic acid) and Omega-6 (linoleic acid). These must be obtained from the diet or from supplements.

Omega-3 and Omega-6 oils are both necessary for the healthy functioning of the body, especially for the heart, brain, and cell membranes. They are the precursors of substances that regulate many body functions, including the immune system and the ability to fight infection. They also help maintain body temperature, insulate nerves, cushion and protect the tissues, and are vital to metabolism. They promote adrenal hormone production, skin and hair health, make calcium available for tissue use, elevate the calcium level of the bloodstream, and aid in weight reduction by burning saturated fats. Both are involved in the regulation of cholesterol and triglycerides in the body and in the formation of many hormones.

An unborn child requires Omega-3 fatty acids for the development of the brain and to form the membranes that protect cells from invasion. Essential fatty acids are exactly that—essential. Life without them is impossible and when you have a deficiency you can expect health problems. The average person now receives only a fraction of the "good" fats that were present in the diet of our ancestors. A deficiency can lead to an astonishing array of physical problems, including the symptoms of attention deficit syndrome with or without hyperactivity (ADD or ADHD).

ADHD and EFA Deficiency

The Hyperactive Children's Support Group in England has researched and found the connection between this problem and the deficiency of essential fatty acids. Their research has led them to suspect that hyperactive children might have a problem with an important pathway in the body that converts EFAs to prostaglandins—tissue-like hormones that control all bodily functions at the cellular level. The group's survey reveals that many children cannot metabolize nor absorb EFAs normally. Their requirements are higher than normal. An EFA deficiency results in some serious symptoms—many of which look like ADHD. Other common symptoms are eczema, asthma, and allergies. The following points suggest the involvement of essential fatty acids in ADHD-like behavior:

- Hyperactive male children outnumber females by three to one. They require two to three times more EFAs than females to prevent the signs of deficiency. Supposedly, boys have more difficulty converting EFAs to prostaglandins.
- About two-thirds of children with EFA deficiencies have abnormal thirst. Thirst seems to be a key feature.
- Asthma, eczema and other skin problems are more common in hyperactive children. This is because of the defective formation of these prostaglandins.
- Many children with ADHD are zinc deficient. Zinc is required for the conversion of EFAs to prostaglandins.
- Wheat and milk can adversely affect some children. These foods can block the conversion of EFAs.
- Some families have only one child with hyperactivity, while other siblings eat exactly the same diet and appear normal. There may be a deficiency or a defect in essential fatty acid absorption in the hyperactive child causing them to need a much larger amount.

Fatty acids must be converted in order to be used. Diet plays a key role in the process because it takes adequate zinc, vitamin E, vitamin C, niacin (B3), and pyridoxine (B6) to convert Omega-6 fatty acids to Omega-3 fatty acids. Other factors that can interfere with this important conversion process are chronic illness, stress, and eating large quantities of saturated fats and hydrogenated oils.

The finding that hyperactive children have an EFA deficiency also correlates perfectly with the Feingold diet. Dr. Ben Feingold describes a large number of natural food substances and non-natural food additives that may precipitate symptoms in children with ADD. These include natural salicylates and other coloring materials. Many of the agents described by Dr. Feingold are known inhibitors of the conversion of EFAs to prostaglandins, or are chemically related to such known inhibitors. One of the worse offenders is yellow dye. It inhibits prostaglandin formation when essential fatty acid levels are very low, but has little or no effect when essential fatty acid levels are high. This suggests the possibility that children with normal levels of EFAs are not affected. Adding EFAs to the diet of children with hyperactivity may be necessary to correct the symptoms. See the chapter on the Feingold diet.

CIS-FATTY ACIDS AND TRANS-FATTY ACIDS

When polyunsaturated oils are hydrogenated and heated at high temperatures, they form into oils called trans-fatty acids. Natural plants have their oils in a "cis" formation, but chemically altered oils have a "trans" configuration. This type of configuration was not a part of our diet in the past. Trans-fatty acids are harder to metabolize and cannot be used in the synthesis of many hormones and important chemicals the way natural fats can.

Good quality cis-configuration oils play an important role in a well-balanced diet. They provide the EFAs the body needs to protect cell membranes and form prostaglandins. Highly unsaturated EFAs (such as flaxseed oil) combined with high-quality proteins work to counteract toxic and poisonous accumulations in all body tissue. Understanding the benefits of EFAs is understanding that the body has many healthy uses for good quality fats.

Fats of bad quality, on the other hand, are extremely detrimental. Trans-fatty acids change the permeability of cell membranes, disrupt the vital functions of the EFAs, and interfere with certain enzymes needed to detoxify insecticides. They can increase EFA deficiency by interfering with their transformation into other important molecules.

What Foods Contain Trans-Fatty Acids?

We get trans-fatty acids mostly from margarines and shortenings made from partially hydrogenated vegetable oils. Hydrogenation uses strong chemicals that remove most of the vitamins and mineral from the product and results in many altered, unnatural substances that interfere with normal biochemical processes. In Holland, it is prohibited by law to sell margarine containing trans-fatty acids, but in the U.S. hydrogenated margarines and shortenings are found in most processed foods—bread, rolls, crackers, pies, pretzels, cookies, donuts, bread sticks, muffins, bread crumbs, stuffing, pop tarts, biscuits, pancake mix, quick breads, potato chips, candy bars, non-dairy creamers, peanut butter, salad oils, fast-food shakes, baked and canned goods, packed-in-oil products, and fried foods at restaurants. The annual consumption of trans-fatty acids is almost twice as much as the total intake of all other unnatural food additives put together.

Lost Nutrients

Manufacturers continue to use hydrogenation because it keeps their product from spoiling for months. What they do not acknowledge is that the nutrients lost during the hydrogenation process are the very ones that are most necessary. For this reason it is best to avoid hydrogenated or partially hydrogenated vegetable oils.

Agricultural methods have also decreased our intake of EFAs. Caged chickens and their eggs, as well as feed-lot-raised cattle, are producing much lower levels of Omega-3 and Omega-6 fatty acids than their free-range counterparts. The same has happened to fish. In the wild, fish eat other small fish, shrimp, algae, insects, and insect larvae that are high in EFAs. Now fish are being farmed and fed soy meal and other less nutritious foods.

In our diets today there has been a substantial increase in drugs and pharmaceuticals, sugar, caffeine, alcohol, and refined carbohydrates that block EFAs and their conversion to the vital prostaglandins. Add to this mix the increase in toxic food, water, and air, plus the lack of breast feeding, and clearly the average diet is just not going to contain enough EFAs unless an effort is made to find good quality sources. Not only are we not eating enough of the right types of essential fats and oils, but we are increasing our intake of the harmful ones. For the good of our children, and for our own health, we must make some changes.

Sources of EFAs

Because fatty acids are extremely perishable and quickly become rancid, it is best to obtain them from fresh foods such as cold-water fish (Omega-3) and leafy green vegetables (Omega-6). Omega-6 fatty acids are abundant in other plant sources such as the seeds of sesame and sunflowers and their oils. Other products containing high levels of Omega-6 fatty acids are borage oil, evening primrose oil, and black currant oil. Omega-6 is also present in safflower and corn oil, as well as in walnuts, almonds, tofu, avocados, barley, cashews, garbanzo beans, peanut butter, and rice.

There are two major sources of Omega-3 fatty acids. Fish oils, especially cold-water fish such as salmon, mackerel, halibut, albacore tuna, cod, and sardines, are an excellent source. The richest plant source is fresh-pressed organic flaxseed oil that contains 50 to 60 percent of Omega-3 by weight and approximately 20 percent Omega-6 fatty acids. This oil contains almost twice as much Omega-3 as fish oils. Other good sources of Omega-3 fatty acids are nuts, pumpkin seeds, walnut oil and walnuts, wheat-germ oil, soybean oil, soybean lecithin, tofu, common beans, seaweed, safflower and canola oils, avocados, barley, cashews, garbanzo beans, and corn.

Which Omega-3 Fatty Acids Are Best?

The oils derived from the seeds of the black currant and borage plants have much more Omega-3 fatty acid than flaxseed oil or evening primrose oil. However, there is a difference. Only a very small amount of an important prostaglandin is formed from black currant and borage oils, as compared to flaxseed or evening primrose oils.

FLAXSEED OIL

Flaxseed oil contains both Omega-3 and Omega-6 fatty acids. The suggested dosage is from one to two tablespoons of raw flaxseed oil daily. Use it in salad dressings, pour it over vegetables and potatoes, or take it in capsules. You could grind two tablespoons of flaxseeds in a coffee grinder and mix them with juice, water, soy milk, rice milk, or add them to food. The seed mixture will thicken quickly so drink or eat the combination soon. In order for the Omega-3 fatty acids in flaxseed oil to unfold properly the other essential nutrients (proteins, vitamins and minerals) must be present in the diet in adequate amounts. Vitamin B6 and magnesium must be present for the body to convert EFAs into the beneficial end products. Dr. Donald Rudin, co-author of *The Omega-3 Phenomenon,* believes that a deficiency of Omega-3 oils is partially responsible for widespread illnesses, including the increase in emotional and behavior disorders.

Aspirin Decreases Assimilation of EFAs

There are various health problems associated with aspirin. For one thing, it inhibits an enzyme needed to assimilate Omega-3 fatty acids. Another problem that occurs when aspirin is taken every day is that little or none of a substance that rids the lungs of breathed-in dust and bacteria is produced. People who suffer from allergic disorders may benefit from avoiding aspirin and other nonsteroid anti-inflammatory drugs while taking essential fatty acids each day.

What Are EPA and DHA?

Eicosapentaenoic acid (EPA) and docosahexaenoic acid (DHA) belong to a particular class of polyunsaturated fatty acids. EPA and DHA are associated with clean arteries and the absence of fatty degeneration diseases. They can both be produced by the healthy human body from Omega-3 fatty acids, but they are produced very slowly. They are essential as structural components of all cell walls, are necessary for proper brain and eye development, and are required for the proper functioning of the immune, reproductive, respiratory, and circulatory systems. They are also precursors to prostaglandins, which are also essential for overall health.

EPA and DHA can be found in fish oils. There is not a reliable vegetarian source of the two acids. Claims have been made that it is available from vegetable oils such as flaxseed oil, but research shows those sources of EPA may not be bioavailable to the body. The best supplemental source is from fish tissues (as opposed to fish liver). The best sources are cold-water fish such as salmon, sardines, cod, trout, and mackerel. If the fish come from fish farms, the amounts of Omega-3 fatty acids are greatly reduced.

If you take supplements, it is best to divide the doses and take them with meals. Find products that also have added vitamin E to reduce the possibility of the oil becoming rancid. Be careful with products that have vitamin A or vitamin D added, however, because they can become toxic to the body in large doses.

HOW MUCH FAT SHOULD BE CONSUMED?

If you followed the U.S. Department of Agriculture's (U.S.D.A.) food-guide pyramid to daily food choices, you would eat six to eleven servings of bread, rice, cereal, and pasta. These foods, however, contain few EFAs. If you get the proper kinds of fat, your total fat intake should be about twenty percent of your daily calories. Many experts believe the higher the Omega-3 fatty acid consumption, the better it is. It may not be necessary to increase the Omega-6 levels because there is already an over-consumption of Omega-6 from refined oils and margarine. The average person consumes up to twenty times more Omega-6 fatty acids than Omega-3. A healthy balance seems to be a one-to-one ratio.

Low-Fat Diets—Not For Children

Low-fat diets are not for everyone. They even may be dangerous for infants and children. Growth requires the energy of concentrated calories such as those we get from fat. Calcium and some vitamins require fat for absorption. Even breast milk is high in fat content. Growing children are fast oxidizers and require more fat and oil in their diet than adults. Many children with ADD and hyperactivity are eating precisely the wrong diet for their body type. Parents are being told that all fats and oils are bad and often give the children inadequate amounts. This only aggravates symptoms and speeds up the oxidation rate. It is important to add adequate quality fats to the diet.

Storing Oils

Omega-3 and Omega-6 oils are fragile and easily destroyed by light, air, and heat. Their sensitivity is precisely what makes these oils precious to human health. Natural oils will keep four to six months if properly stored. Safflower, sunflower, and corn oils (polyunsaturates) become rancid more quickly than olive oil (a monounsaturate). The best place to store fats and oils is in a tightly capped, dark bottle in your refrigerator. The only exception is olive oil. It has its own anti-oxidants that keep it from turning rancid. Store olive oil at a cool temperature in a dark cupboard. When the temperature edges up into the 70s or 80s, refrigerate it. To reduce the chances of rancidity, add vitamin E to your oils immediately after opening. Put a hole in the end of a vitamin E capsule and squeeze the oil into your container. You may want to buy oils in smaller bottles to insure freshness.

Flaxseed oil only retains its Omega-3 fatty acids unspoiled for about four months. Light, oxygen in the air, and high temperatures destroy it very rapidly. Once opened, consume flaxseed oil within three to six weeks. The container must not encounter light. Add flaxseed oil to foods just before serving, not before cooking. Heating oils can destroy vital fatty acids.

A Caution For Consumers

A label that pronounces a product is "made with 100 percent pure vegetable oil" is a signal for the buyer to beware. When making unsaturated fats into saturated ones, most vegetable oils undergo a chemical change. The process creates abnormal or unnatural fatty acids. Not only is the body unable to use them as EFAs, but abnormal fats can even block the utilization of the needed EFAs in the body.

Use caution when buying "all-purpose" vegetable oils. They are usually made from pressed cottonseed oil that comes from pesticide-laced cotton plants. Cottonseed oil is a very poor-quality oil. Many sprayed toxins remain on the seeds after the removal of the cotton fiber. Cottonseed oil contains a fatty acid, cyclopropene, that is toxic to the liver and gall bladder and interferes with the functions of EFAs. It also contains gossypol, an irritant of the digestive tract, that can cause water retention in the lungs and shortness of breath. Because cottonseed oil is an inexpensive by-product for food processors, it is often used in many packaged products.

So-called "natural" food oils found in health-food stores are not recommended. Their method of production usually differs very little from that of the highly refined, harmful oils. These oils use the same damaging refining technologies and packaging methods as supermarket brands.

Canola oil is processed rape seed oil, a member of the mustard family. It may contain a substance called euric acid. This concerns some nutritionists because they believe that euric acid may not be healthy and cannot be totally removed by processing. Food companies claim that minute trace amounts will not adversely affect us. Since this seed is often sprayed with pesticides, at least buy a certified organic source.

Who Makes the Best Oil?

Natural and unrefined oils contain a little sediment, plus a distinct aroma and taste. For years I thought buying oils in a health-food store gave some assurance that they were good quality, health-promoting oils for cooking and salad dressings. I was wrong. Even some health-food brands have deceived the public regarding the purity, safety, and nutritional value of their oils. Be assured, however, that there are three companies in Canada and the United States you can trust. Seymour Organic Foods, Flora Inc., and Omega Nutrition all produce oils that meet the highest standards of quality. Flora Inc. and Seymour Organic Foods distribute truly fresh-pressed, cold-processed, unrefined oils and package them in the appropriate dark glass bottles. There is still some penetration with damaging light rays into the dark amber glass causing a certain amount of rancidity. A black glass container would be a better choice.

Arrowhead Mills distributes the full line of Omega Nutrition oils in the United States. They bottle the oils in completely light-excluding containers. They also produce a full line of organic, fresh-pressed vegetable oils that have both Farm Verified Organic and Organic Crop Improvement Association certification. There is a new butter alternative called Spectrum Spread, a non-hydrogenated, non-dairy spread, made by Spectrum Naturals of Petaluma, California. The spread is free of trans-fatty acids and saturated fats. (See "Resources" for the telephone numbers and addresses of these companies.)

CHAPTER 31

Fiber

A diet high in plant fiber decreases the risk of most degenerative diseases of Western society. The current low amount of fiber in most American diets leads to digestive disorders since fiber normalizes or regulates bowel function, aiding in the formation of soft, smooth, easy-to-eliminate stools. A low-fiber diet is also linked to allergies, sensitivies and other chronic health conditions, such as the following:

Varicose veins	Diverticulitis	Heavy metal toxicity
Elevated cholesterol	Hemorrhoids	Chronic headaches
Inflammation of colon	Intestinal gas	Sluggish bowel function
Allergic syndromes	Hypertension	Colon cancer
Atherosclerosis	Candidiasis	

Dietary fiber has no equal as a natural laxative. It doesn't have the problem of gripping, diarrhea, or other complaints often experienced with laxatives. Most people have substantially reduced their natural fiber sources by avoiding foods that contain adequate fiber, by overcooking vegetables, and by not using whole grains. This results in slow movement of the digestive tract. You must consume some form of fiber every day to help prevent many of the digestive problems listed above. The latest studies indicate that increasing fiber by eating more fruits and vegetables, and not grains, reduces the risk of colon cancer.

Fiber is present in all plant foods. Increase the fiber content of your diet in gradual steps to allow the intestinal tract to adjust to the new fiber-rich food supply. The additional fiber may initially cause gas or bloating in some people. Most people in this country consume only 15-20 grams of fiber in their diet daily when they need 20-40 grams. Diet is not only the best source of fiber, but it also provides a wealth of nutrients and is usually low in fat. By increasing the daily intake of fiber, many people could prevent digestive disorders. If there is a medical history of bowel obstruction, avoid any increase in fiber without seeking professional advice.

It is well known that bran has beneficial effects upon digestion and general body health. Bran is the fiber-rich, outer covering of whole grains that the intestines do not absorb. A balanced diet, with ample whole grain products, contains sufficient fiber to promote normal bowel function, and lower the risks of bowel disease. It appears that the fiber of oat bran can soak up more water than the less absorbent bran of wheat. Oat bran is inexpensive and readily available and has healthful effects in regulating the fat levels of the blood. A bowl of oatmeal, or three to six oat-bran muffins during the day may help to lower the blood cholesterol and fat level.

What is Insoluble Fiber?

Insoluble fiber does not dissolve in water. Beans, wheat bran and most other whole grains contain insoluble fiber. This type of fiber includes cellulose, chemicellulose, and lignin, which comes from the seed bran, husks, and stems. Insoluble fiber moves through the digestive tract, largely unchanged, absorbing many times its weight in water and increasing fecal bulk. Pressure increases against the intestinal walls, facilitating and regulating transit through the intestines. In this way, the fiber bulk encourages expulsion of fecal waste material and contributes to regularity.

Foods high in insoluble fiber such as wheat bran, do not bind bile acids or lower cholesterol, but may prevent colon disease. Insoluble fiber has a big influence on reducing bacterial toxins, increasing elimination, absorbing other toxins, softening stool, improving bowel disorders, and reducing appetite. When supplementing the diet with insoluble fiber you also need to significantly increase your fluid intake or the fiber will make you constipated and very uncomfortable. Drink at least six to eight glasses of water each day. This does not mean a lot of tea, coffee, or alcohol. It would be better to cut down on these substances and increase your water intake, preferable the filtered kind. Remember, it is best to drink between meals and not with your meal. Drinking water routinely helps your body flush out toxins.

Diets rich in insoluble fiber prevent other digestive disorders such as irritable bowel syndrome, Crohn's disease, colon cancer, and ulcerative colitis. Insoluble fiber also includes factors that aid in reducing absorption of toxic heavy metals in the intestine. Wheat bran is the richest source of insoluble fiber, but oat bran is less irritating for some bowel conditions. Large quantities of wheat can irritate the lining of the gut and upset sensitive individuals. A high-fiber diet may initially interfere with mineral absorption, but the body usually adapts within a few weeks. High-fiber foods are usually rich in nutrients so a small temporary decrease in absorption is not usually significant. If really large amounts are consumed, then there may be problems with mineral absorption. It is usually better to take supplements at a different time than when having fiber. You may also experience an increase in flatulence. But as your body adjusts to the added fiber, this side effect will decrease.

What is Soluble Fiber?

Soluble fiber holds water, but does not increase fecal bulk and does not prevent constipation. This type of fiber is digested completely and absorbed in the large intestine. Soluble fiber delays gastric emptying and slows the absorption of glucose from the small intestines. This ability to slow absorption makes soluble fiber useful in the management of conditions such as diabetes, hyperglycemia, and hypoglycemia. It also prevents dramatic swings in blood sugar levels. A diet rich in oat bran greatly improves the blood sugar control of diabetic patients.

Soluble fiber also lowers blood cholesterol levels causing a decrease in bad cholesterol (low-density lipoprotein or LDL) and an increase in good cholesterol (high-density lipoprotein or HDL). The gall bladder secretes bile acids to digest the fat you eat. Normally your body absorbs these acids again and recycles them for future use. Bile acids will stick to soluble fiber and pass straight through the digestive tract instead of being absorbed and flushed out of your system with the fiber. Down goes your blood cholesterol level! Soluble fiber not only has a big influence on reducing serum cholesterol and fats and stabilizing blood sugar, but it also makes you feel full longer, as well as reducing bacterial toxins.

Gums, mucilage, pectin, beans, and fruit are good sources of soluble fiber. One cup of cooked beans contains the same amount of soluble fiber as 2/3 cup of oat bran. Other foods high in soluble fiber include: squash, apples, beans, citrus, cauliflower, green beans, peas, lentils, cabbage, carrots, strawberries, potatoes, and many other vegetables and fruits. There is not much difference between the amount of soluble fiber in oat bran when compared to regular oats.

Most plant foods contain both soluble and insoluble types of fiber. Taken in sufficient quantity throughout the day, the mixture of soluble fiber and water fills the intestines with a moist, gelatinous mass that clings to the walls. It soaks and softens the encrusted material on the intestinal wall allowing the body to slough off this hardened build-up.

Guar gum is a mucilage found in most plants. It is a water soluble indigestible carbohydrate. Food processors use guar gum as a stabilizing, thickening, and film-forming agent in the production of cheese. Salad dressings, ice cream, soups, toothpaste, pharmaceutical jelly, lotion, skin cream, and tablets often contain guar gum. It is effective in promoting improved intestinal motility. Guar gum and other mucilages, including pectin, are some of the most potent cholesterol-lowering agents of the gel-forming fibers. They will reduce after-meal glucose and insulin levels in healthy and diabetic subjects. People who diet find that guar gum decreases the feeling of hunger.

Psyllium seed husk is also a mucilage fiber and acts as a bulking and laxative agent. It has many of the qualities of guar gum except that it has a greater laxative effect. Pectin is found in all plant cell walls and in the outer skin and rind of fruits and vegetables. The water-soluble and gel-forming properties of pectin help to lower cholesterol levels in the body, reduce heavy-metal absorption, and aid in detoxification.

There is extensive use of agar as a thickening agent by the food industry. Derived from a sea vegetable, it is also a bulking agent, inhibits heavy-metal uptake in the gut, and acts as a laxative.

Never attempt to increase the amount of fiber into the diet of an elderly person without medical supervision. Giving too much of the wrong kind of fiber to the elderly can cause severe pain, blockage, and other problems. Never give fiber to anyone with a history of bowel obstruction. Diseases such as Crohn's disease, ulcerative colitis, and irritable bowel syndrome usually respond well to dietary changes. If you suffer from any of these conditions find a local holistic practitioner to help guide you.

A Dutch study found that men with low-fiber diets had three times the death rate of cancer than men with high-fiber diets. Fiber protects because:

• fiber helps the body eliminate potentially toxic waste in the colon.
• fiber absorbs a large amount of water that dilutes potential cancer-causing agents in the intestines or the stool.
• fiber inhibits the production of bile acids that help generate carcinogens.
• fiber-rich foods are naturally rich in antioxidant nutrients that neutralize the free-radicals that can damage healthy cells.

The bowel transit time for healthy people is twelve to eighteen hours. For too many people in Western cultures, it takes two to three times longer. The longer the transit time, the greater the possibility that putrefaction will generate toxic waste products in the colon, including carcinogens. Insoluble fiber is crucial for healthy bowel function. Regular elimination with large, soft stools, will reduce the risk of diverticulosis, appendicitis, hemorrhoids, varicose veins, irritable bowel syndrome, Crohn's disease, and gallstones.

Iron is available from plant foods, but some vegetable-based foods such as uncooked grains (European muesli) contain phytates. These phytates bind up minerals including iron, like a magnet. The iron is not absorbed and passes out with the stool. Eat cooked or sprouted grains, but limit the amounts of unleavened bread, especially if you have iron anemia. Cooking and sprouting destroys most phytates. The addition of Vitamin C helps to reduce the action of phytates on iron absorption. Dietary phytates also adversely affect the uptake and utilization of calcium and zinc. The following is a list of foods divided according to their phytate levels:

NONE	TRACE LEVEL	MILD LEVEL	MODERATE LEVEL	HIGH LEVEL
apples	broccoli	blackberries	artichokes	beans
bananas	carrots	figs	potatoes	cereals
celery	green beans	strawberries	sweet potatoes	grains
mushrooms				nuts
prunes				
pineapple				
spinach				

CHAPTER 32

Grains

Grains have been in our diet throughout history. They provide high fiber, complex carbohydrates, minerals, B-complex vitamins and are low in fat and sodium. Grains consist of bran, germ, and endosperm. During refining, the bran and possibly the germ are stripped away. The bran contains fiber, B-vitamins, proteins, fats, and minerals. Bran also promotes good bowel health and helps to stabilize blood sugar levels. The germ supplies us with B-vitamins, E, and A, as well as proteins and fats. What is left after milling—the endosperm—contains complex carbohydrates.

Whole grains are miniature storehouses of important nutrients. As long as they are intact and not ground, cut, cracked, rolled, puffed, or bleached, grains have life-giving nutrition readily available to us. Be sure to store your whole grains in air-tight containers. Keep them dry and in a cool place. The refrigerator is fine, but grains need to be at room temperature if you intend to grind them. Whole grains keep well, but they are still perishable foods. Only grind the flour you intend to use right away, because the nutrients begin to deteriorate and the oils are prone to becoming rancid upon grinding. Unfortunately, the average grocery store is not the best place to shop for whole grains. Instead, shop at the health-food stores if you want your grains whole and free of chemicals and pesticides. If you soak and then simmer whole grains they will retain much of their nutrient content. Sprouting grains and seeds, and then eating them raw, is one of the most nutritious ways to consume them.

Commercially prepared breads, cereals, and baked goods contain harmful chemicals, preservatives, and rancid oils. White flour that has lost its vitamins, minerals, and fiber-rich bran layer, and is just not as nutritious as whole grain. Some white flour products, especially breads, have been fortified with certain nutrients, (usually only the B vitamins and iron) and may have added vegetable gums. But even these additions don't make them nutritionally equal to whole grain breads that contain approximately twenty different nutrients.

Organically grown grains are preferable for several reasons. They do not have the chemicals, pesticides, and herbicides found in nonorganically grown grains. Become familiar with the many healthy kinds of grains available today and add them to your diet unless you have a food sensitivity. The increased variety and rotation of grains ensures more nutrition and minimizes your exposure to any potential grain sensitivity.

Grain Glossary

Berries: the hulled, whole kernels.

Bran: the outer coating or husk, or the grain that is scraped off during processing.

Bulgur: steamed, parched, and cracked wheat berries.

Cracked: whole grains that are steel cut into coarse pieces.

Couscous: granular semolina or millet.

Farina: flour or meal from cereal grains with the germ removed.

Gluten: a protein found in certain grains; forms the elastic-like structure in bread.

Grain allergy: do not use grain vinegar or grain alcohol if sensitive to grains.

Grits: hulled grain that is very coarsely ground.

Groats: hulled, whole kernels of whole grain.

Gruel: thin porridge made by boiling cereal and water or milk.

Hull/Husk: dry, outer layer of a seed.

Kasha: simmered, softened whole or coarsely ground grain usually made from buckwheat.

Kernel: whole seed grain.

Meal: edible part of a grain, coarsely ground.

Porridge: softened grain made by boiling.

Pilaf: vegetable and grain dish that is fried, steamed and seasoned, usually with curry.

Semolina: granular form of milled durum wheat; usually the basis of pasta.

Most whole grains are generally cooked in the same way. The raw grains should first be rinsed well under cold water to remove surface grit and excess starch. It also starts the swelling process. Bring the proper amount of liquid to a boil. Add the grain(s), stir, and leave to simmer. Add additional flavors by using meat or vegetable stock to the cooking grains. All grains expand two to four times their original size when cooked. The following are descriptions of some of the most beneficial grains available for consumption.

AMARANTH

This ancient grain of the Aztec people was recently rediscovered and is now available in health-food stores. It is gluten-free and available organically. The tiny amaranth seed, about the size of millet, is light-colored and can be bought as a whole grain, puffed, or as flour. The unusually high protein content of amaranth is absent in most other grains, except for quinoa. It is especially high in the amino acids lysine and methionine, as well as calcium and iron. Three tablespoons of amaranth flour have more protein and calcium than half a cup of milk. This grain is the highest in fiber having more than twice the amount as wheat. Amaranth is low in leucine, an amino acid abundant in most common grains, making it an excellent complement to other grains.

Use amaranth flour to make a variety of quick and nonyeast breads or use with any baked goods. It adds a sweet nutty flavor and a rich moistness. It is a fine substitute for wheat, but does have an unusual flavor and texture. After cooking as a grain, it remains fairly sticky rather than fluffing up. This makes it a perfect grain for cooked cereal or as an addition to other grains. The best use of this grain is combining it with conventional cereal products such as puffed rice. Cookies, quick breads, muffins, pancakes, and waffles can be successfully made with 100 percent amaranth flour. Amaranth is one of the world's most promising foods.

BARLEY

This ancient grain is seldom at our dinner table. Barley has a high level of malt, which is used as a sweetener in many food products. Malting uses over 30 percent of the harvested barley and more than 50 percent is used as animal feed. Grind this mild-flavored, nutritious grain into a fine, white flour and use in gravies. Combine it with another gluten-containing flour for a lighter bread. Choose the pot barley instead of the pearl variety.

BUCKWHEAT

Buckwheat, a native to Russia, has a very distinctive look and flavor. The name "buckwheat" comes from the Dutch word "bockweit," meaning beech wheat and reflecting the fruit's physical resemblance to beechnuts. Buckwheat may be called wheat, but is not related to wheat. It isn't even a cereal grain, but the fruit of an herb plant related to rhubarb. It is thought of as a grain only because it is cooked and eaten like a grain. It does have the nutritional properties similar to grains and is one of the better sources of protein for a cereal-type food. Buckwheat is comparable to other grains in calories, contains no fat, and is rich in B-vitamins, vitamin E, potassium, phosphorus, iron, calcium, and fiber. Do not use buckwheat as a substitute for wheat or any other grains that contain gluten if you are gluten intolerant.

Buckwheat seeds are light or dark brown, fairly large, and three-cornered. Purchase it in its whole form, groats, and cook and serve like rice. This grain's flavor is distinctive and it can be roasted or left raw. You can store whole unroasted buckwheat for more than a year if kept cool, dry, and in an airtight container. Buy roasted buckwheat in small amounts. Use the flour for baking such as in buckwheat pancakes.

Buckwheat has a fairly strong flavor so mix it with a more bland grain such as rice, corn, or millet. This herb cooks quickly, in about fifteen minutes, making it ideal for last-minute meals. It is available as a spaghetti-like pasta called Soba noodles, a hearty noodle traditionally made in Japan. Another name for buckwheat is "kasha." This is buckwheat without the hull. Buckwheat is nourishing, easily digested, good for the intestines, and ideal for soothing the intestinal tract when there is diarrhea.

CHIA

Chia is an ancient grain used by the Aztecs. They called it "Indian running food" because hunters carried it with them for nourishment on long treks. It is black in color and almost flavorless. Chia grows in the Southwest and Mexico. This high-protein grain (about 20 percent) also contains essential omega-3 fatty acids.

CORN

Corn is the most widely used grain in this hemisphere and the only one containing vitamin A. Grits are coarsely ground corn. When corn is milled into grits and meal, this involves removing the hull and germ resulting in a loss of nutrients. When using cornmeal, make sure it is fresh. Corn is an addition to many foods in the form of a sweetener such as dextrose, high fructose corn syrup, corn syrup, or nutritive dextrose. Many artificial sweeteners contain corn, usually as dextrose.

Other varieties of corn are flint or dent corn. These are the basis for cornmeal, mush, tortilla, and polenta. Blue corn has more protein, iron, manganese, and potassium than any other variety. It is also higher in the amino acid lysine. Corn combined with legumes provides a complete protein (containing all the essential amino acids).

KAMUT

Kamut is the ancient Egyptian name for wheat. It originated in the fertile crescent of Mesopotamia around 4000 B.C. and is a relative of modern durum wheat. This large kernel grain has remained free from the manipulation of modern plant breeders whose priorities often sacrifice flavor and nutrition for disease resistance and high yields.

This type of wheat makes a very tasty whole-grain pasta. It is a satisfying, rich grain with a nutty flavor. Kamut did not receive real notice until the macrobiotic community learned about it. It is higher in eight of the nine minerals usually found in common wheat, and contains up to 65 percent more amino acids. It is also higher in lipids and protein than the wheat used in regular breads. The results are a higher energy and more nutritious grain than any other type of wheat. Kamut contains a unique type of gluten that is easier to digest.

MILLET

Commonly used in Europe, Africa, and Asia, this bland flavored grain has similar uses to corn or rice. It is a delicious, mild-flavored, yellow-colored grain. It is also very versatile in recipes. Millet is one of the most nutritious foods, high in protein, and has a good balance of essential amino acids. It is also high in magnesium, iron, calcium, phosphorus, iron, potassium, manganese and copper, but low in sodium. Millet has a low starch content, is easily digested, does not cause gas, and will assist in regulating the bowels. This is an important grain to consider for people with food sensitivities because it is seldom a problem. It is the only alkaline-forming grain. Cooked or roasted, it is a wonderful, nutritious food.

Cultivation of millet is largely restricted to the Eastern Hemisphere, especially those areas with dense populations that do not have mechanized agricultural practices. Millet grows well where other grains won't grow, because it is tolerant of poor soil. Millions of people in the world eat millet. It is the staple grain of the northern Chinese, many Africans, Indians, and the Hunzans, the long-lived people of the Himalayas. Millet was the staple food grain in America until wheat became economically more feasible. The early colonists planted this grain and used it like corn. Popularity faltered, and now it has been relegated to the lowly ranks of bird and poultry feed. Millet is tasty and nutritious and really deserves a more respected place in our diet.

OATS

This common cereal grain has many uses besides oatmeal. Oats are easy to digest and a good source of the B vitamins. They contain the highest percentage of sodium and unsaturated fat of any grain. Oats also contain an antioxidant that delays rancidity. High in protein, oats have an amino acid content similar to wheat. They are one of the richest sources of silicon making them good for the hair, skin, eyes, and nails.

It is especially helpful to use oats as fiber (see the chapter "Fiber"). Pure oat bran has more concentrated fiber, but all forms of oats contain soluble fiber. Eating oats and oat bran in recommended amounts seems to lower serum cholesterol, especially if the diet is also low in fat and cholesterol foods. Be aware that some oat products (cookies, cereals) contain substances that are high in saturated fats and can actually raise blood cholesterol.

Unlike other grains, when oats are milled only the inedible hull is discarded. So they retain more of their original nutrients than processed wheat products. Cooked oatmeal is filling, but low in calories. The following is a description of the different types of oats available:

- Oat groats have the outer hull removed. This edible form is the most nutritious way to eat oats. The oat groat is the oat's natural state with its complete whole-grain goodness. It is used in breads and muffins, with rice, or as hot cereal. Try adding groats to vegetables or as a thickener in bean soup.
- Steel-cut oats are groats that are sliced into pieces with steel blades. Since they are not processed or heated, they retain all their nutritional value.
- Old-fashioned rolled oats are sliced groats that have been steamed to soften some of the starch. The oats are then flattened by rollers into flakes and allowed to dry. This increases the surface area so they can cook in a short time. Quick-rolled oats are produced in a similar manner to regular rolled oats, but the groats are cut more finely and rolled until they are quite thin. This process decreases the nutritional value.
- Oat flour consists of oat groats milled with the bran included. Oat flour is sweet and produces a cake-like crumb that makes it an excellent addition to cookies, pie crusts, yeast breads, and muffins. Oats contain very little gluten. Use this flour in soups and sauces.
- Oat bran is the outer layer of the rolled oat grain. Use oat bran in baked goods, breading, and toppings.

QUINOA (PRONOUNCED KEEN-WAH)

This ancient, grain-like fruit comes from the Andean mountain regions of South America. It was anciently used as a staple along with corn and potatoes. Quinoa contains more complete protein than any grain, making it close to an ideal food. It can supply most life-sustaining nutrients. Researchers call it the "super grain" because it contains up to 50 percent more protein than other common grains. Its essential amino acid balance is close to the ideal set by the United Nations Food and Agriculture Organization.

The tiny and light-colored seed expands four to five times its volume when cooked and can be served like rice. It substitutes for most grains in recipes and has a light and satisfying quality. Combined with other grains or legumes it increases the protein value. This easy-to-digest grain is low in gluten and has a mild taste that complements vegetables, poultry, or fish. It is also high in linoleic acid and contains high levels of calcium, phosphorus, iron, and the B-vitamins.

A note of caution is important when cooking with quinoa. The seeds are naturally coated with a bitter substance called saponin. Quinoa that is available in the United States is washed by hand before being imported from South America, but the seeds still have sufficient saponin to give an unpleasant bitter taste to the cooked grain and to dishes prepared with it. Taste a few of the seeds and if they leave a sharp and bitter taste on the tongue, wash them again. To prepare the seeds for washing put the quinoa in a bowl or pan and add cold water. Rub the quinoa between your hands and drain it in a fine-mesh strainer. Repeat until the fresh water no longer foams. Sudsing is sign of saponin left from inadequate washing.

To cook quinoa, rinse thoroughly, place one cup grain and two cups water in a 1/2-quart sauce pan and bring to a boil. Then reduce to a simmer, cover, and cook until all water is absorbed (ten to fifteen minutes). When all the grain has turned from white to transparent, it is done.

RICE

Rice is a staple food for more than half of the world's population. This common grain comes in long, medium, and short-grain varieties. Brown rice has the indigestible husk removed, but the whole kernel is still intact. It has a pleasant, mild flavor and a chewy, satisfying texture. It is rich in vitamins B and E, as well as iron, fatty acids, and protein. Rice is one of the easiest grains to use. It is very versatile and comes in several shapes and sizes. White rice is less nutritious because of the removal of many outer layers, including the husk and the germ. The following is a description of the different types of rice available:

- Instant rice is a precooked rice with the outer coating removed. It lacks protein and has a much reduced mineral and vitamin content.
- Polished white rice is a very refined, white rice with the hull, bran, germ, and endosperm removed.
- Converted rice is soaked and steamed before the milling process to retain more of the nutrients.
- Brown rice results when the outer husk has been removed, but much of the nutrition has been retained.

- White-rice flour is made from polished white rice so the nutritional value is low and has little taste.
- Brown-rice flour has more nutrition and a little more taste than white rice flour.
- Rice polishings are brown rice with the bran and other materials removed to make polished rice.
- Wild rice is not a true rice, but a member of the grass family. It is nutritional with a lot of taste, but more expensive than other types of rice.

RYE

Rye's strong, rich flavor is a pleasing alternative to the milder, lighter grains. This hardy, annual grass can thrive in poor soils and cold, wet climates. During the Middle Ages, rye was finding its way into the cultivated wheat fields and forcing farmers to harvest the two grains together. As a result, rye soon became the choice of cooks and bakers all over the world. The people in Eastern Europe produce and eat more rye than anywhere else in the world.

Rye contains little gluten and produces a more compact, heavier bread. Rye berries, the whole form of rye, are also edible. Use rye flour to vary breads. Add the flour as a thickener to soups and gravy. Today, whole or rolled rye berries, flakes, meal, grits, and flour add a strong and distinctive flavor to breads, cereals, and other baked goods.

For those who are sensitive to rye, it is important to be able to identify it in products. You can find rye is some multi-grain breads and some granolas. It is also in gin, vodka, and scotch whiskey.

SPELT

This is a grain related to wheat and one of the oldest natural grains known to man. Spelt was the staff of life in early Europe. The husked kernels were eaten as a whole-grain staple. After nourishing Europe for decades, this grain nearly vanished from use. With the coming of the industrial revolution, spelt became old-fashioned and out-of-date because of its long straw, and thick, heavy husks. Compared to regular wheat, it produces a lower yield and has to be mechanically hulled before milling. This is why it has fallen into disuse since the nineteenth century. Only on a few farms high up in the Alps did this grain continue to grow. Then the current health movement rediscovered it.

Substitute spelt flour in any recipe using wheat flour. It is easily digestible and often requires less liquid in recipes. Even people who have a wheat sensitivity usually can tolerate spelt. Be sure to try a small amount first if you have a problem with wheat. If there is a gluten sensitivity, then you probably need to avoid spelt. Spelt is rich in complex carbohydrates and fiber. It also tops wheat in protein, amino acids, minerals, and vitamins B1 and B2. This easily digestible, gluten-containing grain is available as pasta, flour, and whole berries. Order the grain and the recipe book called *The Wonderful World of Spelt* from Purity Foods, Inc., 2871 W. Jolly Road, Okemos, MI 48864-3547, (517) 351-9231.

TEFF

Teff is also known as "lovegrass." This leafy, quick-maturing plant is an important cereal food of Ethiopia and the eastern African highlands. Teff is a traditional grain used to make Injera, a large flat bread that is an Ethiopian staple. Teff adapts easily to these harsh and arid areas and has been the staple grain for thousands of years. It seems that most people suffering from wheat and corn allergies may safely eat teff.

It takes approximately 150 grains of teff to weigh as much as one kernel of wheat. This small size adds to teff's nutritional content. It seems that most small seeds are more nutritional than large seeds because of the concentration of nutrients. It is rich in minerals, especially calcium, iron, zinc, and copper. It contains almost three times as much calcium as hard winter wheat or whole oats.

Make teff flour at home with a grain, coffee, or nut mill. This grain is available in white, red, or brown varieties. Each has a pleasing, almost nutty flavor. The mild white teff is chestnut-like in taste. The darker colors are more earthy and taste like hazelnuts. Brown or red teff makes a rich, rustic breakfast porridge, whereas white teff makes a more delicate creamy cereal. When cooked into a soup or stew for thirty minutes or more, teff provides additional body and flavor. This pleasingly light and uniquely flavored whole grain will add more nutritional quality and variety to your family's diet. Since this grain is unrefined, it still contains its vitamin- and mineral-rich outer bran layer. This includes a good amount of thiamin and soluble fiber.

TRITICALE (PRONOUNCED TRIT-UH-CAY-lee)

This is a winter-hardy hybrid grain derived from a cross between wheat and rye (secale). Triticale has a stronger flavor than wheat, though not as strong as rye. Its protein content is higher than wheat and it contains all the essential amino acids. You can sprout the berries or use them as a substitute in rye or wheat recipes. Triticale, in the form of flakes and flour, is often available in health-food stores. It is high in protein and a good source of vitamins B and E, as well as the minerals zinc, selenium, magnesium, iron, and copper.

WHEAT

This grain comes in hard and soft varieties. Hard wheat contains higher levels of protein and the soft variety contains more carbohydrates. Whole wheat contains most of the B-vitamins, vitamin E, protein, essential fatty acids, and trace minerals. Even though it is nutritios, wheat is more likely to cause a food sensitivity than any other grain. Even if you are not sensitive to this grain, it is still a good idea to minimize its use. Substitute with one of the other grains when possible.

Coarse milling is what makes cracked wheat. Pasta is made exclusively from durum wheat, whereas semolina is refined durum flour. Couscous comes from either durum wheat or millet. Bulgur wheat is partially cooked and toasted cracked wheat. Refined white flour has the nutritive properties removed in the milling process to produce a finer flour. It produces a product that has a long shelf life in the grocery store, but is low in nutrients. The milling and bleaching process used to make enriched, bleached white flour destroys a large amount of niacin (B3) and pyridoxine (B6) and significant amounts of other B vitamins.

Food processors in the United States use the process called "70 percent extraction" whereby 30 percent of the wheat is discarded, including most of the germ and bran. The bran (containing the first three layers) is first removed. Then the aleurone, rich in protein, minerals, and useful essential fatty acids, is removed. The germ also contains a high percentage of the protein, natural sugars, wheat oil, and large amounts of minerals and vitamins. Nearly all of the natural and valuable nutrients of the wheat are lost. Fortifying them with synthetic vitamins and iron does not produce a wholesome product. At least 23 factors are depleted in the processing of white flour. At best, some eight are restored. Today's highly processed bread has about the same nutritional value as sawdust.

Sprouted wheat breads are healthier than breads made from wheat that has been refined and ground into flour. They contain more nutrients per unit than any food. When a grain of wheat is sprouted, it retains all the original nutrients of the wheat berry. Breads made from sprouted grains digest more easily than whole grains or flour. This can be important for wheat-sensitive bread lovers.

CHAPTER 33

Protein

WHAT IS PROTEIN?

Amino acids make up more than 1600 different compounds in the body, primarily proteins and neurotransmitters. Proteins composing the human body make up the skin, tendons, muscles, cartilage, and even the hair and nails. New proteins form enzymes, hormones, and antibodies to replace old cells; build new tissues, and transport nutrients in and out of cells. Protein is not only the basic structural component of all body parts, but is itself the biochemical structure of all enzymes. Without adequate protein, the body cannot make adequate enzymes that act as catalysts. Catalysts speed up chemical reactions that otherwise would not take place or would take place too slowly.

The adult human body cannot synthesize nine out of the total twenty-three amino acids needed to sufficiently meet physiological needs, including the proper building of protein. These nine amino acids are "essential" and must be derived from food. All of the essential amino acids that make up a complete protein must be present in the digestive tract at the same time for proper assimilation. If even one essential amino acid is missing, the necessary protein cannot be made. These amino acids will pool in the body for 12-18 hours. That is why it is important to get adequate and good-quality protein from the diet every day.

Allergies and Amino Acid Deficiencies

Amino acids are often deficient in modern diets due to certain food processing and a tendency away from meat and dairy. The body cannot store these essential amino acids, but must obtain them daily through diet or supplements. There are links between amino acid deficiencies and many common disorders such as immune dysfunction, connective-tissue breakdown, PMS, chronic fatigue syndrome, depression, and insomnia. Many of the symptoms of these disorders can be mistaken as allergies or sensitivities. The need for protein increases up to five times during stress or trauma.

It is important to realize that while a food may contain all the essential amino acids, this does not mean it is available to humans through digestion. This is true of some legumes that have an anti-enzyme factor called phytates. They can block or inhibit the proper assimilation of amino acids. For more information on phytates see the chapter "Fiber."

THE IMPORTANCE OF PROPER PROTEIN DIGESTION

It is not difficult to acquire the necessary grams of protein per day on a simple diet. Every amino acid needed to build human protein is available in fruits, nuts, seeds, and vegetables, including legumes. The average protein consumption in the United States is anywhere from 75 to over 100 grams of protein per day. Overdosing with protein may be harmful due to the complex digestion process required to utilize protein. If you are ingesting adequate calories, you are probably getting enough protein from your diet.

Protein foods are everywhere, but the trick is to eat them in a form your body can use. The body can manufacture fourteen of the twenty-three amino acids it needs to make protein. The other nine must come from the diet and in proportions that your body can mix and match. "Perfect protein," symbolized by the egg, provides your body with the exact amount needed by the body so that all is used and none is wasted. Most other foods from nonanimal sources are not so well balanced.

PROTEIN FROM PLANT SOURCES

Many people believe that if you try to live on a plant-based diet, you would soon perish from lack of adequate protein. It is rare that anyone eats just grains, just beans, or just a single vegetable. These foods are usually taken in combination with other foods so that the amino acids absent in one food are supplied by those present in another. At least two-thirds of the dietary proteins should be derived from plant-based foods. Whole grains, legumes, soy products, nuts and seeds are primary protein sources in a plant-based diet. Nearly all vegetables contribute to the daily protein needs.

Typical menus around the world are based primarily on grains, vegetables, and legumes with only 1/10 of the protein coming from meat, milk, and eggs. A diet sufficient to supply 2,500 calories would supply 50 percent more protein than needed by most of the population. For most adults, it is difficult to eat a mixed vegetable diet that produces a significant loss of body protein without resorting to eating high levels of essentially protein-free foods.

The most important point for aspiring vegetarians is to lay off the junk food. Coke and Pepsi with French fries may be vegetarian, but they replace

other essential nutrients. A vegetarian diet can be very nutritio
foods with empty calories are avoided; these include sugars, refined sta
es, refined fats and oils, and alcohol. If you eat these foods in large
amounts, you might find it necessary to resort to meat as a concentrated
source of protein despite its disadvantages and liabilities. Meat does supply
the protein, but ordinarily at the expense of considerable fat. Grains,
legumes, and soy foods are bulky and filling, yet contain virtually no fat.
They provide a feeling of fullness that keeps the body fueled and satisfied
for hours. Plant-based diets are also high in fiber.

Is Protein Stored in the Body?

Since the body does not store the essential amino acids that make up a
complete protein, you must eat the right amount and quality every day or
many problems will follow. If you eat a restricted diet for weight loss then
vital tissues begin to break down. The body requires carbohydrates to keep
the blood sugar stable. Certain organs, such as the brain, demand the use
of carbohydrates for fuel rather than fat. The body cannot make carbohydrates from fat and will use proteins for fuel unless there is an inadequate
supply.

How Much Protein is Necessary?

The recommended daily allowance is 0.36 grams of protein per pound
of body weight. A 160-pound man needs about 58 grams of protein a day
and a 120-pound woman needs about 43 grams. Pregnant and lactating
women need considerably more protein as well as those recovering from
severe trauma or surgery. Infants and children need more total protein per
body weight than adults and the protein must be of high quality and rich
in amino acids. An athlete's requirements would be higher.

Which Foods Provide "Complete" Protein?

The word *protein* makes many people think of meat, eggs, dairy, fish,
and fowl. These foods usually contain all the essential amino acids in
approximately ideal proportion and are "complete" or high-quality proteins. Plant foods are not. There are good complete protein choices available from animal sources that are low-fat products. Some of the worst
choices are hard cheeses, butter, and other full-fat dairy products, as well
as meats. Remember, once your body has satisfied its need for protein, the
excess becomes fat.

If you eat protein from animal sources, fish is one of the easiest and
most enjoyable ways to improve health because it is low in calories and fat.
Haddock is the lowest in fat of all the flake fish. Other fin fish are only a

tiny bit higher. Shellfish are the highest in fat content and best used as a treat rather than as a steady diet. Oysters have high levels of zinc. Sardines are a super-rich source of minerals.

Just as there are foods that supply complete protein, there are those that provide "incomplete" proteins; these proteins lack some of the essential amino acids and are unable to sustain life if eaten alone. Amino acids must be present in certain proportions to be well utilized by the body. Plant-based proteins are usually lacking some of the amino acids. Soy protein is one of the exceptions, as well as the grain quinoa. They are closer to the ideal protein and become valued in meatless dishes. The proteins of corn and wheat are not adequate by themselves.

Kidney beans are deficient in amino acids that contain sulfur, and in tryptophan. Rice is low in isoleucine and lysine. When you combine beans and rice, the amino acid strengths of one make up for the weakness of the other. They add up to a very good protein source and called "complementary" proteins. Other good combinations are grains and legumes, peas and wheat, seeds and legumes.

Legumes are deficient primarily in the amino acid methionine. Grains, on the other hand, usually contain ample amounts of methionine but are limited in lysine, another of the essential amino acids. Putting these two foods together provides a more ideal balance and makes the protein easier to assimilate. When combined in the right proportions, the protein of the grain and the legume become more useful gram for gram than either of these proteins alone.

For any grain and legume combination, a certain proportion is optimal. For example, when one eats four times as much rice as black beans in the diet, this is a good combination. If you are eating corn bread and peas, as they do in the southeastern United States, the more ideal proportion is half and half. Generally, the best results occur when there is more grain than legumes. The most successful ratio is about two to one.

Previously, the belief was that complementary foods must be eaten in the same meal. The current belief is that the amino acids will find each other as long as you eat a varied diet over the course of a day. Amino acids that don't form a complete protein survive in the body for twelve to eighteen hours. Eating a variety of foods throughout the day is the key. If you are eating enough high-quality foods and enough calories, you are probably getting adequate protein.

Amino acids are found in considerably less quantity in fruits and vegetables than in legumes, grains, or dairy products. The diets of vegans and fruitarians offer no source of complete proteins. Vegetarian diets will be nutritionally sound if they include a wide variety of nuts, legumes, grains, fruits, and vegetables. It is important to use complementary proteins that will together form a complete protein.

Possible Deficiencies Resulting from a Vegetarian Diet

Vitamin B12 supplements or yeast-containing B12 may be necessary if you omit all traces of dairy and eggs, as well as meat. Vitamin B12 is necessary in the body. Since meat and meat products are the chief sources of this vitamin, vegetarians may need to supplement. If you need a good source of calcium, see the chapter on "High-Calcium Non-Dairy Foods." Otherwise, use supplements to provide calcium.

How can Protein Affect Moods?

Proteins play a major role in the food-mood chain. The brain needs the amino acid tryptophan to create a vital neurotransmitter called serotonin. Low levels of serotonin play a major role in such disturbances as depression, insomnia, and anxiety. Tyrosine is another amino acid available in foods. It is essential for building the neurotransmitter dopamine. A lack of dopamine appears to play a major role in some mental disease such as schizophrenia. It also plays a role in the sex drive. In fact, chronic depression is often treated with tyrosine. There have been substantial improvements in a person's mood with the control of this chemical. Sometimes, the problem is not too little, but too much of the wrong amino acid. Too much of one amino acid can result in lower levels of another.

Amino Acid Combinations

The following list contains some recommended amino acid combinations. Each grouping (e.g. "legumes and rice" or "soybeans, wheat and sesame seeds") contains the complementary foods necessary to making a complete protein. Eating these foods together provides a balance of total protein without eating animal products. Sprout any seed or nut to activate an abundance of amino acids.

Food Group   Examples of Complementary Proteins

Legumes/beans:
legumes and rice
soybeans, rice, and wheat
beans and wheat
soybeans, corn, dairy
beans and corn
barley and kidney beans

soybeans, wheat, and sesame seeds
soybeans, peanuts, sesame seeds
soybeans and almonds
soybeans and Brazil nuts
kidney beans and sesame seeds

Grains:
rice and legumes
corn and legumes

whole-grain bread and nut butters
wheat, sesame seeds, soybeans

	wheat, peanuts, dairy millet and kidney beans rye and lentils (sprouts) rice and dairy whole grains with beans wheat and legumes	brewer's yeast and rice oatmeal and wheat germ wheat, sprouts, potato flour rice with nuts and sesame seeds flour combination: wheat, barley, beans, lentils, millet, and spelt

Vegetables:	combine seeds and nuts
	  with vegetables
	dates, sprouts, and leafy
	  vegetables
		lima beans and brown rice

Nuts and seeds:	sesame seeds and beans peanuts and dairy peanuts, wheat, dairy almond and buckwheat buckwheat and cashew trail mix: almonds, cashews, peanuts, coconut, and soy	sesame seeds, soybeans, wheat peanuts and sunflower seeds cashew and peas brazil nuts and garbanzo beans peanuts, sesame seeds, soybeans

Note: Spelt or quinoa can be substituted for wheat; this means those who cannot have wheat have another choice of grains and know they can select another grain.

CHAPTER 34

Washing Your Food

One of the most overlooked steps in food preparation is that of washing food before consumption. Proper washing can help remove some of the pesticides, toxins, mold and other substances that can act as allergens. Some product labels state that they can rinse away virtually all toxic chemicals with just a couple squirts of the liquid, but they can't eliminate poisonous pesticides in food despite marketing claims. They make some of the products from water and soap combined possibly with alcohol, citric acid, baking soda and oleic acid. These sell in grocery stores and mail order catalogs as the "safe" way to remove pesticide residues, wax, dirt, and bacteria. Even if you eat organic foods, you may still want to remove mold, dust, or any other substance used to deter pests on the food.

Studies show that washing produce only minimally affects the pesticide levels. This is because pesticides can usually cross through the outer skin of the food and be inside where no rinse can reach. In 1992, *Safe Food News* reported a USDA study that indicated washing and peeling fruits and vegetables left pesticide residues of nearly 60 percent in over 5,700 samples tested. The study found that the tested produce had anywhere from four to twenty-five pesticides.

The only safe choice is to buy foods free of pesticides. This means buying organically grown food. For the money you pay buying products that probably do not work very well, you could invest in certified organic foods. If you still want to buy and wash pesticide-laden foods the following are some suggestions that will help.

When you arrive home after shopping at the grocery store, you can clean all your food at once. Fill the sink with about a gallon of pure filtered water. If you don't need a gallon of water to wash your foods, then reduce the amount of the water and the food wash accordingly. Use tap water if that is the only available water source. Add the food wash of your choice. Use a vegetable brush on the more sturdy vegetables and rub the other vegetables with your hands. When using a food spray instead of a bulk wash, you will need to spray your foods well, rub gently, and rinse well. There are several methods for washing your food listed below:

- Add seven to eight drops of liquid grapefruit-seed extract to one gallon of water and use as your food wash. This excellent vegetable and fruit rinse can be bought at most health food stores. Its potency as a bactericide and fungicide will help kill what is consuming, decaying, or contaminating your food. Various tests using grapefruit-seed extract in low concentrations have extended the shelf or transport life of fruits and vegetables by as much as 400 percent.
- Dilute one tablespoon of 35 percent food-grade hydrogen peroxide in one gallon of water and wash all of your foods in this.
- Dilute two ounces of freshly squeezed lemon juice, with rind included, in one gallon of pure filtered water and use this as your food wash.
- Buy a food wash from your health food store. There are several varieties available. See their instructions for use as a spray or as a bulk wash.
- Scrub all fruits and vegetables with a food-grade soap and water, then rinse well.
- Place the fruits, vegetables, or fish to be treated into the food bath. The thin-skinned fruits and leafy vegetables will require ten minutes, as will the fish. The root vegetables and heavy-skinned fruits will require fifteen to twenty minutes. Make a fresh wash for each group. Remove the food and place them into a fresh water bath for ten to fifteen minutes.
- Regardless of what food wash you use, dry the food carefully, preferably with 100 percent cotton dish towels. Wrap them in dry dish towels for storage to prevent moisture accumulation. (Keeping foods in plastic or paper bags will shorten their shelf-life.) Now the food is ready to be put into storage.
- There are several advantages to using this treatment. Fruits and vegetables will keep longer. The wilted ones will return to a fresh crispness. The flavors will be greatly enhanced, tasting almost fresh picked from the garden.
- Peeling root vegetables may remove some of the mold, but it also just spreads it around, so scrub before peeling. Clean melons before slicing them. When you cut into the melon the knife blade drags the mold into the flesh of the melon. The same applies to squash, pumpkin, avocado, oranges, etc.

CHAPTER 35

Healthy Snacks and Lunch Ideas

Cooking healthier meals is great, but what about brown bag lunches and snacking? Are you still reaching for that bag of cookies or eating fried potato or corn chips? These simple tips can help you improve your snacking habits and still enjoy a great treat.

- Food safety is important when you don't refrigerate your food for several hours. Bacteria grow rapidly on food at room temperature and up to about 110 degrees. A healthy lunch could become a live colony of harmful bacteria in a period of three to four hours if the environment is warm. If there is no way of keeping food cold or hot, it may be difficult to take some foods with you. Here are some suggestions—invest in a lunch box that you can insert blue ice or a frozen packet to keep the food cool; you can freeze many beverages and place them in the lunch box; and wrap a frozen drink in newspaper or foil to keep it cold until snack time or lunch.
- The best time to pack the next day's lunch is right after the evening dinner. Put leftovers in small containers and refrigerate or freeze until needed the next day. Wrap the container up in newspaper or foil before placing it into the lunch box.
- Bring a hot lunch of soup, stew, or perhaps a casserole, in a wide-mouth insulated thermos.
- Canned seafood such as sardines, tuna, salmon, and shrimp make a good snack. Put them on crackers, bread, or on a slice of vegetable such as a carrot or cucumber round.
- Ask your child's teacher to let you know when food will be served in the classroom. Then you can prepare something special for your child to take that day. If there is a refrigerator available, then make use of it.
- Dried, assorted fruits make a good snack. Try to find the organic type that is free of preservatives and additives.

- Emergency foods may be needed as an extra snack at school or office. Package bags of nuts and seeds, crackers, and other non-perishable foods.
- Fresh whole fruits such as pineapple or banana slices, grapes, berries, or peaches usually make a good snack. They can be threaded as fresh fruit chunks on a stick. Fruit combinations are a nice change for breakfast or blend fresh fruit into smoothies.
- Fruit ices that do not contain milk are available at some stores. Keep a supply of fruit ices, popsicles, Rice Dream frozen desserts, juice ice cubes, Ice Bean made from soy or rice, or frozen fruit smoothies on hand in the freezer when others are having ice cream. Sorbet is also a nice treat.
- Granola or cereals added to yogurt gives a crunch to the snack.
- Hot dogs made from soy, chicken, or turkey and combined with vegetarian-style beans make a meatless version of franks and beans.
- Lettuce and sprouts need to be packed separately from any sandwich or filling to avoid wilting. Use a variety of sprouts for fun and variety.
- Nut butters can be mixed with all sorts of finely chopped vegetables, sprouts, nuts or seeds. Spread this mixture on acceptable crackers, bread, or rice cakes.
- Nuts and seeds make delicious and unusual cakes and quick breads. Use ground Brazil nuts, almonds, sunflower seeds, and soy grits instead of wheat flour. Fresh and raw nuts and seeds make great snacks such as pumpkin, sunflower, sesame, walnuts, pecans, cashews, or almonds. The most nutritious seeds are flax, sesame, sunflower, and pumpkin. Almonds are the most stable of all nuts and keep well in a sealed container. Store nuts and seeds in the refrigerator.
- Package and freeze individual quantities of meats, poultry, and spreads. They will be fresh and cold, but thawed by lunch time.
- Pancakes with toppings make a good snack. Prepare an extra batch of pancakes ahead of time and fill with a variety of spreads. Roll or stack them for variation. Mix spreads with chopped vegetables, sprouts, nuts, or seeds.
- Rice cakes, oat cakes, rye or rice crackers, flat breads, or sprouted breads with a variety of toppings make a good snack. Use toppings such as almond spread, avocado, sprouts, vegetable slices, hummus (chickpea spread), falafel spread, guacamole, or egg salad.
- Roast garbanzo beans with added garlic powder and tamari. Slow cook for twenty minutes on a lightly oiled cookie sheet or until the beans are crisp on the outside and slightly tender on the inside.
- Salad vegetables placed in a sealed plastic container make a good snack.

- Seasoning popcorn with brewer's yeast, chili powder, garlic salt, or your choice of savory herbs is a quick and easy snack.
- Soup broths make a different kind of drink. Use a thick soup as a topping to serve on potatoes, rice, or other starch foods.
- Soy milk or rice milk can be added to cereals instead of cow's milk.
- Spreads made from soybeans, black beans, and refried beans are delicious on vegetables.
- Turkey slices or chicken can be curled up with some type of spread or stuffing inside. Stuff potatoes, olives, avocados, eggs, or celery with nut butters or a tofu spread.
- Unsweetened applesauce makes a good between-meal snack.
- Vegetable juices are an excellent snack item.
- Vegetable sticks (fresh) can be made from carrots, celery, zucchini, cherry tomatoes, broccoli, cucumber, cauliflower, or turnips.
- Whole-grain pita bread layered with sauce, sauteed vegetables, and a sprinkling of soy cheese or beans makes a great lunch pizza.

There are many new healthy snacks being added to grocery store shelves. Check with your local health-food store for additional wholesome treats and lunch ideas. Recent available items include rice puffs, salsa made from corn and beans, frozen treats made from rice or soy, and a wonderful tasting cheese derived from almond milk.

EATING OUTSIDE THE HOME

The following are some good suggestions for knowing exactly what you're eating when you go to a restaurant or other establishment:

- Ask questions when you eat out. How do they prepare the food? What thickening or breading agent is used (corn starch or wheat), and what spices, sugar or food additives are being used?
- Choose a restaurant with a large variety of food so you will have choices. You can call before going to the restaurant to ask questions about the food and their methods of preparation.
- You may need to bring your own salad dressing, crackers, or bread when going to a restaurant.
- It is difficult to get fast-food restaurants to reveal a list of ingredients, so be careful. There are many hidden sources of allergens at these types of places.
- Cafeterias may be a solution to eating out, but they also use additives, sugar, and MSG to improve the taste of foods.
- A la carte choices on the menu can give you the best flexibility in choos-

Section 4

ALLERGIES AND THE ENVIRONMENT

CHAPTER 36

It Could Be Something You're Breathing

Every spring, summer, and fall, millions of people sneeze, wheeze, drip, and sniffle with the common symptoms of hay fever. More people suffer today than ever before. These allergies and asthma symptoms are usually triggered by foods, airborne pollens, or chemicals absorbed into the blood through the lungs, skin or intestines causing a hyperactivity of the immune system.

This hyperactivity of the immune system may be the result of a chronic state of inflammation in the body. There may be many factors, environmental pollution being one of them. The average adult breathes in and out approximately twelve to fifteen times per minute. This results in an air exchange at the rate of 10,000 liters per day, bringing toxins from the environment into constant contact with the membranes that line the respiratory tract. With this continual contact, the defense system of the body attempts to deal with these toxins. Allergies or sensitivities are often the results of a hyperactive or inflammatory state.

As millions of people know, these allergic reactions are caused by growing levels of grass, tree and weed pollens. Household allergens like dust, pet hair and other factors also can cause or exaggerate the allergic episode. The following is general information on pollen and allergen seasons and levels.

- The pollen seasons overlap one another, but usually occur in somewhat the following order: trees first, then grasses, followed by weeds. The weeds usually cause more trouble in the summer months.
- Molds are especially troublesome close to the shower area and in homes with damp basements. Eradicating mold accumulation may require a do-it-yourself fumigation. They also grow on moist vegetation, alive or dead. Molds can spread over a great distance every time the lawn is cut, leaves are raked, or when the wind blows. Some of these molds are more prevalent at certain times of the year.

- House dust is one of the most important year-round offenders. Symptoms increase when the furnace is turned on in the fall.
- Other inhalants such as animal hair, dander, rug materials, feather pillows, and synthetic fabrics can cause trouble all year.
- It is usually necessary to correct the diet, remove any food sensitivities, and improve digestion. This can go a long way to decreasing the total toxic load on the body and the immune system.
- Symptoms from pollen are more commonly present in the daytime. Dust and molds often cause more symptoms in the morning and evening. When the wind blows, extra treatments may be necessary.

CHAPTER 37

Multiple Chemical Sensitivity

The typical description of a multiple chemically sensitive (MCS) person is someone who is repeatedly exposed to any number of different sensitizing chemical agents. The agents themselves don't have to be definitely poisonous, or present in overwhelming doses, to cause a reaction in susceptible people. In a vulnerable individual almost any chemical can tax the body's immune system beyond its normal adaptive capabilities. People suffering from this problem have a variety of responses to very low levels of environmental chemicals. Symptoms range from subjective symptoms to recognizable syndromes affecting many body systems.

A person becomes chemically sensitive to multiple substances when the body's adaptive mechanism finally becomes overwhelmed. There is a general breakdown in the body's ability to rid itself of toxic substances. People who were sensitive to only one or two chemicals begin to react now to several chemicals in their environment. This causes the immune system to gradually become compromised and over time produces a wide variety of physical and mental symptoms. Symptoms generally become worse with the passage of time and can lead to being a universal reactor. This is someone who reacts adversely to virtually all synthetic substances in their immediate vicinity.

Causes of Multiple Chemical Sensitivities

Some of the more common chemicals that can initiate multiple sensitivities include: volatile glues, aromatic hydrocarbons, pesticide sprays, automobile exhaust, cigarette smoke, and perfumes. On a regular basis we are exposed to chemicals. Modern life exposes us to thousands of different substances that are capable of causing environmental illness in susceptible people. This hidden chemical assault will almost certainly overwhelm the defense mechanisms of most people. When you add to this burden any emotional stress, along with a poor diet and lack of exercise, then it is not surprising to find people with compromised immune systems. One of the body's first areas to break down is its ability to tolerate foreign chemicals. The body is dependent upon a constant supply of good nutrition to keep the immune system working, protecting, and healing itself.

ARE THESE CHEMICALS REALLY SAFE?

Do not assume that because our government has authorized the sale of these toxic substances that they are safe to use. Look at the case of DDT. Our government has banned DDT in this country, but allows manufacturers to produce and sell it to other countries. We then import foods from that country sprayed with DDT. We often have no idea how they will affect us until much of the damage is already done. To deal more effectively with chemical sensitivities, our society needs to place a major emphasis on education.

WHEN DO CHEMICAL SENSITIVITIES BEGIN?

Many chemically sensitive people begin having their problems within one to three years after a major stress in their life. Symptoms may begin after a move into a renovated office, a brand new home, after a root canal, or following repeated pesticide exposure. It is important to know when a person who is now ill with chemical sensitivities was last feeling really well. What was his or her lifestyle like (diet, home, and work environments) at the time of becoming ill? Were there any unusual stresses? It is important to sift through other exposures for clues such as hobbies, home furnishings, hidden pesticides, cooking utilities, industrial and traffic exposure.

WHY DO SYMPTOMS VARY WITH DIFFERENT INDIVIDUALS?

The total burden of toxins on the body is never the same at any two moments. Symptoms may fluctuate and appear inconsistent. Also, two people may have very different symptoms to the same environmental toxins. There can be problems depending on which chemical exposure occurs on any given day. Any number of defects or deficiencies can keep the body from ridding itself of these toxic chemicals and leaving high levels that might not cause any symptoms to another individual. There might be throat spasms after being exposed to auto exhaust in traffic. The environmental overload from the car exhaust is just one factor. If the individual wasn't also deficient in magnesium, the resulting symptoms probably would not be spasms.

Diet and Chemically Sensitive Persons

A major factor affecting the chemically sensitive individual is the diet. Food sensitivities have a profound influence on symptoms. They may be due to digestive enzyme activity, acid-alkaline balance, a nutrient deficiency, and abnormal gut flora. Chronic prostatitis and vaginitis, colitis, arthritis, and many more symptoms often improve after the identification of hidden food sensitivities. People appearing to be chemically sensitive may find out that the real cause of their problem is dust or mold. Once you are supersensitive, it only takes a toxic overload to set you up for the next chemical exposure.

Many people with various forms of severe arthritis have a reduction in pain and symptoms after avoiding all red meat and the nightshade family (potatoes, peppers, tomatoes, eggplant, chili, paprika, pimento, cayenne, and tobacco) for one month. Chronic nasal and chest congestion usually decrease or disappear after the discontinuation of all milk products and wheat. Many symptoms disappear with the elimination of fermented and aged foods, as well as sugar, from the diet. For milder forms of chemical sensitivity, a change in diet may be all that is necessary.

Starting Treatment

Learning how to reduce the total toxic burden on the body can have a major role in determining whether any symptoms manifest. The best treatment for chemically sensitive people is an education in avoidance, environmental controls, attention to the diet, inhalant desensitization such as to dust and mold, along with the correction of identified nutrient deficiencies. Some deficiencies take longer than others to correct since frequently more than one mineral is abnormally low. With improved education, other health problems usually improve as well.

Chemically sensitive people are often deficient in taurine, a common amino acid. Supplementing taurine can make a dramatic difference in some heart problems, seizures, recurrent infection, or inflammation. Other nutrients and amino acids can help the body detoxify from paints, solvents, adhesives in new carpet glue, gasoline, and room deodorizers. This is a solid treatment program for most people and can bring a respectable number of chemically sensitive people some relief within a few weeks or months.

The body becomes depleted of nutrients from all the chemical exposures. It has trouble ridding itself of this overload of toxins resulting in more sensitivities. Having sufficient nutrients is important to the detoxification of the body. Recovery also depends on how much damage there is to the detoxification pathways that carry these toxins out of the body (lungs, kidneys, intestinal tract, etc.). The earlier the recognition of chemical sensitivities, the less time it takes for recovery. Often, these cases have their diagnoses delayed by years because of physicians untrained in this field and their unwillingness to consider this type of treatment.

This may seem like an attempt to oversimplify chemical sensitivities, but it can be this simple. The first thing to do is remove the sufferer from the known offending substances. To heal, the body needs to rest by reducing the total burden on the body. This is the time for exposure to clean air, clean food, and clean water. That isn't easy to find these days, but following suggestions found in this book can help. Remember, you usually do not have to remove all the allergens, just reduce the total toxic burden on the body. Often, the diagnosis is the treatment. As you reduce the total load of stressors on the body, your symptoms will begin to decrease and recovery will begin.

CHAPTER 38

Dust, Mold, and Dander Control

HOUSE DUST

House dust may cause allergic symptoms, the same as pollens and animal dander. It is a complex mixture composed of the breakdown products of plants, animal dander and furs, synthetic material, molds, and fabrics. Allergic reactions may also be due to fragments of mites and their feces found in house dust. Keeping the house dust-free helps. Mattress stuffing, pillows, overstuffed furniture, comforters, quilts, and stuffed toys often contain large amounts of dust. Avoid damp and dusty places, especially attics, basements, closets, and storerooms.

The allergy-producing properties of dust increase after prolonged storage, even if the stored materials have been in wrappings for a long time. House dust can produce year-round symptoms, but usually the problem is worse during months when the house is closed and the furnace is operating. Reducing the quantity of dust in the house will effectively control your allergy problem.

You should have at least one dust-free room. The bedroom is usually best. It should contain a minimum of furniture. Fewer problems usually result when the furniture is made from wood, metal, or plastic. Bare floors and windows are preferable or use washable rugs and curtains. Avoid mattress pads, chenille-type bedspreads, comforters, fuzzy or wool blankets, heavy rugs, drapes, Venetian blinds, excess books and papers, stuffed toys, open bookcases, or old upholstered furniture. Avoid bedding or pillows that cannot be washed. Everything should first be taken from the room including floor coverings (if possible), curtains, drapes, etc. Take everything out of the closet.

If you have a hot-air heating system, you will need to cover the register outlet in the wall with several layers of glass or nylon. This will make a room-level filter. Wash the filter every few weeks. Replace furnace filters three or four times during the heating season to reduce dust. If there are no filters, then shut off the furnace to the allergic person's room and heat the room by other means. An alternative is to use cheese cloth or an old pantyhose to cover the vent, but change them frequently.

Initially, thoroughly clean the room including walls, woodwork, ceiling and floor. Clean the closet. Clean all surfaces with a moist or oiled cloth. Wax the floor with a thin layer of oil to hold down the remaining dust. Keep doors closed and put only washed clothing in the closet. Set up a clean bed in a cleaned room. Encase the mattress, pillows, and box springs in dust-proof covers. You can obtain these products from department stores or order from the companies listed in "Resources." Alternatively, use dacron pillows. Do not use feather-filled bedding.

It is preferable to clean the room every day, but if this is not possible then clean it at least twice a week. Use only freshly laundered linens. Wash blankets and bedspreads each week. Vacuum cleaners without exposed bags are more satisfactory since house dust can pass through the bag of the usual vacuum cleaner. Avoid using a broom or duster. Keep the windows and doors of your dust-proof room closed, if possible. Remove clothes and shoes before entering the room and store them somewhere else. Showering and washing the hair is also helpful before entering an allergen-free room. The following recommendations will help you to further minimize your exposure to house dust.

Suggestion 1: Vacuum regularly with a water-trap vacuum cleaner.
Reason: Water will trap dust picked up by the vacuum and prevent it from being discharged back into the air.

Suggestion 2: Clean air conditioning filters and vents often.
Reason: This will prevent dust build-up and dust distribution throughout the environment.

Suggestion 3: Use a damp or treated cloth when dusting.
Reason: A dry dusting cloth transfers dust from a surface into the air.

Suggestion 4: Clean the chimney regularly.
Reason: This reduces build-up of soot and dust that can cause allergic symptoms.

Suggestion 5: Use smokeless fuels and avoid burning wood.
Reason: This will reduce your exposure to dust, smoke, and mold spores.

Suggestion 6: Discourage smoking in your home, and avoid other smoke-filled environments.

Reason: Tobacco smoke aggravates allergy symptoms to dust and other inhalants.

Suggestion 7: When driving, close your windows and use air conditioning if necessary.

Reason: This reduces your exposure to environmental dusts, pollens, exhaust, and fumes.

Suggestion 8: If you must do the house cleaning, cover your mouth and nose with a damp handkerchief or a dampened surgical mask tied with strings.

Reason: When the dust is at a level high enough to cause symptoms, these masks can filter out most of the particles.

Suggestion 9: Use a bedspread to cover your bed during the day and remove it from your bedroom before going to bed.

Reason: This will keep the dust on the bedspread and not collect on your sheets and pillows.

Suggestion 10: Do not store things under the bed.

Reason: They collect dust.

Suggestion 11: Avoid open book shelves; enclose in glass.

Reason: Books collect dust and mold.

Suggestion 12: Avoid any food sensitivities.

Reason: This reduces the total allergen load on your system.

DUST MITES

Dust mites have droppings that contain a digestive juice that is a very potent allergen, making them one of the most common causes of allergy, along with animal dander, cockroach droppings, and grass pollen. Unless the dust mite levels are controlled, the allergy will be hard to treat. It is estimated that 30 million people have dust mite allergies and it may be a factor in 50 to 80 percent of asthmatics, as well as in cases of eczema, hay fever, and other allergic ailments. Some sufferers have sneezing episodes first thing in the morning, when making the beds, or doing housework, but feel better when going outside. Others have stuffed-up ears, especially during the winter.

A typical used mattress may contain from 100,000 to 10 million mites inside. They are so small that thousands of mites can be found in a single gram of house dust. These microscopic organisms feed on flakes of human skin and food debris in the dust. They also live in carpets and other furnishings, but beds are their prime habitat. They like warm, moist surroundings such as the inside of a mattress when someone's lying on it. A typical mattress is well stocked with skin flakes, fungi, and other foods fit for a mite.

Mites are related to the spider and tick. Under optimal conditions, the mites can grow from egg to adult in a month and live for about another month. They are most abundant in wet, moist areas, and least likely in very high and very dry areas. Steam cleaners can kill the mites. Commercial mite-killing fluids don't always get to the mites deep inside the mattress. Air ionizers also appear to be ineffective in dealing with them. The best solution seems to be lining the mattress and pillows in special plastic covers to separate the mites and sleeper. Clean the rugs weekly with a vacuum equipped with a good filter. Remove any bedroom carpeting or other mite-friendly furnishing. Avoidance is the key to dealing with any allergy problem, including dust mites.

Suggestion 1: To control dust mites, buy cotton or polyester covers for mattresses and pillows.
Reason: The highest concentration of dust mites is in the bedroom, especially in mattresses, carpeting, and pillows. These covers offer the comfort of sheeting with a dust- and mite-proof barrier.

Suggestion 2: The single most important factor in curbing dust mites is controlling the humidity.
Reason: Heat and low moisture appear to be the best prevention, and hot water washing will destroy mites in bedding. It is not the live mites that are inhaled, but the feces and carcasses. House dust contains an abundance of this material.

Suggestion 3: Use tannic acid and benzyl benzoate powder to kill mites.
Reason: Some chemicals are effective, but mites are often resistant to chemical measures. Sensitive individuals may not be able to tolerate these products.

Suggestion 4: Sleep on synthetic pillows.
Reason: Dust mites like synthetic pillows as much as those made from feathers or foam, but synthetic pillows are easier to wash.

Suggestion 5: Buy washable rugs, toys, and fabrics to use in the house.

Reason: Hot water kills dust mites and washes off dust. Remove carpets from the bedroom or use rugs that are washable. If carpets cannot be removed, spray them with a solution to deactivate the dust mite allergen. Be sure to wash bedding, including mattress pads, bedspreads, and blankets weekly in hot water. It is one of the best ways to kill dust mites.

Suggestion 6: When cleaning, cover your mouth and nose with a dampened surgical mask tied with strings.

Reason: When the dust is at a level high enough to cause symptoms, these masks can filter out most of the particles from dust mites.

MOLD

Airborne mold spores are more numerous than pollen grains. When inhaled, they can produce allergic reactions. High humidity and warmth encourage mold growth. Keep the humidity below 35 percent. Use an exhaust fan to remove the excess humidity that results from cooking and showering. The most common place to find mold is in the basement and near the shower.

If you have sensitivity to mold, but not a chemical sensitivity, a fiber-filled pillow such as terylene, kodel, or dacron is better than foam. Foam pillows tend to become moldy. You can protect the pillow with allergen-proof encasing. If you have a problem with dust or mold, and are also chemically sensitive, then use a double pillow case. Wash pillow cases two times a week or daily if your symptoms are very severe.

Hot steam automatically kills molds; cold steam does not. Using a hot-steam vaporizer eliminates the mold problem. Be sure to use distilled water. Since heating systems rob air of vital moisture, humidifiers are important to correct this problem. However, these can also become mold- and dust mite-spawning areas. Be sure to check and clean mold from humidifiers and vaporizers. Wear a face mask if there is no other way to avoid exposure.

If someone awakens in the morning having symptoms such as a headache, nasal congestion, bronchitis, or asthma, then expose a petri dish in the bedroom. Take the petri dish to your doctor who can have a laboratory grow and identify the fungi causing the problem. The following recommendations will help to minimize your exposure to mold: .

Suggestion 1: Eliminate dampness in your home. Check walls and roof for leaks. Waterproof walls and ceilings before painting. Check outdoor rain spouts for good drainage away from the house.

Reason: Mold thrives in damp conditions. Garbage pails, shower curtains, and damp basements are ideal places for mold. Any place where it is damp, warm, or dark with poor ventilation probably contains mold.

Suggestion 2: Do not wallpaper; paint instead. Mold-resistant paint can be obtained from Sherwin-Williams.
Reason: Mold grows on wallpaper and in wallpaper paste.

Suggestion 3: Avoid carpets as floor covering. Replace carpets with wood floors, vinyl, ceramic tile or terrazzo. Do not use carpeting in the bath-room.
Reason: Mold grows in carpet pile. Carpets also trap dust that can cause allergic reactions.

Suggestion 4: Allow good air circulation in closets. Leave space between hanging clothes and check leather clothing, belts, shoes, and luggage for signs of mold growth.
Reason: Mold grows in damp, enclosed environments, especially on leather items.

Suggestion 5: Keep bathrooms and laundry rooms well aired. After taking clothes from the washer, dry them as soon as possible. Spread out tow-els and washcloths for fast drying. Ventilation is extremely important in controlling household mold.
Reason: Mold grows rapidly in damp conditions and on damp fabrics.

Suggestion 6: Regularly inspect bathrooms and laundry rooms for mold growth. Look for evidence of discoloration in the tile grout and caulk-ing. Don't forget to check under sinks, around the commode, shower curtains, and shower-door runners. Pick up bath mats and dry after use.
Reason: You probably realize by now that mold thrives in damp environ-ments. Dissolve white vinegar or borax in warm water to clean surfaces containing mold.

Suggestion 7: In humid conditions use air conditioning or a dehumidifier.
Reason: Mold does not grow well in dry environments. Indoor mold levels are proportional to the relative humidity. It is amazing how much water will be eliminated each day with the use of air conditioning or a dehumidifier.

Suggestion 8: Avoid foods that contain mold or are related to mold such as mushrooms, yeast-containing foods, fermented meats and pickles,

smoked fish and meats, or blue cheese. Other foods to avoid are fermented beverages, dried and candied fruits, cheeses in general, and vinegar.
Reason: Inhalant allergy symptoms can be aggravated by foods that are related to or contain mold. Also, avoid any food intolerance to reduce the total allergen load on the system.

Suggestion 9: Look for mold growing on the leaves or in the soil of house plants. Charcoal can be sprinkled on top of the soil to control mold. Clean and dust leaves regularly.
Reason: Greenhouses, sunrooms, atriums, or other areas of the house that contain house plants are major sources of mold.

Suggestion 10: Avoid old dust found in attics and unoccupied buildings.
Reason: Old layers of dust are full of mold. Throw out any old newspapers, magazines, or old furniture that might harbor mold. Avoid anything that smells musty because this smell is produced by mold.

Suggestion 11: Clean and check the basement regularly for mold. If the basement humidity exceeds 50 percent, use a dehumidifier.
Reason: Basements are notorious for the presence of mold. Correct any situation that causes standing water.

Suggestion 12: Check the drip pan of self-defrosting refrigerators regularly. Check for mildew on refrigerator seals. Clean these areas at least monthly.
Reason: Refrigerators are often forgotten sources of mold. Certain bacteria thrive in the drip pan under frost-free refrigerators and in the front grates of air-conditioners and humidifiers. Do not allow molded fruits, vegetables, or leftovers to remain in the refrigerator.

Suggestion 13: Do not keep fireplace logs in the house.
Reason: Tree bark has mold growing on it. The rough surface probably harbors dust and pollens.

Suggestion 14: Never put damp clothing or towels into a hamper or closet. Do not leave wet clothes in the washing machine. Keep the lid of the washing machine open when not in use.
Reason: Soiled, damp clothes in hampers or washers can produce mold.

Suggestion 15: Check for leaks under waterbeds.
Reason: The rugs and flooring beneath waterbeds are prime spots for mold growth.

Suggestion 16: Do not use a humidifier unless absolutely necessary.
Reason: Humidifiers frequently grow mold and dispense spores into the surrounding air. The humidifier should be cleaned frequently.

Suggestion 17: Avoid storing upholstery, sleeping bags, pillows, mattresses, and bedding in areas that are exposed to dampness.
Reason: The chances of being exposed to mold on these items are high.

Suggestion 18: Remove your shoes or clothing when entering the house.
Reason: Mold is frequently brought into the house on work clothing, shoes, and boots. The work clothes should be removed and left outside the house or removed and put inside a container for transport to the washing machine.

Suggestion 19: Avoid outdoor activities such as raking, burning, or jumping in leaves. Do not spread compost, hay, or sawdust. Avoid cleaning debris from gutters, mowing grass, or other clean-up chores in the yard. Yet, keep the exterior of the home free of leaves and debris. Have someone else do these chores. If you must rake leaves, do so when they are damp from dew or rain to avoid stirring up the mold and dust on them. Dampening any area of the garden where you plan to work will hold down dust and mold in the air. Of course, it will contribute to more mold growth.
Reason: Exposure to a high level of yard mold could bring on allergic symptoms.

Suggestion 20: Avoid sweeping porches, basements, and garages.
Reason: Approximately one-third of cement dust contains mold.

Suggestion 21: Do not store things under the bed.
Reason: Mold easily collects under the bed.

Mold Inhibitors

Use soap and water and wash thoroughly, scrubbing with a brush if possible. Bleach will kill mold, but people who are sensitive to chlorine or other chemical sensitivities should avoid it. If your mold allergy is severe, you may need to change your sheets twice a week, the pillowcases daily, and wash clothes after each wearing.

Impregon is a mold inhibitor especially useful for mold allergies. Use Impregon solutions for fabrics such as diapers, shower curtains, small rugs, towels, bedding, clothing, and drapes. Also use it on surfaces such as shower stalls, bathtubs, shoe linings, air conditioning filters, lockers, tile, concrete and hardwood floors, wallpaper and fixtures. Zephiran will kill mold for up to three months. A suggested dilution is two tablespoons to one gallon of water. It has no odor when diluted and is available at drugstores. All chemically sensitive persons will need to use caution when applying products for dust and mold control. The manufacturers do not usually consider that chemically sensitive people may need to use their products.

An excellent vegetable and fruit rinse is grapefruit-seed extract. It is a bactericide and fungicide. Using grapefruit-seed extract in low concentrations will extend the shelf life of fruits and vegetables by as much as 400 percent. For home rinsing use seven to eight drops of the extract in a gallon of rinse water.

Charcoal on top of the dirt in house plants will help retard mold growth. Buy charcoal at fish aquarium supply stores or in health-food stores. Add taheebo (an herb) as a tea to house plant water to retard mold in the potting soil. Taheebo is also available at health-food stores. Borax sprinkled in moldy places will retard mold growth. Mix borax and water in a spray bottle and wash the walls of your shower or bathroom. Let it dry on the walls to prevent mold growth.

ANIMAL DANDER

Animal hair may not be the cause of your sensitivity, but is instead caused by flakes of dead skin called dander. Animals, including humans, shed their dander into the air. It is light, airy, and floats about freely. Even days after the removal of the animal, dander may remain in the area. There can be a sensitivity to animal saliva as well. Symptoms could include difficulty breathing, hives, headaches, loss of voice, sneezing, and itching or watering eyes.

Suggestion 1: If possible, keep all household pets outside.
Reason: This reduces your exposure to allergy-causing dander. Cat and dog dander and saliva are extremely potent allergens. Many people develop symptoms after being licked by an animal. Saliva can even cause a reaction after it dries on the fur.

Suggestion 2: Vacuum regularly, preferably with a water-trap vacuum.
Reason: This removes dander from the immediate environment.

Suggestion 3: Avoid clothing made from animal fur.
Reason: Animal skins shed dander even after being made into clothing.

Suggestion 4: Avoid feather or down-stuffed clothing, pillows and comforters.
Reason: Feathers contain bird dander that can cause symptoms. Many people are sensitive to chicken, goose, and duck feathers. The feathers of
canaries, parakeets, pigeons, parrots, turkeys, and sparrows rarely produce reactions.

Suggestion 5: Bathe your family pets regularly.
Reason: It is best to begin regular baths when animals, especially cats, are
very young. Never groom animals in the house and never by the person
who is having the symptoms.

Suggestion 6: Air cleaners remove animal dander and hair from the air.
Reason: Animal dander can spread throughout the house by forced heating
or cooling systems. Homes that never housed animals can still contain
dander. Because of the lightness of dander, it can drift long distances and
contaminate your environment.

Suggestion 7: Try fish and reptiles for pets.
Reason: If you are allergic to most pets with fur then perhaps a pet without
fur would be appropriate. Some dogs have hair or dander that cause few
problems. There are also cats available without much, if any, hair.

FILTERS & AIR CLEANERS

Replace or clean furnace filters three or four times during the heating
season to reduce dust. Use air filters made with activated charcoal, metal,
or glass wool (untreated), but without hexachlorophene or oil derived from
petroleum. If the furnace has no filters, it would be best to shut it off to
the allergic person's room and heat that room by other means. If this is not
possible, use cheese cloth or an old pantyhose to cover the vent. Changing
the covering frequently can provide some relief. If this doesn't help, seal off
the heat vents and use an electric hot-water portable heater. The most
highly regarded mechanical filter is the HEPA (High Efficiency Particulate
Air), or "absolute" filter. These filters have a deep bed of randomly posi-
tioned fibers with a very large total thickness. The air flow passages are not
straight, but very tortuous with twists and turns. Particles adhere to the
fibers causing the passages to become smaller and filtration efficiency
increases. These filters do not degrade in efficiency through use. They are
capable of filtering over 99 percent of all bacteria, pollen, and dust particles. The operating life of these filters is two to five years. This makes
HEPA filters the most desirable of all air filters.

Another method using HEPA filters is the duct-cleaning system. Once the duct system has been cleaned at the source by a technician, they reseal' all access holes and your ducts are returned to "like new" condition. Check with your local heating and air-installation people for more information.

Central air conditioning poses a difficult problem because of the duct systems. Metal ducts may be lined with fiberglass that are sealed at joints and attached with very volatile adhesives. Do not use plastic or plastic-lined duct work, fiberglass duct work, oil-treated filters, or hexachlorophene filters. Exercise great care in the selection of materials for the air conditioning of the home, and buy window units equipped with filters that do not use volatile oil or chemical agents.

Many people are using air cleaners to protect themselves from inhalant allergies. Many firms are producing these products. A reputable manufacturer will provide a written money-back guarantee or a free trial period. Get a unit that filters out the smallest particle size from the air; less than .3 microns, if possible. Charcoal doesn't filter out formaldehyde.

Electronic air cleaners are the most common type of cleaner. Many newer electrostatic air cleaners will help keep dust and mold from accumulating in central air systems. They are also very effective in removing pollens, yeast, bacteria, viruses, and fungi from the breathable air. They work even better when used in conjunction with charcoal filters to remove small chemical particles. These filters use alternate polarity and self-charging layers of substaces, such as polypropylene filtration media, to attract very small particles. Reports vary on the effectiveness of this type of cleaner. The following facts may make these units less desirable than the HEPA filters:

• The efficiency of home units can decrease over time.
• Their efficiency decreases with larger particles such as plant pollens.
• Electronic units produce ozone that may have negative effects.
• They must be cleaned and replaced frequently to preserve efficiency.
• Particles that pass through the unit, without being captured, are electrostatically charged and cause additional problems in the room.
• Every time there is an electrical arcing, efficiency is lost and particles are released into the room.
• Air filtration systems only affect the air that passes through them. Much of the air will not get to the filter on a regular basis.

Negative ion generators produce negative ions that are dispersed into the room, they combine with particles in the air, imparting a negative charge to them. These charged particles are attracted to and held by walls, floors, or anything that carries a positive charge. They share some of the inconveniences produced by the electrical systems mentioned above.

There is another type of air cleaning device that works by combining radio frequency ionization with activated oxygen. It is called "Living Air" by Alpine Industries. The claim is that activated oxygen, or ozone, is a natural disinfectant that kills bacteria, mold, yeast and fungi. When ozone is at very low and safe levels it can keep the air healthy and pure. The ozone interacts with moisture and makes small amounts of hydrogen peroxide, also a disinfectant. This provides a double disinfectant benefit. Ozone is also an oxidizer. Many chemicals and hundreds of other substances are rendered safe by this breakdown. Its action breaks down smells and reduces pollutants. These units also remove particulate matter, but not through filtration. It uses ionization. The process involves energy pulses (radio wave ions) emitted from within each purifier unit. These units charge particles/molecules as the power wave passes them, up to sixty feet away. These newly-charged ions have a magnetic-like attraction to nearby pollutants making the combinations too heavy to stay in the breathable air and the pollutants begin to settle to the floor. These waves are not harmful to humans, animals, plants, or other electronic devices. See the sections "Resources" for more information on Alpine Industries.

Chemical filters act upon chemical substances in the air such as ozone and other gases, vapors, and irritants. Activated carbon or charcoal makes the best known chemical filters. They remove certain offending chemicals by trapping them on the charcoal's surface area. Use activated charcoal filters to control minute chemical odors. They absorb fumes from cooking, tobacco, and perfume, but perform less effectively against pollen or mildew. Charcoal filters are almost worthless protection against powerful odors such as formaldehyde. Avoid filters made of fiberglass or asbestos. In the kitchen it helps to have an efficient fan, filter, and vent system.

Face masks can be a life saver. You can also get cartridge masks that protect against a specific irritant. An air cleaner protects most other members of the family from illness after painting or cleaning, if there is good ventilation. It does not protect the person working directly over the fumes, so a face mask may be the answer. Safety supply companies listed in the yellow pages will assist you in selecting the right equipment for your needed protection.

VACUUM CLEANERS

Vacuum the house daily. Give special attention to the bedroom of the allergic person. Cylinder or canister vacuum cleaners are more useful for dust-allergic people because the upright air bag type may leak dust back into the air. To check for dust leaks, run the vacuum cleaner in a dark place and use a flashlight to sight any escaping dust. The following are other hints to follow when vacuuming:

- Replace the vacuum cleaner bag frequently.
- Do not ask a dust-sensitive person to vacuum. They should be out of the room, and ideally out of the house, when the vacuum cleaner is on.
- Dusting should be done with a vacuum attachment.
- Damp mopping and damp dusting may collect whatever the vacuum missed.
- Watch for deodorant pads on vacuum cleaners (Electrolux, for example) that contain perfumes.

Buying a good cylinder vacuum is an excellent idea, but there are also some interesting "alternative" vacuums on the market:

- The Filter Queen was invented during World War II to clean up radium dust. It has an inside cone that does not permit dust particles to travel.
- The Rex-Air Rainbow catches dust in water rather than in a conventional bag. The dust cannot escape and is removed with the water. Use the Rex-Air Rainbow as a humidifier and deodorizer. Finding a local distributor may be a problem.
- Central vacuum systems are ideal. Permanently install them in the house. They contain a powerful motor with a dust-free central collection exhaust. This directs the dust outdoors into a container.
- Regina Electric is an inexpensive solution. It keeps dust from flying out by collecting it in a plastic cup, not in a bag.

Most cities now have services available for cleaning duct work for forced air furnaces. This not only helps keep walls and curtains from becoming soiled quickly during winter, but it also helps alleviate dust sensitivities. Consult your yellow pages under "Furnaces--Repairing and Cleaning." Spring is the ideal time to have this type of work done since the furnace is not being used. The demand in autumn for service is usually high.

The HEPA-Aire method is a technician-hired method to clean your ducts with a portable power vacuum and the Aire-Sweep compressor. This system can reach and thoroughly clean your entire duct system. It pulls dislodged contaminants 1/300 the diameter of a human hair and returns filtered "hospital grade" air to your home. After cleaning your duct's system, they reseal all access holes and return your ducts to like-new condition.

Check with your local heating and air conditioning installation people to see if they provide this service.

VAPORIZERS AND OTHER AIDS

Many people find that cold-steam vaporizers help during an asthma attack more than hot-steam vaporizers. Before using a cold-steam vaporizer, be sure to clean it with a fungicide; otherwise you will be distributing mold into the air. Hot steam is usually helpful for chemically sensitive patients. Remember, hot steam automatically kills mold and cold steam does not. Be sure to use distilled water.

Don't forget that heating systems rob air of vital moisture. This is especially bad for those with respiratory ailments. Humidifiers are important to use. Remember to check and clean mold from humidifiers with a mold inhibitor like Zephiran.

There is a type of furnace called a converter that works like a refrigerator's coil. In warm weather, it collects hot air and releases it outside. In cold weather, it collects cold air and releases it outside. It is effective to 20 degrees Fahrenheit. Use supplemental electrical heat for lower temperatures.

Air conditioning is effective at reducing pollen in the air. It is also helpful with dust mites and mold because they do not thrive in a low humidity atmosphere. Keep the unit and filter clean to discourage the growth of mold. Catalytic converters or other emission-control devices can be added to wood stoves and kerosene heaters.

CHAPTER 39

Indoor Air Pollution

I ndoor air quality is the single most significant environmental issue we face today. The EPA says that indoor air pollution is more of a threat to good health than outdoor pollution. Indoor pollution levels can be up to 100 times greater than outdoor air. When buildings are air tight, the air inside becomes toxic. This toxic air can lead to an increase in absenteeism, behavior problems, reduction in learning, multiple chemical sensitivities, and other illnesses. Such results come mostly from volatile organic chemicals such as formaldehyde present in carpeting, paneling, cabinets, fabrics, and paint. Reduce pollution with the proper air filtration system, better ventilation, or inform yourself about less toxic products. The quality of the indoor air we breathe has become an increasingly important environmental concern. Authorities in environmental pollution have determined the following facts:

• People are spending 60-90 percent of their time indoors.
• Polluted indoor air is aggravating or causing half of all illnesses.
• The reported number of people suffering from allergies is more than 50 million.
• Fungi or bacteria in airduct systems may cause allergies in one out of every six people who suffer from allergies.
• Asthma is on the increase in this country, numbering from 10 to 12 million people.
• The elderly and children are most affected by polluted indoor air.

Since most people spend the majority of their time indoors, it is more likely that toxins in your house will make you sick. The worst pollutants in the home are gas and oil heat, pesticides, formaldehyde, foam rubber, and dry-cleaned clothes. The typical house harbors over 100 chemicals at concentrations up to forty times greater than outdoor levels. The average house also contains hundreds of toxic construction materials. You need to care for your house's health as you would for your body's health.

Dust, smoke, mold, odors, and mildew are just some of the indoor pollutants easy to see and smell, but there are substances such as gases, pollen, and bacteria that are difficult to detect. After the energy crisis of the 1970s, buildings were insulated and sealed more tightly. This may have saved energy, but it trapped many pollutants inside. Perfumed air sprays and air wicks were then introduced to cover up the odors produced by these airtight environments.

This pollution has an impact on productivity, health, and the well-being of many people. The risks posed by inhaling the air at home, at school, in public buildings, or at work can exceed the limits used to regulate pollutants in outdoor air. Respiratory allergies offer a challenge occurring with greater and greater frequency for those who live in cities. It affects the respiratory passages and immune system and contributes to many days lost from work. It causes a decrease in vitality that has a significant effect on the economy and personal well-being. The EPA says indoor pollution is one of the top ten health hazards in some areas.

Where Does Air Pollution Come From?

Indoor air pollution originates mainly from the volatile organic chemicals present in carpeting, paneling, cabinets, fabrics, and paints, as well as from building materials, furnishings, and other consumer products. A very high percentage of pollutants comes from the materials used in newly constructed or remodeled buildings. Materials such as particle board, carpet glue, adhesives, caulking, sealants, and finishes add fumes to the air. These are joined by pollutants from pesticides, waxes, polishes, disinfectants, deodorizers, solvents, office machines, and cleaning materials. The three most common pollutants are formaldehyde, benzene, and trichloroethylene.

We are also exposed to tobacco smoke and combustion appliances that are not operated and vented properly. This causes substantial build-up of indoor air contaminants. Other major indoor air pollutants may be radon, asbestos, carbon monoxide, nitrogen oxides, biological aerosols, particulate matter, and carbon dioxide. When these pollutants combine with other synthetic materials, cleaning agents, pesticides, perfumes, or printing and copying devices, the indoor air quality quickly becomes a hazardous place.

Volatile organic toxins have one important thing in common. They are all fat or lipid soluble. This means they have an affinity for the fatty tissues of the body, of which the brain is the prime target. There are now about 70,000 chemicals used in commerce; several hundred are known to be toxic to the brain and the nervous system. Symptoms might include dizziness, forgetfulness, headaches, mental fogginess, and poor coordination. Many people also have symptoms of anxiety, social alienation, poor concentration, and learning and memory impairment. It is common to find fatigue, lethargy, hyperactivity in children, and irritation of the eyes, ears, nose, and throat. Symptoms may be flu-like illnesses, nausea, and skin irritations. Overall, these chemicals decrease the immune function and increase your susceptibility to other diseases.

Sources of Carbon Monoxide

Carbon monoxide (CO) is an odorless, invisible, and potentially deadly gas, responsible for about 1,500 deaths each year. Any appliance that burns fuel can be a source of carbon monoxide, including the gas clothes dryer, kitchen range, gas or wood-burning fireplace, furnace, and portable heater. Toxic levels can build up from clogged chimneys, leaking fuels, and disconnected vent pipes.

This gas readily replaces oxygen in the body. Symptoms connected to low levels of carbon monoxide poisoning can resemble the flu or produce nausea, headaches, dizziness, and fatigue. If several members of the household feel ill at the same time, or if you feel better when away from the house for several hours, suspect carbon monoxide gas. Levels of about 40 percent can cause brain damage and death.

SICK SCHOOL SYNDROME

Many of our schools today are suffering from "sick school syndrome." It is sad to think that the institutions which nurture our children may be a culprit in their learning disabilities. Poor grades don't always reflect learning and teaching skills. Each day, students and teachers are unnecessarily exposed to hundreds of hidden chemicals. Cleaning products, pesticides, paints, and perfumes contain substances that can trigger serious behavior, health, and learning problems. All chemicals used in construction, furnishings, housekeeping, maintenance, pest control, food services, and classroom activities can and do affect indoor air quality. This affects the health of the students and teachers. Indoor pollution, as the real source of illness, usually goes undetected or incorrectly diagnosed.

In 1984 in Chicago, students became sick from pesticide fumes. In Palm Beach in 1986, thirty-five children became sick from pesticide fumes causing the school to close for a while. In 1987 a school in Indiana closed because of "sick school syndrome." By the next year even more schools had health problems because of pesticide use. By 1990, there were articles in all the major papers about children becoming sick from pesticides or other pollutants found in and around the schools. How do children learn in an environment that can also make them sick? Symptoms vary from feeling faint, headaches, black-outs, eczema, fatigue, numbness, inability to concentrate, slurred speech, irritability, multiple chemical hypersensitivity, asthma, insomnia, sore throats, depression, disorientation, and respiratory problems.

More and more schools now install synthetic carpeting without realizing how it contributes to poor indoor air quality. Carpets will outgas formaldehyde, toluene, xylene, benzene, styrene, mold inhibitors, fire retardants, dirt-repellent coatings, pesticides, and other potent chemicals. This outgassing may continue for years after installation. Carpets also support the growth of mold and dust mites. Janitorial supplies often receive little scrutiny in the schools. One of the schools investigated used as many as twenty-eight different products. More than sixteen products routinely used during school hours emitted toxic fumes.

We place our children in these classrooms and buildings for eight hours a day, five days a week. During this time, they breathe in chemicals, paints, pesticides, toxic cleaning fluids, office machinery fumes, molds, etc. Add to this mix the poor diet that most children eat today. Their bodies and brains are starving for nutrients. Chemicals, heavy metals, and contaminated air and water can all cause a child's immune system to become damaged which, in turn, can increase their sensitivity to certain foods. Should we be surprised when the child develops a learning disability?

Environmentally hypersensitive children often have many symptoms that defy diagnosis. Conventional physicians do not receive training to detect environmental factors that can change a child's behavior and energy level. They do not understand, nor accept, that an allergy or sensitivity can affect any organ or body system, including the brain. That is why it is very important that concerned parents and teachers educate themselves about classroom dangers and the symptoms they cause. Special workshops can empower educators, parents, and students with the needed skills to make schools safe. Their workshops teach how to identify the types of chemicals present in the schools and their potential threat to a student's health and learning. They also help you develop practical strategies to cure the contaminated classroom. For more information about workshops contact Irene Ruth Wilkenfeld at (219) 271-8990 or write to her at 52145 Farmington Square Road, Granger, Indiana 46530.

SICK BUILDING SYNDROME

Formaldehyde is the most common cause of "sick building syndrome." When it is emitted from manufactured goods in its gaseous form, it is a pollutant of indoor air. Plywood, particle board, carpets, fabrics, and many other products contain formaldehyde.

The EPA pointed out that high energy costs encourage the development of tight buildings with poor ventilation. The use of so many chemicals, along with synthetic materials, cleaning agents, pesticides, perfumes, and printing and copying machines can cause "sick building syndrome."

In "sick building syndrome," look for buildings that have high occupant density. Improper ventilation along with a high occupancy causes high levels of carbon dioxide levels in work areas and not enough oxygen. If new carpets are installed with no fresh-air ventilation, some people will not be able to work without getting sick. Poor indoor air quality may affect 800,000 to 1.2 million commercial buildings in the United States. About one billion dollars are lost every year due to sick leave, lost earnings and productivity.

Control the Source of Pollution

The most effective control method of indoor air quality is source control. This means the elimination, isolation, reduction, containment, or removal of the source of the pollution. It is important to identify and avoid the aggravating agents and correct the underlying susceptibility to these reactions. It also involves the removal by exhaust ventilation of pollutants generated within the building and an increase in a healthy air supply. You need some sort of filtration system to remove particulate or gaseous contaminants and to keep ventilation systems and furnace filters clean and well maintained. Other important sources of indoor air pollution come from outdoor air. They include dust, pollens, mold, animal dander, insect parts, and fumes from vehicles and industries. High indoor humidity increases the levels of dust mites, molds, and microbes. Other possibilities are the lack of full-spectrum lighting, stress, or being exposed to different electromagnetic radiations (x-ray, microwave, television, radio, computers). It often takes much investigation to pinpoint what is making an individual sick.

Every day the average person breathes in an average of two heaping tablespoons of dust, pollen, bacteria, viruses, and other airborne pollutants. The most efficient forced-air heating and air conditioning units only remove about 7 percent of the dust that flows through it. The remaining 93 percent of the dust, and almost all of the bacteria and other micro-pollutants, are recirculated through the building. Installing efficient air filters may be the only solution.

Store any odor-producing products in a separate building away from the living quarters. This includes products such as paints, solvents, insecticides, glues, cleaning supplies, wood and shoe polish. Substitute safer products and store toxins far away from your living area. Tightly seal storage containers. Don't leave your car running in an attached garage.

It is difficult to compile facts concerning what housing should be like for the allergic and chemically sensitive individual. Each sufferer has particular needs and tolerances. What may be just right for one person may not be helpful for another. The following information may be helpful in determining the sources of indoor pollution that affects you.

Basements: Radon gas can accumulate in sealed basements. High humidity increases mold and mildew.

Bedroom: Remove as many allergens as possible from your bedroom: carpet, shoes, cosmetics, dry-cleaned clothes, foam cushions, vinyls, and soft plastics.

Building Materials: Stainless-steel counter tops are preferable in the kitchen, but Formica tops are usually tolerated by the majority of people. A standard cement is acceptable for use with Formica and usually does not cause problems if the seal is good. Formica cabinet facing could also be used or hardwood cabinets.

The best flooring is terrazzo or ceramic tile. Some ceramic tile floors need a filler or surface treatment. Avoid these types. The next best type of flooring appears to be a hardwood floor with a varnished surface. The varnish will cause less trouble if it is allowed to dry thoroughly before the house is occupied. It may take nine to twelve months to gas out completely so it can be a real problem for a severely sensitive person. Avoid all floor waxes.

The next best type of flooring is a vinyl floor, but it does give off vinyl chloride. This type of flooring does not need waxing, but it requires an adhesive. Do not use any tar or smelly adhesives or sponge-rubber sealer. Since environmental products are becoming more available, search for adhesives that are less toxic or without odors. Be careful when using adhesives with floors containing heating elements. This includes upstairs floors where there are heating elements in the ceiling above the first floor. They will evaporate into your breathable air for years.

Buy interior paneling that is made from non-odorous conifers. The use of a good grade of pine studding for walls seems satisfactory, but avoid knotty pine or other odorous woods. Do not use adhesives to attach paneling to walls because it may take up to two years for the glue to evaporate. Plywood used in sub-flooring, wall paneling, counter tops, kitchen cabinets, and furniture usually contains formaldehyde.

The use of plaster is better than dry wall because of the formaldehyde and other chemicals in the paper part of the dry wall. It would take three coats of an oil-based paint to help, but this takes months to completely dry. If dry wall is used and not sealed properly it will take time to gas out. Wallpaper that can be wiped clean has a plastic coating. Flocked patterns are synthetic. Commercial wallpaper paste contains fungicide and mold retardant chemicals.

Carpet: There should not be carpet in the bedroom of an allergic person. If you must use carpeting in the house, consider putting it in the living room only, but not in the bedrooms. It is the single largest source of allergens, mold, dust, and dander.

Charcoal: There are different types of charcoal. You may be allergic to any one or all of them, and unable to tolerate them in any filter or unit. Samples may be obtained from the company and tested for tolerance in your doctor's office (if they do this type of testing).

Cleaning Supplies: When cleaning, avoid all aerosol sprays. Use vinegar (one tablespoon per quart of water) for cleaning glass, mirrors, and stainless steel. It will remove detergent residues in shampooing or laundering. A damp or oiled cotton cloth is excellent for dusting. To disinfect use the antifungal and antibacterial product Zephiran diluted in water. Use biodegradable products for dish washing. See the "Resources" section for companies that supply nontoxic cleaning supplies.

Obtain organic fruits and vegetables whenever possible to avoid insecticides and pesticides. If this isn't possible, soak your produce thoroughly in products such as Shaklee's Basic H or Neo-Life Green. Put in warm water and rinse thoroughly.

Cooking Utensils: Use heat-resistant glass, stainless steel or cast-iron cookware. Avoid aluminum, copper or Teflon-coated types.

Emission Control: Control emissions where they originate. Choose less-volatile materials by buying solid wood furniture that contains much less formaldehyde than "wood-product" furniture made from particle board or chipboard. Loose cushion furniture with solid wood, metal, wicker or rattan frames will produce fewer emissions than fully upholstered furniture. Further reduce emissions by using tightly woven, washable, natural-fiber fabrics.

Read the labels on all products used in your home and follow directions. If they recommend use only with ventilation, then use only at a time when this direction can be followed. Usually, the more warnings on the product label the more risky the product. Look for less hazardous ones. Try to reduce the number of cleaning products used in the home. Don't use scented products to cover up odors, but ventilate instead.

Ducts, Filters, and Vents: A dirty duct system may be the major source of indoor air pollution. Dust, dirt, pollen, animal dander and other airborne contaminants are pulled into your duct system every time the furnace or air-conditioner runs. These contaminants build up inside the ducts over time and can help make your duct system an ideal breeding ground for mold spores, bacteria, fungus, mildew, and other microbes.

Fireplace: A fireplace is a collector of dust, wood molds, and smoke. Use a glass screen. Wood fires may backdraft when a door or window is opened, pulling smoke and gases back down the chimney and into the house. Fumes can even seep into your house from under the eaves from your neighbor's house.

Foundation: Do not use insecticides or oils under the foundation of the house. These products can be harmful to the people living inside. Avoid any cement containing calcium chloride. If cement blocks are used, be sure they do not contain synthetic materials. Radon gas from the soil may be present and stone foundations can allow the gas to seep into the house.

Garage: Under no circumstance should there be a passageway between the garage and any portion of the house. It is best to enter the garage by first going outdoors and then entering the garage. There should not be a common attic over the garage and the house. If the attic extends over both, a tight partition extending to the roof and separating the house from the garage is necessary.

Chemicals, solvents, garden supplies, and paints can produce contaminants that can be pulled into the house if it is attached to the garage. Store these volatile materials, as well as any detergents, cleansing agents, mops, insecticides, herbicides, waxes, bleach, and other odorous materials in a non-attached garage or other storage unit away from the house. If your garage and house are attached, don't let your car run while in the garage. The fumes are very toxic and can enter the home.

Heating Systems: Use electrical heating or a combustion of fossil fuels that are burned outside the living quarters of the house. Some units provide a gas forced-air furnace where the entire unit sits outside the house. An unattached garage is a good place. The stack of the chimney should be higher than the rest of the house or fumes from the chimney will enter the house. Gas or vapors will penetrate anything.

The type of fuel used can also cause problems for the chemically sensitive. Do not use gas, fuel oil, or coal in any area of the house. This means the basement, attic, or any portion of the house. If you have forced-air gas, it would be better to change to forced-air electric. Furnaces are prime problems for the allergic person because they create a lot of dust. Older gas furnaces can leak carbon monoxide. Kerosene heaters and gas appliances that are not vented properly can contribute nitrogen dioxide, carbon monoxide, and fine particles that cause respiratory illness.

House Site: If your house site is near a marsh or brook, expect mold.

Having a basement increases the risk of dampness and mold. Profuse vegetation surrounding the house can contribute to increased pollens. Landscape the yard with products and plants that do not increase your risk of allergens. A house built in an area of high winds can yield a very high pollen count.

A home located in a non-industrial area without major sources of air pollution is best. If the house is near an industrialized urban region, it needs to be on the windward side of such an area. Find a house set as far back from the road as possible. It would be best to have a house built on a side road with less traffic and not near a stoplight intersection.

Insulating Materials: Fiberglass and rockwood are good insulating materials, but the papers that surround these materials are often impregnated with undesirable substances. Black papers are not suitable. Never use polyethylene or plastic insulation. Do not use injected insulation because of high levels of formaldehyde fumes. Asbestos was used to insulate hot water and steam pipes, heat ducts, and furnaces. It may still be found in wall insulation, shingles, siding, and roofing. Asbestos is in some cements, ceiling tiles, old flooring, and commercial insulation.

Motors: Some people do better if the motor of refrigerating equipment is in a special utility room rather than sitting out in the kitchen.

Paint: When considering what type of paint to use, check with your environmentally friendly store to see what is the latest in nontoxic paint. If you can't find any information on these types of products, then at least avoid latex or other rubber-based paints as well as vinyl or acrylic paint. They are volatile for several months so do not use under any circumstances. The alkyl-based paints seem to cause the least trouble and are not diluted with mineral spirits or turpentine solvents.

If enamel paint is used inside the house be sure that it is allowed to dry thoroughly before occupancy of the house. Enamel paint used on woodwork must air out for some time. Paint should not contain moth repellents or anti-mold compounds, but it often contains mercury as a fungicide. Wall paints release solvents such as toluene, xylene, and benzene. Old paint on the walls, paint chips and dust containing lead may still be present in older homes. This could be a factor when moving into or renovating an older home.

Plants: Reduce pollution with certain plants. Many plants are effective air purifiers. NASA has done studies to find out which plants could remove toxic chemicals from the air in space stations. If you want to use them to clear the air then you need to put many of them into your home or work place. The plants that topped their list in clearing the air of formaldehyde, benzene, and trichloroethylene are:

Mass cane (*Dracaena massangeana*)
Banana (*Musa oriana*)
Ficus (*Ficus benjamina*)
English Ivy (*Hedera helix*)
Chinese Evergreen (*Algona* "silver queen")
Pot mum (*Chrysanthemum morifolium*)
Bamboo palm (*Chamaedorea seifrizii*)
Gerbera daisy (*Gerbera jamesonii*)
Marginata (*Dracaena marginata*)
Peace lily (*Spathiphylum* "Mauna Loa")
Mother-in-laws tongue (*Sansevieria laurentii*)
Janet Craig (*Dracaena deremensis*)
Green spider plant (*Chlorophytum elatum*)
Heart-leaf philodendron (*Philodendron oxycardium*)
Warnecki (*Dracaena deremensis*)

Roofs: Asphalt roofs directly outside windows with a southern exposure are often troublesome. Most slate shingles, wood shingles, ceramic tile, metal shingle, or metal roofs are satisfactory materials.

Ventilation: Adequate ventilation is critical in keeping pollutants under control. Pollution indoors can come from vapors, fumes and particles, carbon dioxide and other gases, or shedding hair and skin particles from pets. It can also come from scented and aerosol products, hair processing chemicals, hobbies, and even cooking. The products you use to rid your home of pollution and dirt can add other pollutants to the area. The new odors of fresh paint, new furniture, new carpet and other furnishings can cause enough vapors to cause severe symptoms. If you must add a new odorous product to your home, use extra ventilation to dilute and disperse the odor and vapors. Do not decorate at a time when you can't provide the proper ventilation with a continuous flow of fresh air.

The stove and clothes dryer must be ventilated. Exhaust fans can prevent the spread of moisture and product emissions. Do not use the kind of fans that simply blow emissions around indoors or circulate them throughout the house through the ventilating system. Vent all the way outdoors; don't just dump the pollutants into the attic or air return. Prevent mildew with heat, dryness, and fresh air circulation. It is important to the health and well-being of yourself and your family to have a well-ventilated, clean home. The home is the place where you can most easily control environmental exposures and protect your health.

Walkways and Driveways: Blacktop sidewalks and drives are more prone to creating volatile fumes, especially if the fumes can be transmitted into the house. Cement or gravel is far preferable.

CHAPTER 40

Environmental Toxicity: A Problem With Chemicals

The founding editor of *Prevention Magazine,* J.I. Rodale, once wrote that only those who protect themselves from the steadily increasing burdens of toxic environmental chemicals would survive in coming times. Environmental pollution is a serious problem facing us today. In the last 100 years we have witnessed the progressive poisoning of nature with the chemical by-products of modern agriculture, industry, power generators, and transportation. These chemical changes are not confined to just the local area of release. There is evidence of pollution everywhere on earth, from the largest cities to the remote South Pole.

Congress has passed a series of laws that seriously damage years of valuable health and environmental laws and regulations. They have seriously diluted the Clean Water Act, the Clean Air Act, the Safe Drinking Water Act, and the Meat and Poultry Products Inspection Acts. These laws are meant to protect the environment, thereby protecting us.

You may think that bad conditions don't exist in the United States, but they do. In 1993 hundreds of thousands of people fell ill from the bacteria cryptosporidium, which infected the city water system in Milwaukee. More than one hundred people died. In 1994 the Pacific Northwest had an incident of contaminated hamburger meat containing *E. coli.* Hundreds of people became ill and two children died. These incidents are happening more often in the United States. America needs stronger environmental laws and regulations to help protect our health and our future, not less. Congress is making it much harder to enact desperately needed new environmental regulations.

No toxicity data is available for over 39,000 commercially used chemicals. Of the 70,000 chemicals now in use, less than 10 percent have been tested for toxic effects on the nervous system. The Environmental Protection Agency (EPA) can provide safety assurances for only 6 out of 600 active pesticide ingredients that are under their control. The United

States Geologic Survey reports the presence of herbicides in rainwater samples taken in 23 states.

Some of the most common factors contributing to illness are the overuse of antibiotics, cortisone, birth control pills, and other drug-induced nutritional deficiencies. The constant exposure to chemicals, heavy metals, mercury amalgam fillings, toxic building materials, formaldehyde, cigarette smoke, pesticides and insecticides, and industrial toxins deplete our body's immune system. Low levels of toxins usually accumulate in the body over time. Increasingly, more people use and abuse recreational drugs, eat poorly, and experience constant mental, emotional, and spiritual stress. A compromised immune system causes more nutrient depletion leading to chronic disease and organ damage. Allergies and sensitivities are becoming much more common as a result.

Exposure to chemicals may only cause minor symptoms at first. Each health complaint usually gets treated as an isolated ailment instead of recognizing the underlying chemical poisoning that is really causing all the symptoms. If treatment of the underlying cause is delayed, the damage will continue. With the addition of suppressive drugs, the condition that started out with a simple solution has now become a serious problem. To give another chemical to an already compromised system just does not work. It just adds to the toxic load on the body. It is essential to find the underlying cause. The continued depletion of nutrients from the diet along with continued exposure to these toxins can only lead to illness.

Donald Dudley, M.D., in Seattle Washington, is researching the brain mapping of the chemically sensitive person. He can identify actual injury in the brain of sensitive individuals when exposed to common chemicals. He discovered that smelling something can obviously affect the brain. Chemically sensitive individuals can have a reduction in thinking, concentration, and memory. They may struggle with depression and fatigue, muscle weakness, as well as emotional problems. Unfortunately, the "medical authorities" have not wanted to look at his research. Their reluctance causes difficulty getting this information into the public forum. Contact the Well Mind Association for more information (see the "Resources" section).

The minimum time of exposure to a toxic substance to get a change in brain function is about thirty minutes, but the time to get over the exposure can take weeks. Being exposed every day to these toxic substances can cause continuous symptoms. Houses and buildings are more air tight then ever before increasing our exposure to toxic chemicals. You do not have to be aware of a chemical odor for damage to occur. Carbon monoxide is just as lethal without perception of its presence. Toxic scents are everywhere.

They are in cosmetics, household items, detergents, magazine advertising, body-care products, etc. There are over 5,000 components available to create fragrances. The majority of these ingredients have minimal testing for human toxicity, and some are never tested. The National Academy of Sciences reported that 95 percent of chemicals used in fragrances are synthetic compounds derived from petroleum. Many of these chemicals cause allergic reactions, birth defects, cancer, and central-nervous-system dysfunction. Methylene chloride is one of the twenty most common chemicals used in the manufacture of fragrance products. It is a known carcinogen and may cause autoimmune disease.

You really don't know what toxic chemicals, if any, are in some products. Most household products found in retail grocery stores contain harmful chemicals. Many cleaning products are so toxic they are regulated by the Federal Hazardous Substances Act. Many are toxic when absorbed through the skin or inhaled. Washing clothing or bedding in these household products is another source of contact. About 15 percent of this country's population experiences hypersensitivity to chemicals found in common household products. According to the National Institutes of Health, allergic reactions and hypersensitivity affect 35 million Americans.

The increasing burden of toxic chemicals in our air, food, and water is rapidly increasing both in frequency and severity. The immune system is being challenged in ways we never imagined. The body will store many of these toxins in the body reaching a toxic overload. It may be necessary to explore the possibility of chemical toxicity. Toxic chemicals can block your body's self-regenerative processes so that you can not achieve total wellness.

Because of the huge number of chemical toxins in our environment, the identification of a single chemical toxin in the body is almost impossible. There are over 70,000 chemicals in daily use in this country and specific testing is only available for about 250 of them. This forces us to rely on symptoms, basic blood work, and some other tests to identify a chemical overload. Some of the most common conditions and symptoms are:

Heart palpitations	Skin problems	Anxiety	Insomnia
Airborne sensitivities	Nerve problems	Joint pains	Depression
Food sensitivities	Nerve Pain	Mood swings	Fatigue
Chemical sensitivities	Abdominal pain	Ear congestion	Headaches
Low immune function	Tremors	Asthma	Nausea
Respiratory infections	Impaired thinking	Eczema	Constantly sick

Chemical toxins may trigger autoimmune problems. This is when the body builds antibodies against itself and then attacks itself. This includes diseases such as lupus and rheumatoid arthritis. Toxins can also affect the endocrine organs: the thyroid, adrenal glands, ovaries, and testes. There is a link between several cancers, such as sarcomas and certain types of lymphomas, and regular exposure to broad-leaf herbicides.

Environmental Toxins and Children

Children and developing fetuses are more vulnerable to the damaging effects of chemical poisons. A fetus could be as much as ten times more sensitive to chemical toxicity than an adult. Since children also have a greater ability to recuperate from injury than adults, there may still be hope that they can recover from such toxic overloads.

When fathers have occupational exposures to organic solvents, petroleum and chemical products, there may be an association with brain cancer and leukemia in the children. This may be the results of malformations in the sperm. Sperm and ova begin their maturation processes approximately three months before conception. The two most vulnerable periods to the developing sperm are about 90 days before conception when sperm replication is at its peak. Exposure to chemicals or radiation during this time increases malformation in the offspring as well as increasing cancers such as leukemia. The other period of vulnerability occurs immediately before conception. Drugs taken at this time can cause malformation, low birth weight, and stillbirths. Sperm can be a carrier for drugs such as cocaine. This can result in the malformation or birth mishaps to the fetus. It is important to avoid environmental chemicals during the preconception period.

Cancer of the testes has increased significantly. Environmental exposure to solvents such as benzene and butadiene may have contributed to these changes. Also, the use of cocaine, marijuana, and alcohol is associated with reduced sperm counts. As environmental pollution gets worse, infertility is likely to increase as well. The ultimate cost of not cleaning up the environment is that fewer children will be conceived.

Chemical Culprits

The following is a list of chemicals found in and around the home. They are often the culprits that cause the allergic symptoms.

ADHESIVES

Avoid cements and other adhesives. This includes fingernail polish and remover, shoe polish (use olive oil to remove marks and shine shoes), paint remover, and airplane or toy adhesives. Also avoid adhesives for floors that contain tars.

ALCOHOL

The following is a list of different alcohols and their uses:

Ethyl alcohol:
• forms as wine or hard cider by the fermentation of any sweet fruit juice
• may be made from molasses, potatoes, or grains; usually made from corn into industrial ethyl alcohol
• is an ingredient in tinctures and many toilet and drug preparations
• is used as body rubbing alcohol
• is used in making ether and sterilizing surgical instruments
• is used in making rubber

Amyl alcohol:
• is made from ethyl alcohol
• is used as a solvent

Isopropyl alcohol:
• is used in the manufacture of antifreeze, rubbing alcohol, and solvents

Glycerol:
• is used for sweetening and preserving food
• is used in the manufacture of cosmetics, perfumes, inks, and certain glues and cements
• is used in medical suppositories and skin preparations

Menthol:
• is used in perfumes, confections, liqueurs
• is used in medicine for colds and nasal disorders because of its cooling effect on mucous membranes

Alcohol is used in the preparation of:

• anesthetics	• explosives
• cleaning fluids	• formaldehyde plastics
• flavoring extracts	• rubber tires
• preservatives	• rubber overshoes
• acetic acid	• synthetic chemicals
• hand lotions	• paint, varnish and shellac
• perfumes	• rayon/nylon textiles
• Bakelite products	• toothbrushes
• dyes	• drugs
• photographic film	• soaps
• printer's ink	• disinfectants

AMMONIA

All-purpose cleaners, including window cleaners, may contain ammonia. It attacks the lungs when you breathe in the ammonia mist. Ammonia is a poison, but glass cleaning products do not carry any warning on the label. When chlorine, another common ingredient is also present, the combination can form a deadly chloramine gas.

CADMIUM

This heavy metal is a contaminant of tap water. Zinc used for galvanizing iron (tin roofs, pails, water storage tanks, iron pipes, gutters, nails and a variety of other products) can contain up to 2 percent cadmium. Zinc and copper smelters, as well as refiners, release more than two million pounds of cadmium into the air annually.

Cadmium is a neurotoxin suspected of causing mental retardation. Only a small amount of cadmium absorbs into the body when swallowed, but when we breathe in cadmium, about half is retained by the body. The cadmium in cigarettes is probably the primary source. Women who smoke during pregnancy have increased levels of cadmium in the placenta. This may be one of the causes of lower birth weights. There has been some speculation about a link between high blood pressure and cadmium toxicity.

CLEANING AND LIGHTER FLUIDS

If you are having your carpets cleaned, it is best to stay elsewhere for several days. Dry-cleaning chemicals can be a problem for sensitive individuals. Aerate clothes in the sun after picking up dry cleaning. Do not use lighter fluids in the house. Check natural product companies for less toxic chemicals whenever possible.

CHLORINATED SOLVENTS AND CHLORINE

Twelve million tons of chlorine are produced annually with sales of chlorine-dependent products at about $71.4 billion in 1990. The use of chlorine is prevalent in plastics, organic chemicals, pulp and paper, inorganic chemicals, waste-water treatment systems, and in drinking water. There are also chlorine-dependent jobs. In states bound by the Great Lakes there were over 100,00 jobs provided in 1990 because of this one pollutant.

The original reason why drinking water was chlorinated was to reduce certain infectious disease. After years of using chlorine in our water supply and products, we need to evaluate what is safe. It may be the same old story. If you take in enough chemicals that are foreign to the body, something bad will certainly happen.

Chlorine is the chemical most commonly found in homes. The resulting vapors are released into the air from showering, drinking water, steam-heating systems, washing dishes and clothes. The skin absorbs chlorine readily during bathing and showering. It is best to take short, warm, not hot showers. Hot showers open up the pores to absorb more chlorine.

There may be a link between a class of chlorine compounds called organochlorines and breast cancer. They are present in products manufactured for industrial and home use. Polyvinyl chloride is such a substance and used in vinyl products, including plumbing material. Scientists recently posed the possibility that organochlorines and hydrocarbons can mimic the effects of estrogen, or trick the body into producing a bad form of estrogen, contributing to breast cancer. Other exposures to chlorines are the wearing and storing of dry-cleaned clothes. Methylene chloride is a common solvent found in many products, especially paint strippers.

An eight-hour exposure to chlorine is equivalent to a normal lifetime dose. Many all-purpose cleaners contain chlorine. The combination of chlorine with ammonia results in a deadly chloramine gas. Finding chemical-free sources of meat and poultry is becoming more important because of the practice of spraying them with chlorine to eliminate salmonella. Studies suggest that some of the most toxic products derived from chlorine are causing health problems, particularly among fish-eating populations. This toxic chemical may cause up to 9 percent of bladder cancers and 18 percent of rectal cancers.

COSMETICS

Cosmetics contain substances that are relatively safe for most people, but cause a hypersensitivity reaction in some. About 85 percent of those with allergic conditions are unaware that cosmetics are causing some of their problems. Men commonly have allergic reactions to women's perfumes, lipstick, and hair spray, and women have reactions to men's after-shave lotions and hair-control sprays. Babies and children can react to their parents' cosmetics, and so can pets.

Just because a product's label says non-allergic or hypoallergenic doesn't mean you won't have a reaction to it. These terms just mean that the product is less likely to cause a reaction. There can be a great variation of substances from one product to another. The biggest problem with cosmetics seems to be the perfume. It is best to buy unscented products. If you cannot tolerate spray propellants, buy hair sprays and deodorants in squirt-type applicators. It could also be the sponges or brushes causing the problem.

Cosmetics can cause respiratory problems such as hay fever and asthma. Some people have sore throats, coughs, and sinus problems. Symptoms may only appear at certain times of the year because you've reached your allergic threshold. Add several different allergic factors together such as exposure to ragweed pollen, perfumed face powder, and eating dairy, and you are more likely to have a reaction.

The symptoms of a cosmetic allergy are similar to the symptoms of other allergies. The most common is contact dermatitis. It usually manifests as redness and itching, dry scaly rash, and possible puffiness or swellings on the skin. Other symptoms can be hives, bloodshot eyes, blisters, styes, loss of eyelashes, canker sores, or dry, cracked, and/or weeping skin lesions. It is usually easy to pinpoint the problem if you apply common-sense reasoning to what cosmetic is in contact with the affected part of the body. A red, itchy rash in the armpit usually indicates a problem with deodorants. If your eyes are itchy, the problem may be from both the eye make-up and nail polish. Nail polish can touch the eyes when applying make-up or at other times when the hands touch the eyes.

One important cause of reactions is the overlooked mold and/or bacteria allergy. Eye shadows are good places to incubate molds or bacteria. To avoid this problem, store make-up in your refrigerator and never let anyone else touch or use your cosmetics. If it smells rancid or goes watery, throw it away. Sometimes soap or a chemical house-hold product in combination with make-up can irritate the skin enough to cause a reaction. An irritation reaction is not an allergic reaction, but the outcome may look the same. Sometimes your problem stems from the container holding the cosmetic. Plastic or metal containers can contaminate cosmetics and cause reactions.

Remember, cosmetic allergies can happen at any time. A reaction may appear after trying a new cosmetic, or when a new ingredient is added to your regular brand. It could appear after using the same product for years. Cosmetic manufacturers are not helpful to the allergic individual. They usually do not list the ingredients, but you can write requesting information. Another serious problem is that cosmetic firms test their own products. It saves money for the government, but how do we really know if the product is safe?

Stop using all cosmetics if you suspect a cosmetic sensitivity. After the reaction has stopped, you can experiment with cosmetics using only one at a time, each for a week. If you have a reaction, discontinue the product's use. Keep a record of each cosmetic tried, its manufacturer, reactions, and the ingredients, if known. In some types of allergies your doctor can desensitize you with "allergy shots." In some cases homeopathic medications may help. Sometimes reactions will disappear when the total toxic load on the body is reduced.

Another point to consider is that many cosmetic products simply cover up the symptoms of vitamin, mineral, and other nutritional deficiencies. Examples are dandruff, facial blemishes, oily skin, brown spots on the skin, white spots on the nails, unhealthy hair, dry skin, bad breath, and premature aging.

CREOSOTE

Creosote is one of several phenols obtained from the distillation of heating wood products. Wood smoke makes a thick deposit of creosote (an oily liquid by-product of coal tar) in the chimney. The odor will often come into the house if there is no glass fireplace screen. A wood stove will ordinarily cause less trouble than a fireplace because it burns the wood hotter and produces less smoke. Dry wood produces less creosote than green wood.

DETERGENTS, BLEACHES, AND CLEANING PRODUCTS

Detergents can cause a variety of problems. Some people have reactions because of inhalation and some through actual contact. It is hard to remove detergent from your environment if every item of your clothing is washed in it. Many people find the perfumes in detergents overpowering. People with chronic allergic symptoms are usually sensitive to many other home environment factors such as fuels, plastics, and cleaners.

If you have a skin reaction, the location of the rash often helps to point out the cause. If detergents are the culprit, you will need to switch to soap flakes and wash soda. If you are only having a mild reaction, then double rinsing may be enough to eliminate the detergent film. Try using gloves if you suspect dish detergents. Rubber gloves bother a number of people, but lining them with a pair of cotton gloves can help. Stop using detergents and bleach until the rash clears. Then experiment carefully using only one of the suspected products at a time.

Most dish washing liquids are detergents, not soaps. Detergents cause more poisonings of children than any other product. Automatic dishwashing powder contains harsh detergents as well. They also may contain high levels of phosphates. When released into lakes and streams, phosphates kill fish and other aquatic life. Many laundry products are still non-biodegradable detergents made from petroleum and usually contain chemical additives such as artificial fragrances and colors. Even phosphate-free, biodegradable detergents can contribute to water pollution. The most tolerated detergents available are Safesuds, Ivory Flakes, Snow, White King soap, Arm and Hammer laundry detergent, Amway, Neo-Life, or Shaklee products. Look for naturally-derived or glycerin-based soaps whenever possible. More environmentally safe products are available on the grocery store shelves each year.

ELECTROMAGNETIC FIELDS (EMF) AND EXTREMELY LOW ELECTROMAGNETIC FIELDS (ELF)

Electric and magnetic fields exist wherever a flow of electricity exists. An electromagnetic field is a charged field that radiates out from where a current flows through a wire. Unfortunately, when the current flowing through the wire increases, the strength of the electromagnetic field also increases. Fortunately, their forces drop rapidly over distance. The strength of a magnetic field is measured in units of gauss (a unit of measuring the intensity of magnetic flux) or tesla (1 tesla = 10,000 gauss). A milligauss is 1/1000 of a gauss.

Electromagnetic radiation in our environment has increased tremendously in the past forty years. We are assaulted by power lines, television, microwave ovens and a variety of time-saving devices. Each of these creates an imbalance, ultimately shortening our lives and reducing its quality. These devices may cause cancer and other health problems, but there is no conclusive proof.

Unlike some environmental hazards, ELFs are virtually everywhere. All electrical devices, from transmission lines to clock radios, create electromagnetic fields. Magnetic fields can zip right through metal, walls of buildings and the human body, making avoidance difficult. These magnetic fields localize near plumbing in houses and under streets, and their strength appears related to the types of wiring configurations nearby. A major location is around power stations, welding equipment, subways, and movie projectors.

Directly underneath some electric utility poles the magnetic pollution registers seven to ten milligauss. Beneath wires at the transformer station down the block the milligauss is above 10. Expect homes near power lines to have higher readings. The electrical wiring system in many homes create high electromagnetic fields with the average magnetic-field strength in the homes surveyed at 0.35 milligauss. The most significant finding was that 10 percent of the homes had an average of 3.7 milligauss present and 1 percent of the homes had levels as high as nineteen milligauss. The causes of the high readings were faulty wiring, grounding problems, unbalanced circuits, or stray currents coming from water and gas pipes. A faulty circuit-breaker panel in the house across the street can be the source of the high reading in your home. Professional EMF testing can identify and eliminate the sources of these high fields. Often an electrician can lower house-generated fields for a small cost. Some homes have excessively high levels in one room and normal levels in adjacent bedrooms due to defective electrical circuits.

In the living room your stereo amplifier is putting out 5-7 milligauss, the television around 3-5 milligauss. Under the electric blanket exposure is over 10 milligauss. In front of the electric stove 5-7, the coffee grinder will be above 10, and the toaster 1.8. Near the wall where the electric feed comes into the house the reading is above 10. A gas stove does not produce any EMF. Your car, at the dashboard, is above 10, and at the front seat there is anywhere from 3.5 to 5. A heating pad puts out about 30 milligauss while an electric shaver exposes the user to 100 milligauss, and electric watches register at 2 milligauss. Magnetic fields used in stores for security systems can measure more than 200 milligauss.

At a distance of only three feet the magnetic fields drop on your television to less than 1.25 milligauss. A computer at 12 inches produces up to 3.5 milligauss, but if you sit back at 24 inches your exposure drops to less than 1.8. Fairly strong fields exist at all control panels of washers and dryers, but fade rapidly with distance. Readings from both the compact disc player and radio are affected by the volume of the sound; the higher the volume, the higher the reading.

A microwave oven not only generates a strong field, but can extend this field a long distance into the room. Strong fields emitted from a baby monitor can expose the child unnecessarily to this radiation. Many products, whether connected to an alternating current outlet or battery operated, will still put out an electromagnetic field. Check them with a gauss meter to know how much output there is. Even if they are not turned on, some items such as radios and electric blankets put out a strong field, as long as they are plugged in. A clock radio gives off a strong field all night long. Since distance decreases the field significantly, just move the radio at least two feet away from your head.

There do not seem to be any safety standards on electromagnetic fields. Since there is a rapid decrease in the magnetic field with an increase in distance, the best solution at this time is to decrease exposure. Consider these danger factors when dealing with magnetic fields:

• the strength of the field
• closeness of your body to the field
• how much of your body is exposed
• how long and how often you are exposed

Large energy users are clothes dryers, refrigerators, air conditioners, water heaters, and furnaces. If being around EMFs worries you, the simplest and cheapest method you can take to avoid these electromagnetic fields is to change your lifestyle a little. Relocate appliances such as fans, toasters, and electric clocks further away from the areas where you spend the most time. You could also replace that electric razor and electric toothbrush with a manual type. It is a good idea to monitor your child's use of video games. Since magnetic fields can travel through walls, don't place a bed or a crib on the other side of the wall from these appliances. Consider what is on the other side of the wall next to areas where you and your family spend most of your time.

Water beds and electric blankets are particularly strong sources of EMF because of the close contact with the body for extended periods of time. If you must have a waterbed, some of the new ones are redesigned to reduce fields. That is also happening with the manufacturers of some electric blankets, especially Sunbean's Slumber Rest, and Odyssey blankets. But even with the redesigned products producing much lower fields, there is still some EMF exposure.

At the office, try to space your computer stations several feet apart. Sit further back from your computer monitor to reduce your exposure to EMF. It will help to be two or three feet away if your eyes will permit. If that is not possible, there are companies that sell products for computers that partially or completely eliminate fields. The cost is about $300 to $1000. New machines from Apple and IBM have lower electromagnetic emission. The Rudolph Steiner College in Germany reports that peat moss bibs are effective in blocking harmful radiation from computers.

When you buy products that say they protect you from these harmful electromagnetic fields be sure you read the fine print. One example is the advertising concerning a computer shield that talks about health concerns dealing with electric fields, not electromagnetic fields. Little is known about the ill effects, if any, of electric fields. Be wary if there is only some vague reference to radiation. Magnetic radiation is your concern. Most of the products currently available to put outside your computer will not shield you from magnetic fields.

There is also the question of dose. How much is too much? What are the long-term consequences of exposure, as well as the dangers of brief, intense bursts? How does your own body's electrical and magnetic force react with outside fields? Within two or three feet of an appliance readings drop off tremendously, so why put yourself at risk? Even if no absolute proof exists that EMF or ELF fields cause these health conditions, there is sufficient reason to take a closer look. Be cautious until more proof is available.

Gauss meters, also known as magnetic-field meters, or power-frequency meters, measure EMF in milligauss. Many cities have them available for testing through your utility company. One of the major problems with these meters is that no one knows exactly what constitutes an acceptable or unacceptable dose. The following are some of the recorded EMF measurements:

	Within 8 Inches	At Two Feet
Video display	20-40 milligauss	Less than one milligauss
Electric clock	10-20	Less than one
Refrigerator	20-50	Less than one
Blow dryer	40-100	Less than one

A gauss meter can at least give you insight into the invisible world of electromagnetic pollution. You could buy a gauss meter to help you locate the fields around your house, walls, car, at the office, or your child's school, appliances, and other areas where you and your family spend time. If you buy a gauss meter or have your local utility company supply one, remember that the current you are picking up may be coming from the other side of the wall. A hot spot in front of a kitchen clock can be just as strong on the other side of the kitchen wall.

You can select from several choices of meters on the market today for under $200. They work reasonably well unless you live close to a radio transmitter. Look for a single-axis meter with a display that reads in milligauss. Be sure that it includes a good manual or guide. The cheap multi-axis meters are not reliable. If you buy a meter and find that the reading seems high, don't panic. Test other houses and see if you get similar readings. Some meters just read high. However, if your house is the only one that has these high readings, it might be wise to contact your utility company and have them check the area again with their instruments.

A recent study suggests that homes close to high-power distribution lines (the thick wires on top of street poles) link childhood leukemia to electromagnetic fields. The death rate among children living in homes with high-current wiring configurations is twice as high as children in general. Some of the studies have linked ELF to tumor growth and electrically heated beds to spontaneous abortions and birth defects. In animal studies, EMF have decreased production of certain hormones and disrupted sleep cycles.

The millions of electrical impulses that balance and regulate the activity of every living cell in our bodies are constantly interacting with these man-made electrical fields, probably to our detriment. This can disrupt our normal mechanisms. When human colon and brain cells were exposed to 60 Hertz fields, cancer cells proliferated and became more resistant to immune system attack.

A startling relationship between Alzheimer's disease and exposure to electromagnetic fields may add a new twist to the debate over EMF and health. High-exposure subjects were three times more likely to develop Alzheimer's than people who did not work around electric fields. The highest risk was among tailors and seamstresses, whose machines may expose them to three times as much radiation as powerline and cable workers.

FABRICS

The number of people suffering allergic or intolerant reactions from textile products is on the increase. The advancement in textile technology has drastically affected the health of these sensitive individuals. It is becoming difficult for chemically sensitive people to manage the problem brought on by fabrics. The chemical content of the fabric can vary enough to produce a reaction in one person, but not in another. It is also dependent on the total toxic load of the individual. Reducing the toxic load on the body may reduce the degree of reaction.

A small percentage of people are sensitive to natural fabrics such as cotton, linen, leather, or animal fibers such as angora, cashmere, mohair, silk, and sheep's wool. Other possible offensive substances are pine-tree resins called rayon, or petroleum-based products such as plastics, Acrilan, nylon, and Dacron. It was once easy to identify these natural materials and then avoid them. The problem is more complicated today because they blend most natural fabrics with synthetics and also treat them with chemicals. These treatments include dyes, perma-pressing, sizing, sanitizing, moth-proofing, and scotch-guarding. Manufacturers should show the type of fabric treatment on the label as well as what chemicals are in these treatments, but that is usually not the case. If you think that the fabric treatment is causing the reaction and the reaction is only a mild one, then a couple of washings will usually wash away the residues. If you still have a reaction after washing, you will have to avoid that fabric or the treatment process used. A person with multiple allergies should avoid garments not properly labeled.

When dry cleaning is necessary, locate a cleaner who uses Stoddard solvent. Request that the solvent remains free of soap and your clothes not be covered with plastic. Many people find the hot summer weather brings out the odors from new fabrics and causes more reactions. This may occur in new shoes as well.

Reading labels does not ensure that the material is untreated. Various fabric treatments usually contain chemicals: formaldehyde for perma-pressing; moth proofing as a pesticide; zinc phenolsulfonate and/or hexa-chlorophene for sanitizing; and polyesters for scotch-guarding. The most common fabric reaction seen by allergists and dermatologists is contact dermatitis (itchy red skin). This reaction could occur because of the formaldehyde used to manufacture durable-press clothes or because of the potassium dichromate found in tanned leather. Synthetic fibers give off formaldehyde for the life of the fabric. One study compared two thousand people, half of whom wore synthetic clothing next to the skin and the other half who wore pure untreated cotton clothing next to the skin. The individuals exposed to synthetic fibers had significantly higher blood pressure, a higher heart rate, and more frequent premature ventricular contractions then those who only let natural fibers touch them. The reactions commonly produced by fabrics could include the following:

- Dermatitis: hot, burning rash
- Eczema: scaly, itchy rash
- Hives: swelling of the skin and itching
- Sneezing: with watery eyes and nose
- Asthma: difficulty breathing
- Edema: swelling of the body tissues
- Anaphylaxis: various reactions including loss of motor control to unconsciousness

FLUORIDE

Recent comparative studies show that fluoride is not only ineffective as a preventive for dental caries, but may be far from safe. Don't overlook fluoride pollution as another possible factor in the total toxic load causing disease. We must evaluate the use of fluoride before we become victims to another environmental toxin.

Only a small amount of the total fluoride put into the water supply is ingested by humans. Most fluoridated water is flushed straight down the city sewers with hundreds of tons of fluoride being deposited into the environment each year. It is also coming from industry. Malfunctioning equipment or operator error causes excessive fluoride levels in some water-distribution systems. These and other sources dump fluoride into rivers or coastal waters and lakes. Sewage sludge spread on farmland or in forests can contaminate and enter ground water or creeks. It may end up in landfills where the fluoride leeches into the water tables.

We need more information about what this chemical is really doing to our food chains. Fluoride is estimated to last in ocean sediments for 2-3 million years. Concentrations used in community water supplies is having adverse effects on animals, including fish and humans, as well as on plants and insects. There is evidence that immature fish are more sensitive to fluoride damage than the adults. The damage includes unproductive eggs and bone abnormalities in survivors. These results are similar to the effects on other animals.

The argument that fluoridating water reduces tooth decay is not enough of a reason to add it to our drinking water. Fluoridation may not deserve the major credit. The evidence suggests that the incident of tooth decay may be low in locations where there is no addition of fluoride to the water and several studies have reported higher prevalences of dental problems following the addition of fluoride in the drinking water. It now appears that fluoride's main action as a decay preventive is best when applied to the surface of teeth where it is most effective at high concentrations. This essentially avoids the dangers of exposing our entire bodies and the environment unnecessarily. A study at the University of Arizona links tooth decay in children to the fluoride content in water. They found that children living in a fluoridated community have 11 times the risk of developing fluorosis.

Sodium fluoride is being used to treat osteoporosis. Even though fluoride-stimulated bone is denser, it is structurally unsound. Studies reveal areas of bone destruction and fracture rates, especially of the hip, increase with the extended use of fluoride. It fails to reduce the risk of fractures in women with post-menopausal osteoporosis, and may even increase the risk of occurrence. In three studies hip-fracture rates increased significantly compared to controls. Side effects included joint pain and gastrointestinal symptoms. Sodium fluoride has so many medical complications and side effects that it seems a poor therapeutic medication for post-menopausal osteoporosis.

Other studies in New Zealand, Europe, and the United States show a strong correlation between the use of fluoridation and the increased incidence of hip fracture and osteoporosis. A large-scale study in England found a significant correlation between hip fractures and water fluoride levels when 0 to 1 part per million were used, the claimed optimal level. In Kuopio, a Finnish city, fluoridation of 1 part per million increased significantly the fluoride content of bone as the person aged. The highest fluoride content in bone was in women with severe osteoporosis. There was considerably less change in the bone of people living outside Kuopio not exposed to fluoridated water. At least eight recent epidemiological studies suggest that water fluoridation increases the rate of bone fractures in females and males of all ages across the United States. This country's hip-fracture rate is now the highest in the world says the U.S. National Research Council.

Fluoride is a very potent enzyme poison, even at 1/20 the concentration that is added to municipal drinking water. Its anti-enzyme activity does much to explain why fluoride may be carcinogenic. Fluoride breaks the DNA and disrupts its enzyme-repair systems, setting the stage for genetic damage and cancer.

In 1991 the United States Public Health Service study linked fluoridated water to bone cancer in young males in Seattle, Washington. A New Jersey Department of Health study in 1992 found bone cancer rates among young males six times higher in fluoridated than non-fluoridated communities. The Department of Health and Human Services supports the link between fluoridated water and cancer by stating that more cases of bone, joint, kidney, and soft tissue cancers are occurring in fluoridated areas.

Some cases of fluoride contamination result in physical symptoms such as hives, but other cases may include emotional problems and behavior changes. When some people who are labeled as neurotic are put on fluoride-free water and foods, they recover. Symptoms return when fluoride is re-introduced back into their diets.

The International Society for Fluoride Research held a conference in 1994. They reported at the Conference the ill effects on soft tissues at surprisingly low levels of fluoride. Some were within the range of acceptable fluoride intake in Canada and the United States. They pointed to increased fractures, poor fracture healing, and bone outgrowth (exostoses) as some of the skeletal effects. They sited examples of neurological lesions (paralysis) as the direct action of fluoride. They demonstrated the adverse effects of fluoride on soft tissues such as thyroid dysfunction, heart disease and abnormal electrocardiograms, and cerebro-vascular disease. More studies showed an association of fluoride intoxication and lowered intelligence, chromosomal abnormalities, decreased immunity, increased senile cataracts, and cancer. They reported higher infant-death rates due to congenital abnormalities and higher death rates generally in endemic fluorosis areas. These reports confirmed many earlier findings from India and South Africa.

The Department of Health and Human Services ignores the dangers of this chemical even with all the evidence stating otherwise. Instead, they are the principal endorser. Do not vote for this addition to your community drinking water. Not fluoridating public water supplies would decrease the cancer incidence in this country and reduce the cost of water treatment. There seems to be plenty of evidence that the deliberate addition of fluoride to our drinking water and our diet is a foolish, if not a criminal, act.

FORMALDEHYDE AND OTHER ALDEHYDES

Recently the public has shown a great deal of interest in airborne formaldehyde found in dwellings, particularly in mobile homes. When formaldehyde is emitted from manufactured goods in its gaseous form, it is a pollutant of indoor air. This toxin is one of the top 50 industrial chemicals in this country. Thousands of products contain formaldehyde, especially the resins or glues found in particle board, fiberboard, hardwood plywood, as well as foam insulation. It is often an ingredient in plastic products and some cosmetics and drugs. It is present in car exhaust and cigarette smoke. Emissions from gas stoves, furnaces, kerosene heaters, and power plants contain formaldehyde.

Formaldehyde causes many health problems and promotes a "spreading phenomenon." Overexposure to this chemical can make someone more sensitive to other chemicals. It is almost impossible to avoid formaldehyde entirely. The many uses of formaldehyde are listed below:

• Intermediate in the synthesis of alcohols, acids, and other chemicals
• A tanning agent
• In the formulation of slow-release nitrogen fertilizers
• Added to concrete, plaster and related products to make them impermeable to liquids
• An antiperspirant and antiseptic in dentifrices, mouthwashes, germicidal and detergent soaps, and in hair-setting formulas and shampoos
• Air deodorants in public places and in industrial environments
• The synthesis of dyes, stripping agents and various specialty chemicals in the dye industry
• Used in combination with alcohol, glycerol, and phenol in embalming fluids and used to preserve products such as waxes, polishes, adhesives, fats, oils, and anatomical specimen
• The synthesis of explosives
• Various synthetic resins used in nail polish and undercoating of nail polish
• In insecticidal solutions for killing flies, mosquitoes, moths and as a rodent poison
• In the synthesis of some vitamin preparations
• For improving the wet strength and water resistance to paper products
• A preservative and accelerator for photographic developing solutions
• To make natural and synthetic fibers crease-resistant, wrinkle-resistant, crush-proof, water repellent, dye-fast, flame-resistant, shrink-proof, moth-proof, and more elastic
• Used in making synthetic resins and wood veneers for wall paper
• A component of wallboard used in construction of houses and apartments
• Used in the manufacture of paper products improving wet strength and water resistance

- For artificial aging and reducing shrinkage in wood preservation
- Various specialty chemicals in the dye industry as well as dyed fabrics
- Urea-formaldehyde foam used in insulation materials

Formaldehyde usually accounts for about 50 percent of the estimated total aldehydes in polluted air. The major source of aldehyde pollution is the incomplete combustion of hydrocarbons in gasoline and diesel engines. It is one of the principal agents responsible for the burning of eyes in smog. Aldehydes can react further to form additional products, such as more ozone.

Formaldehyde vapors are irritating to the body's mucous membranes. Symptoms include eyes tearing, sneezing, coughing, difficulty breathing, a suffocating feeling, rapid pulse, headache, or weakness. If this chemical touches you, there may be dermatitis. Ingestion may cause severe abdominal pain, protein in the urine, the inability to urinate, or an overly acid system. Alcoholics have an increased risk of sensitivity to formaldehyde, as do people with excessive yeast, because of the amount of aldehyde already present in the body.

When the indoor and outdoor air contain too much formaldehyde, it may produce skin irritation, watery eyes, burning sensations in the eyes and respiratory tract, coughing, and similar reactions. It bothers some people more than others. Sometimes it is hard to tell what is causing these symptoms because other pollutants or a cold could be the problem. Exposure to high levels of formaldehyde causes cancer in laboratory animals. Minimize formaldehyde exposure by taking the following steps:

- Increase home ventilation, especially in warm weather. In the cold months, don't seal up all the windows and doors. Circulating fresh air is necessary to control indoor pollution and allergens of all kinds.
- Wash permanent-press clothing and sheets before you use them. If you are installing permanent press draperies that you can't wash, try to air them out for a few days before hanging them.
- When buying hardwood plywood and other pressed woods for home-building projects, look for materials stamped with the HUD emissions seal.
- If you buy unfinished furniture or other pressed-wood products, be sure to varnish or paint them with a water-proof finish such as polyurethane to reduce formaldehyde emissions.
- If you already have formaldehyde foam insulation in your home, seal it off with nonporous wallpaper, patch any cracks, or seal wood paneling with varnish.

- Have an adequate ventilation system installed if you buy a mobile home. Mobile homes tend to be worse than other homes because they contain newly pressed wood materials in a compact space.
- Provide good ventilation in a motor home or other recreational vehicle, especially in warm weather. Be sure to air out the vehicle after it has been in storage. RVs don't fall under HUD jurisdiction and may contain hardwood-plywood or particle-board fittings as well as new curtains and upholstery that are all potential sources of formaldehyde.
- Have carpets aired out for several months before installing them, or look for carpets free of formaldehyde.

Some good news about formaldehyde includes a recent reduction by government regulations. Only a maximum of 0.1 percent is currently allowed in commercial products. Permissible air levels are being reduced. Some evidence shows that the sturdy and ubiquitous spider plant can slightly reduce formaldehyde in indoor air.

Consider having the formaldehyde levels checked. Blue Sky Labs in Seattle, WA (206) 721-2583 has a home-testing kit for formaldehyde. This kit can help you find out if formaldehyde poisoning is a problem in your home. Monitors suitable for measuring formaldehyde can be ordered from Air Technology Labs in Fresno, CA, (800-354-2702), and from Air Quality Research International in Durham, NC, (919) 544-2987. If you don't have symptoms, you probably don't need to go to this expense.

FRAGRANCES AND PERFUMES

Perfumes are used in a wide variety of substances, including hygienic products, drugs, detergents, plastics, industrial greases, oils and solvents, foods, and other household products. Their composition is usually complex, involving numerous natural and synthetic sweet-smelling ingredients. Many of the ingredients used in the perfume industry are toxic, yet no testing for toxicity exists. No enforcement is possible due to trade secret laws protecting the chemical fragrance industry. Most of the chemicals used in fragrances are synthetic compounds derived from petroleum. They include benzene derivatives, aldehydes, and many other known toxics and allergens. The National Academy of Sciences targeted fragrances as one of the six categories of chemicals that need high priority for neurotoxicity testing. The other groups were insecticides, heavy metals, solvents, food additives, and certain air pollutants.

Fragrances contain the same chemicals classified as either airborne contaminants or as hazardous-waste-disposal chemicals. Some of these are toluene, methylene chloride, methyl ethyl ketone, ethanol, and benzyl chloride. It is amazing that these hazardous chemicals are being used on an unsuspecting public. Other compounds causing frequent adverse reactions are linalool, a-terpineol, benzyl alcohol, benzyl acetate, and limonene. They are also among the twenty most commonly used in fragrance products tested by the EPA in 1991.

Some disorders thought to result from exposure to neurotoxic chemicals are multiple sclerosis, Parkinson's, lupus, Alzheimer's, and dyslexia. The symptoms of chemical hypersensitivity are identical to some neurological dysfunctions. Could fragrant fabric softeners or detergents cause neurological breakdown by emitting neurotoxic chemicals? Perfumes often contribute to allergic respiratory disorders such as asthma and skin disorders.

Over 2,900 chemicals are used in the perfume industry and 884 of these are toxic substances. Many are capable of causing cancer, central nervous system disorders, breathing and allergic reactions, birth defects, and multiple chemical sensitivities. Other symptoms from the exposure to fragrances may include dizziness, sneezing, double vision, coughing, breathing problems, nasal congestion, headaches, fatigue, seizures, memory loss, poor concentration, nausea, depression, anxiety, restlessness, skin irritation, muscle pain, and irregular heartbeat.

The list of fragrance chemicals known to be toxic and the problems they cause is very long. In 1986 a study by the National Institute of Occupational Safety and Health (OSHA) found 314 fragrance chemicals capable of causing biological mutation; 218 caused reproduction problems; 778 caused acute toxicity; 146 caused tumors; and 376 caused skin and eye irritations. The following is a list of some of the most common chemicals found in fragrance products and the symptoms they can cause:

Acetone: It is on the hazardous waste lists of the EPA and other agencies. Dryness of the mouth and throat can occur when inhaling. Symptoms may include dizziness, slurred speech, nausea, drowsiness, and incoordination. It acts chiefly on the central nervous system.

Benzaldehyde: This chemical is another common ingredient and known to be narcotic. Benzoin causes large lymph nodes and spleens, as well as liver damage in mice. It is a local anesthetic, central nervous system depressant and causes irritation to the mouth, throat, eyes, skin, lungs, and gastrointestinal tract. It can irritate the eyes of people who wear contact lenses.

Benzyl acetate: There is a link between this chemical and pancreatic cancer. The vapors can irritate eyes and the respiratory passages. Benzyl acetate absorbs through the skin causing effects anywhere in the body. Do not flush it down the sewer to pollute the water system.

Benzyl alcohol: It is irritating to the upper respiratory tract causing symptoms such as headaches, vomiting, nausea, dizziness, drops in blood pressure, and depression of the central nervous system. In severe cases there is the possibility of respiratory failure.

Benzyl chloride: Another common ingredient of perfumes is benzyl chloride, a central nervous system depressant. It is irritating to the eyes and mucous membranes. It causes cancer according to the California Safe Drinking Water and Toxic Enforcement Act of 1986. Benzyl chloride, along with toluene, methylene chloride, methyl ethyl ketone, and ethanol are classified as either airborne contaminants or as hazardous waste disposal chemicals.

Camphor: Camphor is a local irritant and central nervous system stimulant and absorbs easily through the skin. It may cause irritation to the eyes, throat, and nose, as well as dizziness, nausea, twitching muscles, and convulsion. Do not inhale the vapors.

Ethanol: Ethanol is made from ethylene gas by the oil companies. It is also made from grain. Petrochemical ethanol is an excellent solvent and its almost limitless derivatives keeps us constantly exposed. Many individuals who become ill from chemical additives and contaminants in foods and water, in addition to fumes and combustion products of petrochemicals, will react to the small quantities of hydrocarbons dissolved in synthetic alcohol. Smog and auto exhaust fumes are one of the most common exposures.

Ethanol vapors are on the EPA's hazardous waste list. They can cause fatigue, irritation to the eyes, and upper respiratory tract symptoms, even in low concentrations. Ethanol can cause similar symptoms when ingested. These include an initial stimulatory effect followed by drowsiness, impaired vision, loss of muscular coordination, and stupor. Room fresheners may contain high levels of ethanol. Other common products are insect sprays, glue, varnish, paint, disinfectants, hair spray, mothballs, deodorants, and detergents.

Ethyl acetate: It is on the EPA's hazardous waste list. It may cause symptoms such as irritation to the eyes and respiratory tract, headaches, dryness to the skin, and damage to the liver and kidneys. Wash thoroughly after handling.

Limonene: This is one of the chemicals listed in the top twenty most common ingredients in perfumes. It is a known cancer-causing agent and has the capacity to cause multiple chemical sensitivities. It is an irritant and sensitizer to the skin and eyes. Always wash thoroughly after using this product and before you eat, drink, or apply cosmetics. Do not inhale limonene vapors.

Linalool: This chemical can cause respiratory disturbances. The testing on animals resulted in the following symptoms: abnormal gait, reduced motor activity, depression, and respiratory disturbances.

Methylene chloride: Methylene chloride is on the hazardous waste list of several agencies, including the EPA. It metabolizes to carbon monoxide resulting in less available oxygen in the blood. Then the body stores it in the fat tissues. Symptoms may include headaches, irritability, fatigue, limbs tingling, and mental symptoms. Methylene chloride is a known cancer-causing agent and may cause autoimmune diseases. It is one of the twenty most commonly found chemicals in fragrance products in the 1991 EPA study. This is really interesting because there was a ban on methylene chloride in all cosmetic and fragrance products in 1989. Since no agency regulates the fragrance industry, there is no pre-clearing of chemicals with any agency. The fragrance industry is exempt from listing ingredients on their products.

A-Terpineol: It is very irritating to the body's mucous membranes. Inhaling the fumes into the lungs can cause pneumonitis or even fatal edema. Other symptoms may include depression of the central nervous system and respiratory system, and headaches. Avoid skin contact.

Toluene: Pulmonary function tests dropped 18 to 58 percent on exposure to toluene, yet its use in the fragrance industry has increased in the past ten years. Perfumed kitty-litter gravel is a possible cause of asthma in humans according to a Danish toxicological journal. Other places to fine toluene are in furniture wax, tires, plastic garbage bags, inks, hair gel and hair spray. In every fragrance sample collected by the EPA in 1991, they detected toluene.

Synthetic fragrance molecules are one of the major contributors to indoor air pollution. You have the right to protect yourself from fragrances coming in the mail and polluting your home. Make a difference! Do the following:

1. Write to the editors of newspapers and complain.
2. Call or write to magazines that contain fragrance strips and complain. Cancel your subscription if they do not stop exposing you to perfumes.
3. File a formal complaint with the U.S. Postal Service against the companies mailing such items if there is a law in your state against such things.
4. Call the FDA at 1-800-858-3760 to report your reaction to the perfumes being used in magazines, mailers, papers, etc., and mailed to you without your consent.
5. Ask your doctor to demand the ingredients of any chemical fragrance

product that is causing you a reaction. Cite the law: 29 CFR 1910.1200 and 1910.20, the OSHA Hazard Communication and Access to Medical Records standards allowing health professionals access to trade secret information.

6. Write to your state politicians urging them to introduce a bill banning these fragrances from coming through the mail.

FUELS

Use electric heat for cooking. Avoid hydrocarbons such as kerosene, coal, oil, and gas. Use dry wood instead of green wood. If you heat your home with electricity, remove motor-driven fans that use oil. Be sure you do not have plastics in the heating ducts.

HYDROCARBONS

Hydrocarbons are organic compounds containing only carbon and hydrogen. The original sources of hydrocarbons are coal, oil, and gas, unless you go back to what created these products, the conifer forests. These compounds make up the bulk of indoor, as well as outdoor air pollution. Aromatic hydrocarbons present a threat to human health. Toluene, xylene, ethyl benzene, and styrene are other important hydrocarbons found in gasoline, combustion products, paints, adhesives, and solvents. Since these are common indoor chemicals they are probably part of the problem causing "sick building syndrome."

Benzene is a human carcinogen based on studies of occupationally-exposed persons. The main source of exposure to benzene for about 50 million Americans is mainstream cigarette smoke. Diesel gasoline also contains benzene. Benzene is so toxic that most American chemical companies have already banned its indiscriminate use by their employees. Scientists, in recently published studies, posed the possibility that organochlorines and hydrocarbons can mimic the effects of estrogen or trick the body into producing a bad form of estrogen, contributing to breast cancer. Sources of hydrocarbons are:

Cigarette smoke	Wood impregnated with creosote
Spray containers	Disinfectants, especially pine-scented
Solvents	Exhausts (such as in diesel exhausts)
Adhesives	Window-washing compounds
Mineral oil	Fuels and their combustion products
Sponge rubber	Evaporating oil from mechanical device
Insecticides	Cleansing powders containing bleach
Alcohol	Various silver and brass-polishing materials

Paints	Food sprays that are oil soluble
Lighter fluids	Foods exposed to gas for ripening/roasting
Newsprint	Refrigerants
Plastics	Varnish
Cements	Burning green wood
Ammonia	Detergents
Cosmetics	Industrial and agricultural chemicals
Chlorox	Food/drugs colored with coal-tar dyes
Natural gas stoves	Hot water heaters
Central heating	Odors from oil furnace
Paraffins	

JEWELRY

According to a study of 1600 allergic patients, the most frequent cause of unpleasant skin reactions come from wearing jewelry made from nickel sulphate. These items are usually inexpensive bracelets, nickel-plated earrings, metal wrist-watch bands, and zippers.

LATEX

Latex is derived from the sap of *Hevea braziliensis*. It contains several potentially allergic fractions. Latex is found in disposable rubber gloves, urinal bags, elastic threads, balloons, condoms, diaphragms, and glue and textile adhesives. Symptoms can range from dermatitis to anaphylaxis.

New experiments suggest that the latex rubber in tires triggers allergic reaction. This may contribute to the rise of asthma in urban areas. The results of experiments with rubber tires suggest that it is possible that tire particles can cause allergies in people, especially those who live near freeways. These people have more antibodies for latex resulting in more cases of asthma than people who live in rural areas.

The number of health-care workers allergic to latex rose as health-care professionals began to use more gloves to protect themselves from infection by HIV. As many as 15 percent of nurses in U.S. hospitals have the antibodies that are the hallmark of latex allergies. According to Timothy Sullivan, an allergist at the Emory Clinic in Atlanta, about 5 percent of the general population many have the antibodies.

At least sixteen deaths have been linked to exposure to latex-tipped tubing used during a barium enema procedure. In some individuals, even indirect exposure to latex can provoke a powerful reactions. Some people have developed asthmatic symptoms just by walking into a room containing an open boxes of latex gloves. Those at the highest risk are children having surgical procedures and operating-room personnel. Latex allergies were unknown until recently. The two likely explanations are: some allergy-provoking chemicals have been introduced into the manufacturing process or the immune system is so compromised that it has become more susceptible to latex.

LEAD

There appears to be an increase of lead in our drinking water. The EPA found that over 800 municipal water systems, serving 30 million people, had lead levels that exceeded federal guidelines. Exposure to lead is considered the nation's most serious environmental threat to the health of children. Water-borne lead exposure could be coming from old lead plumbing pipes or lead solder in the home. Water can also leach lead from new brass fixtures.

Lead exposure even at low levels in children can result in IQ deficits. It has been banned from use in paints, but older houses may still have leaded paint exposed. When these paints get old and start to flake off the walls, small children are especially vulnerable. They are more likely to breathe the dust containing the lead or put the leaded paint flakes into their mouth. It would be wise for home owners to have their paint and water tested for lead contamination, especially if small children are living in the home.

Lead concentrates in the body's liver, skeleton, brain, heart, lungs, kidney, testes, adrenal glands, and thymus. Toxic symptoms include: constipation, diarrhea, nausea, pain, loss of appetite, muscle weakness, tremors, gout, atrophy, insomnia, headache, confusion, clumsiness, restlessness, and mental retardation. Common sources of lead are the urban atmosphere, paints, enamels, glass, printing, insecticides, construction materials, plaster, cigarette smoke, crayons, batteries, imported ceramics and gasoline additives.

MECHANICAL DEVICES

Oil evaporates from any motor. For the sensitive individual this can cause problems. Air filters made of glass wool or fiberglass may contain oil, but they are available without this content. Quaker State oil and lead-free gas are the most odor free.

MERCURY

Another neurotoxin causing many human poisonings worldwide is mercury. In the early 1950s mercury was discharged from a plastics plant into Minamata Bay, Japan, where it was converted to methyl mercury by the action of bacteria living in the muddy bottom. These bacteria were then eaten by plankton that in turn were eaten by fish and shellfish. The families dependent upon the sea for food in the area had a high rate of mercury intoxication resulting in deaths, deformities, and retardation of infants. Other sources of contamination are diuretics, cosmetics, organomercurial pesticides, camera film, antiseptics, plastics, chemical fertilizers, pharmaceuticals, fluorescent lamps, and water-based paint.

The composition of mercury/silver amalgams varies with each manufacturer. A typical formula would be: mercury 48-60%, silver 15-37%, tin 12-13%, copper 0-26%, zinc 0-1%. Dental amalgam and nickel alloys can reduce the immune system's ability to function normally by reducing the T-lymphocyte count. The implications are obvious with regards to AIDS. Other conditions affected by mercury include: disorders of the musculoskeletal and intestinal systems, diseases of sensory organs and the nervous system, disturbances of the vascular system, disorders of the lymphatic system, and allergies (including food allergies).

Mercury concentrates in the brain, kidneys, liver, gastrointestinal tract, mandibular tissue, and lungs. A study of thirty-one patients found mercury still in their urine when they were on a mercury-free diet, but had three or more amalgam dental fillings in their mouth. Even a small amount of mercury in the body damages the cells and can be a factor in chronic illnesses. Toxic symptoms from mercury are loss of appetite, loss of weight, tremors, diarrhea, insomnia, nervousness, dizziness, and protein in the urine. Other symptoms include fatigue, headache, clumsiness, ataxia, impaired concentration, impaired memory, and hearing defects.

Mercury amalgam may be a player in chronic yeast infections and other illnesses due to microbes. It is an antiseptic that attacks microbes in the same way antibiotics do, forcing them to mutate to survive. Microbes learn to defend themselves from such attacks and grow resistant to any treatment that tries to reduce their population.

MICROWAVE COOKING

Atoms, molecules, and cells hit by the process of microwaving reverse polarity over one billion times a second. Molecules are forcefully deformed and their quality impaired. Can any organic system withstand such destructive power without adverse changes? Newly formed compounds are not normally recognized by the body. Microwaving destroys some nutrients and turns some amino acids into carcinogens. The government claims that none of this hurts people, but they have not tested their claims. Many articles are telling us that microwaving is healthier because fewer vitamins are destroyed in the process, but new research has identified free-radical formation in microwave foods. Free radicals are those renegade electrons linked to premature aging, cancer, and more. Maybe we need to hold out for further information before committing all our food to microwaving.

Dr. Hans Hertel of Germany did the first, well-controlled study of the effects of microwaved nutrients on the blood and physiology of humans. The blood of those who consumed microwaved food for two months showed pathological changes compared to matched controls eating food cooked with heat. The changes included a decrease in all hemoglobin values and deterioration in the good cholesterol. Lymphocytes (white blood cells) showed a short-term decrease after the intake of microwaved food, but not after eating normally cooked foods. Warming breast milk in a microwave oven destroyed 98 percent of its immunoglobulin-A antibodies and 96 percent of its liposome activity, reducing the milk's resistance to infectious *E. coli*.

NEWSPRINT

Many people are allergic to the ink used in newspapers and magazines. If you are particularly sensitive to newsprint, you can have someone else open and air out the paper first or have a glass company cut and edge a piece of glass to place over your reading material. Another alternative is to place the item with newsprint in a reading box. You can be desensitized to many allergens such as newsprint with homeopathic medications.

ORGANIC SOLVENTS

Organic solvents easily absorb through the skin and are inhaled as fumes. The main organs affected by these toxins are the brain, nervous system, and cell membranes of the body. The most frequent symptoms are poor concentration and coordination, drowsiness, reduced ability to think, and impaired memory. There is the potential to cause brain and neurologic damage. A study using 400 people and 20 organic compounds detected the substances in the exhaled breath.

Trichloroethylene evaporates into the atmosphere and contaminates air and water throughout the world, generally at nontoxic levels, but ground water in some areas may contain toxic levels. You can switch to mountain spring water for drinking, but remember that organic solvents still penetrate the skin during showering. To really protect yourself from all toxic chemicals in the water, consider putting a good water filter in your house, including in your shower head.

OZONE

Acid aerosols contain fine, caustic droplets formed from gases emitted by coal-fired electric-power plants and other industrial sources. Acid aerosols worsen the effects of ozone on the sensitive tissues lining the airways. Ground-level ozone originating chiefly from auto emissions is a prime source. This pollution may begin in the cities, but it quickly spreads to the suburbs, where levels are often higher than those in the urban area. The American Lung Association claims the EPA's ozone standard of .12 parts per million (ppm) is unsafe and is suing to have the standard lowered. In major metropolitan areas across this country what the EPA calls a safe level is regularly exceeded.

Connecticut has one of the highest ozone concentrations in the entire Northeast. A person can live in a beautiful and wealthy suburb such as the Greenwich area, but the ozone levels can still be high, since the wind carries pollution from New York City into the Connecticut countryside. People who live in suburbs, despite nearly identical exposures to ozone and acid aerosols, seem to suffer less from air pollution's ill effects than their urban center counterparts. The poor nutrition or inadequate health care of inner-city people may play a role in the higher incident.

The danger of ozone to health is still a matter of intense study. The American Lung Association reports that lung disease is now the third leading cause of death and moving up the list. A study found that on days when ozone pollution was greater than .06 ppm, hospital admissions jumped 26 percent. On peak ozone air-pollution days, asthma admissions jumped as much as 24 percent. There appears to be a correlation between acute respiratory problems and increased concentrations of this pollutant in the summer haze that blankets many of our urban centers each year. Levels even below the accepted safe levels are increasing the number of hospital admissions for respiratory problems. Ozone pollution originating in the Midwestern United States was fouling air over Canada, causing a corresponding increase in hospital admissions.

Ozone pollution moves west to east in direction. The further west you live the better. Pollutants are also worse when the sun goes down and before the sun burns them off in the morning. It is worse with fog, in the winter time, and when the nights are longer than the days.

Working around laser printers and photocopy machines exposes a person to as many as ten times the considered safe amount of ozone exposure. The testing of many offices often found the internal filters clogged and emitting unhealthy amounts of the gas. Common symptoms were headaches, nausea, and respiratory problems. The risk is even greater in small areas that have poor ventilation. Apple Computer Company now recommends that the original ozone filter be replaced after 50,000 pages. Hewlett-Packard says that its newest machines produce much less ozone, but suggests changing the filter every 30,000 to 50,000 pages. Currently, there is no safety or health rules governing emissions from this equipment.

PAINTS

Avoid fresh paint, varnish, and wood stain. Paint must be nonodorous. Commercial oil and latex paints may contain many toxic substances, including solvents and fungicides. Vapor emissions continue for months after the paint dries and may cause symptoms.

PETROLEUM

Fruits picked green such as bananas, apples, oranges, and tomatoes, are often exposed to a petroleum-derived gas called ethylene to ensure ripening.

PHENOL

Phenol or carbolic acid is found in coal and wood tar. In dilute solution it is an antiseptic found in Lysol and PineSol. As a phenolic resin, it is found in food can linings. Half of the total production of phenol is used in the manufacture of plastics and one fourth in the production of drugs of coal tar origin such as aspirin and sulfa drugs. It is often used as a preservative in many injectable medications, including allergenic extracts. Phenol, an organic compound, has other names such as hydroxybenzene. Listed below are some of the uses for phenol:

- the starting point for the production of epoxy and phenolic resins, aspirin, and other drugs
- in the manufacture of some explosives
- a constituent of herbicides and pesticides
- in the manufacture of nylon, synthetic detergents, polyurethane, perfumes, dyes, gasoline additives, and photography solutions
- a preservative in medications and for antigen serum in allergy shots
- a phenolic resin, Bakelite, is formed by the reaction of phenol with formaldehyde and is used in molded articles such as telephone parts, thermal-insulation panels, and laminated boards, children's toys, refrigerator storage dishes, and canned goods

Artificial colors, artificial flavors, BHT, BHA, and natural salicylates have the phenol compound in common. Phenols appear naturally as well as in many synthetic compounds. Some natural sources of phenols are tea and vanillin. Vanillin occurs naturally, as well as in synthetic forms, and is a major component of vanilla.

Anything smoked is likely to contain some level of phenol and will be capable of producing a reaction. Hamburgers barbecued with lots of smoke (especially in a covered grill) and smoked bacon may both be potential problems. Smoked bacon cured with nitrates is even more toxic than meat cured with phenols alone. The human skin readily absorbs simple phenol compounds that are contained in smoke.

If you have a problem with phenols, you need to avoid all mint-scented cleaning products containing methyl salicylate. Patients allergic to phenol should consider all salicylate foods and products as a potential problem. Phenol is a common preservative in conventional allergy injections, many other medications, and cleaning solutions. The body has a high affinity for phenol, but a low capacity for tolerance resulting in problems shortly after use. Most wood polishes contain phenol. Its ingestion causes symptoms like skin irritation and in severe cases can cause circulatory collapse. Vapors pollute your home long after the application of phenol-containing products.

PLASTICS

The more flexible and odorous a plastic, the more frequently it contributes to indoor air pollution. Hard plastics like vinyl, Formica, Bakelite, and cellulose acetate are less likely to cause problems from odors. Plastic pillows, combs, powder cases, and shoes can produce symptoms more easily. Avoid plastic air conditioning ducts and plastic kitchenware, but hard types of plastic such as Melmac are usually all right.

Most butchers wrap meat in plastic wrap. Buy meat double wrapped in butcher paper with the first wrap reversed so the wax side is not next to the meat. One side of aluminum foil is plastic coated. When food is heated in foil this plastic will come off on the food. Soft plastic containers are worse than hard plastics, especially for items such as water or other liquids. Tap water may pick up chemicals from plastic pipes. Some people are sensitive to water after storing it in plastic containers. It is best not to store food items or water in plastic containers.

REFRIGERANTS AND SPRAY CONTAINERS

If a refrigerator, freezer, or air conditioner is not working properly, there can be a slow escape of freon gas. This can cause trouble for many sensitive people. There are new propellants on the market replacing aerosols. They are isobutane, propane, and butane. They might not be toxic to the ozone layer but they can be toxic to the body, especially to the heart and central nervous system. Avoid perfumes, hair sprays, and other cosmetics that use propellants. If you must use a spray, consider a pump dispenser.

SPONGE RUBBER

Odors can come from sponge-rubber pillows, mattresses, upholstery, rug pads, seat cushions, typewriter pads, and the rubber backing of rugs.

Avoid contact with these products if you have symptoms such as insomnia, restlessness, or night sweats.

TALC

Talcum powder may be dangerous to your health. It is a very soft mineral called magnesium silicate. Talc is chemically similar to asbestos, a known cancer-causing agent. Once it is pulverized, purified and perfumed, it shows up on the drug-store shelf as baby and body powder. People tend to inhale considerable amounts of this powder when dusting the body. It may be wiser to use lotions and spare your lungs the trouble of dealing with this additional pollution.

Talc is used on surgical gloves to make them easier to put on and keep the latex material from sticking to itself. Dental dams are often coated with talcum powder to keep a tooth dry. It has been used on just about every baby's bottom for the past fifty years, making you think it was one of the safest products around. Apparently, that is not the case.

Talc is a known sclerosing agent. It irritates body tissue on a microscopic level and causes it to thicken and harden. Doctors have suspected that talc deposited in body cavities from surgical gloves might be partially responsible for small nodules and adhesions following surgery.

A recent study at Harvard Medical School reported that women with direct exposure to talc on the genital area, undergarments, sanitary napkins or diaphragms had an increased risk of cervical cancer. The risk was significantly increased among women who used it as a body powder for years. Many more studies are beginning to confirm this suspicion. Other researchers suggest that problems such as endometriosis, chronic inflammation of the ovaries and cervix may have started early in life from childhood exposure to talc.

It is being suggested that many of the problems associated with silicone breast implants were caused by talc instead. The most serious problem associated with silicone breast implants is the hard, inelastic, thickened capsule that forms around the implant. It was thought that the leaking silicone gel was responsible. Now, researchers think it might be possible that during the surgical procedure some contaminant was introduced into the area. When the skin and implants were removed from 41 women and examined for contaminants, talc was found present in the surrounding skin and tissue of 71 percent.

Severe obstructions of the urinary tract and adhesions within the chest and abdominal cavity have resulted from small amounts of talc entering the area during prior surgeries. Many glove manufacturers realizing that the talc from coated surgical gloves was causing these problems switched to cornstarch. Unfortunately, cornstarch seems to cause the same problem. If you are having surgery and have concerns about the use of talc, discuss it with your doctor beforehand. You can request that non-powdered gloves be used. Avoid using talc for personal use and powdering your baby's behind. Condoms can introduce talc into the female reproductive system.

TERPENES

This class of compounds includes several of the most popular scents used in room air fresheners, cleaners, polishes, and bathroom deodorants. Added to many products, including foods and beverages, are limonene (lemon scent) and pinene (pine scent). At the top of the indoor pollution list is limonene. Terpenes could be a problem if you happen to be sensitive to them.

TUNG OIL

Widely used in varnishes and paints, tung oil produces rapid drying or hardening and other desirable properties. Unfortunately, it also contains toxic substances. The widespread exposure to products containing tung oil could cause a major public health and occupational problem. It seems that tung oil seriously damages the immune system. Instead of furniture polish containing tung oil, make a lemon wax by mixing one teaspoon lemon oil with one pint mineral oil. Tung oil uses include:

Wood oil or wood wax for furniture	Varnishes
Many polyurethanes	Some lacquers
Water and proofing fiberboard containers	Insulating varnish
Laminates	Putty
Wood filler	Wood-panel filler
Acrylic-latex paint	Exterior house paint
Anti-corrosive iron and steel paint	Resins and plastics
Waterproof concrete paint	Pressboard
Photocopying paper coating	Floor tile
Resins for making circuit boards	Some nail polishes
Glossy coating on rubber	Linoleum manufacture
Coating on new shoe soles	Rapid-drying inks
Permanent-press coating on garments	Tobacco flavoring
Binder/coating for herbicide granules	Coating for interior of metal cans
Products requiring a drying oil	Deck sealers
Quick-drying varnishes	Some shellacs
Electrical insulating	Caulking compounds
Oil paints	Car paints
Synthetic rubber	Wall board
Car brake shoes	Shrink-proofing wool

MISCELLANEOUS POLLUTANTS AND CONTAMINANTS

Toxic fumes and odors can come from detergents, soaps, ammonia, Clorox, cleansing powders containing bleaches, some silver- and brass-polishing materials, and from prolonged use of television sets and office copier equipment. Avoid highly scented soaps, toilet deodorants, and disinfectants (especially pine-scented). The smell of pine really affects some people, so avoid pine Christmas trees, pine in wood-burning fireplaces, and creosote odors. Most disinfectants contain toxic chemicals including phenol, formaldehyde, cresol, ammonia and chlorine. The fumes from these chemicals can cause a variety of health problems. Be cautious about the new deodorizing, sanitizing chemicals on sanitary napkins and tampons. Dyes in toilet paper are a problem for some sensitive people. White is usually the safest color in these types of products. You can also find unbleached, undyed, and unscented products.

Gloves are a mixed blessing. You can use gloves to protect yourself from the allergenic substance, but sometimes you can become sensitized to the glove itself. If you are the allergic type, then limit the time you wear them. Some people apply skin care or protection before putting on gloves. Others find powder helps. It may help to wear cotton gloves underneath the rubber gloves. Light vinyl gloves are helpful to those needing gloves, but who are allergic to rubber.

Buying a house introduces special considerations. Check the wind direction and location of any air-contaminating factories close by. House owners should get a complete five-year history on any work or exterminating. The garage should not be under or near bedrooms. Plaster walls are better than wallboard if the house is less than five years old. If there was any redecorating, what did they use for glue, coated surfaces, and wall paper? Is there a history of any additional insulation and what kind? Are hardwood floors under the carpeting? How close is the house to heavy traffic? A house over five years old with electric heat is best.

If the construction is at least three years old with treated finishes that do not wash off, wallpaper any walls to prevent chemical exposure or apply two coats of semi-gloss or three coats regular paint. For new wallboard construction apply three coats of oil-based paint because formaldehyde takes five to six years to gas out and is strongest for the first few years.

If you have hardwood floors, use a wood sealer instead of varnish, because it is not as thick and will gas out sooner. If you need to use varnish, use any brand of urethane. This is a plastic product, but tends to dry harder, causing fewer problems. It may still take nine to twelve months to gas out the urethane. Refinish hardwood floors with linseed oil. This may be better tolerated than varnish and wax.

Have any products you might use tested for sensitivities. Also carefully evaluate any materials used in your hobbies. If you are knitting, use wool that has not been moth proofed. You may need to alter or change some hobbies; change to water-color painting if oil paints cause problems. Pianos may have a highly toxic pesticide used on them to prevent moth damage.

People who work around toxic substances may seem well during the work week, but on the weekend, when they are away from the chemicals, they may start to experience withdrawal symptoms or begin to detoxify. These symptoms can be in the form of headaches, muscle aches, and some inability to function normally for the next few days. As the body becomes more and more loaded down with toxins, other products may begin to cause symptoms that were not a problem previously.

When buying new upholstered furniture, make sure that the wood used for the frame does not smell. New furniture will gas off the finish and perhaps the glue for a long time. New leather is usually better than vinyl or naugahyde, but nylon may be better. Soft vinyl has extremely toxic plasticizers in it to make it soft. New cotton batting is treated, so you may have to recycle the batting from some old furniture. You must be able to tolerate the fabric, synthetic or natural. Check for used furniture or new floor samples that have been sitting in the store for months. The outgassing of any toxic chemicals would be further along in older furniture. Hard plastic chairs may also be a problem because of the outgassing of toxic chemicals.

At Christmas time do not use chemical snow sprays. Wash any fabrics before using them for decorations. Buy more glass or wooden ornaments than plastic. If you invite guests to your home, discuss perfume and smoking ahead of time. Get a branch from different kinds of Christmas trees to test for tolerance before buying a large tree. If you find that you are allergic to real trees, then a fake tree may be a better choice. Some plastic trees are not tolerated, especially if new. Floodlights with colored plastic discs give off fumes. Here are more suggestions to reduce environmental toxicity in the home:

• Do not use anything but 100 percent cotton sheets, unless cotton is a problem. Be sure chemicals have not been added to make the sheets permapressed, flame-proofed, etc.
• Change or cover the sleeping pillows if necessary.
• Consider the mattress as a potential problem.
• Remove all soft plastic from the room and any other synthetic items.
• Remove all perfumes from the room.

- Remove all synthetic clothing.
- Take any synthetic rugs out of the room if they can be removed easily, or clean them with a steam machine until the water is clean.
- Take down synthetic drapes and use cotton for curtains. If dust is not a health problem, then mini blinds may be another choice.
- Use a wooden chair to sit on instead of overstuffed furniture or plastic.
- Remove house plants if you are mold sensitive.
- Remove from the home all chemical cleaners, laundry products, or any chemical product used for any purpose.
- Purchase several all-cotton outfits, cotton pajamas and a cotton robe.
- Do not wear synthetic slippers. Any natural fabric will probably do unless you know that you are sensitive to it.
- Remove moth proofing from clothing by washing, if possible.
- Eliminate all cosmetics and try to use products made from natural or hypoallergenic substances.
- Store pollutants away from the house or away from areas where people spend any time.
- Add catalytic converters or other emission-control devices to wood stoves and kerosene heaters.
- Buy bottled water or buy a good water-filtration system. Avoid chlorinated water. Store water in glass containers.
- Buy foods free from pesticides, herbicides, and other chemical contaminants as much as possible.
- Try to use glass-contained products instead of cans or plastic-wrapped foods.
- Store food only in glass or cooking ware, not plastic.
- The more simple and organic the product is, the less likely it is full of toxic substances.
- Do not cook with Teflon. Use stainless steel, Pyrex, or Corningware.
- Carefully evaluate all medications for sensitivities.
- Avoid processed foods contaminated with industrial solvents, artificial flavorings, colorings, preservatives, and antibiotics.

To help yourself, your family, and your environment, make a commitment to rid your home of the dozens of toxic products and replace them with products that are nontoxic and environmental friendly. Part of improving your health involves cleaning up the environment in your home. Toxic products place an additional toxic load on the body. See the "Resources" section at the end of this book for information on companies that supply home and personal-care products that are environmentally sensitive, biodegradable, nontoxic, and packaged in recyclable containers, and not tested on animals. Excellent natural cleaners are available. Read labels carefully to make sure that the product is environmentally safe and non-toxic. If the package doesn't state that it is environmentally friendly, it probably isn't. Some terms to help you select the best products are:

- *Phosphate-free:* If the label doesn't state that it is phosphate-free, it contains phosphates that pollute our waterways. They cause algae to grow at alarming rates, choking out marine plants and animals.
- *Chlorine-free:* Chlorine combines with other chemicals in the environment to create toxic compounds such as chloroform.
- *Rapidly biodegradable:* If microorganisms cannot break down substances quickly, then they accumulate in the environment.
- *Dye-free:* Artificial dyes in cleaners are often toxic and harmful to us and the environment.
- *Free of brighteners:* Brighteners may make our fabrics more white and our colors more vivid, but they are often toxic and harmful to the environment.

What Tests Determine Your Toxic Overload?

The EPA has an ongoing study since 1976 looking for the presence of 150 known toxic compounds in human fat samples. Fifty percent of the chemicals have been present in everyone tested so far. The question is not whether a person is toxic, but how toxic they are and how severely this toxicity affects them. Tests used to determine chemical overloads are:

- A complete blood count to determine the toxin effect on the red and white blood cells
- A general blood chemistry shows the relative health of such organs as the adrenal glands, kidneys and liver.
- D-Glucaric acid test is done with urine to determine the chemical assault on the liver. It will reflect the presence of the most common chemical toxins.
- Caffeine clearance tests show how effective the liver is at breaking down chemical compounds. It lets us know the toxic load on the liver and if there is damage.
- Ask your doctor about the available methods of heavy-metal testing. Blood and urine levels are available for testing solvents, formaldehyde, pesticides, herbicides, chemical inhalants, and other toxins.

WHAT ELSE IS BEING DONE TO OUR FOODS?

Sugar is treated with chemicals of various origins during processing.

There may be a coating of mineral oil and wax on the peel of fresh fruits and vegetables to give them more shine. Chemicals can prevent discoloration of French fried potatoes. Meats may have hormones and chemicals added before slaughter as well as the addition of preservatives and chemicals after slaughter.

Potato skins can pose a health hazard for consumers. They can be a source of human-made toxins because of chemicals used to retard sprouting. Pesticide residue levels are up to four times greater than government guidelines allow. If you have to buy potatoes with chemicals, don't eat the skins. It is best to buy organic potatoes. The major nutrients are not in or near the potato skin, as is commonly thought. The center of the potato has the highest levels of vitamin C. Even without the peel, a baked potato still contains about two grams of fiber. Most of the mineral content thought to be in potato skins actually comes from soil clinging to the peel, but the soil also contains many contaminants. Avoid boiling potatoes because some of the toxins seep into the flesh, whereas baking a potato is less likely to be a problem.

It should also be noted that killing bacteria in our food supply does not remove the toxins made by that bacteria. Irradiated food contains free radicals that form new and dangerous chemical compounds in the food. Some of these are benzene, hydrogen peroxide, and formaldehyde. The process of irradiating our foods does not come close to being adequately tested for safety. It also seems that the irradiation of food destroys up to 80 percent of some vitamins.

The National Academy of Sciences estimates that seventy people per year may die because of penicillin and tetracycline residues in meat, as well as the "super bugs" they encourage. According to random testing by the United States Department of Agriculture, pork and veal are more likely to contain illegal levels of legal drugs than poultry and beef. Some ranchers use illegal drugs to fight livestock diseases. Among the illegal goods the FDA has detected are Chloramphenicol, Carbadox, Nitrofurazone, Dimetridazole, and Ipronidazole. They are all potentially cancer-causing agents. There are also hormones added to beef and milk.

Things are so bad that in 1988 the European community announced a ban on meat raised with hormones in the United States. Salmonella contaminates about one-third of all chickens and causes more than 40,000 reported cases of illness a year. It is showing up in the eggs as well. Salmonella and other bacterial diseases account for about 27 percent of the outbreaks from food-related illness. Nine percent is traced to chemical causes, 3 percent to viruses and parasites, and 60 percent of food poisoning outbreaks remain unsolved.

When the National Research Council in 1987 compiled a list of foods presenting the highest risk of cancer, the tomato was at the top of the list. Beef was second, followed by potatoes, oranges, lettuce, apples, peaches, pork, wheat, soybeans, beans, carrots, chicken, corn, and grapes. This was because of the increased use of pesticides on these foods. Despite the fact that the entire food chain is contaminated with chemicals, there is still good reasons to eat low on the chain. The best reason might be your health. The studies say that those who eat lowest live longest.

We could begin by eating natural foods free of pesticides, herbicides, hormones, and antibiotics rather than the chemically poisoned foods and water that are increasing yearly. We must breathe clean air rather than the chemicals found in modern homes and the pollution that surrounds us. Your thorough understanding of how you can effectively reduce chemical toxicity is vital to good health. We cannot afford to wait before taking reasonable measures to protect ourselves and our families from toxic exposures.

CHAPTER 41

Pesticides

Pesticide use has increased ten-fold since the 1940s, but crop losses from insects have managed to double during the same period. Did the pesticides miss the fields they were suppose to spray or were they just ineffective against the insects they were meant to kill? Pesticides enter the surrounding environment, including the ground water and air. Switching to a nontoxic type of farming helps considerably, but doesn't totally solve the problem. Pesticide residues can still be detected in produce long after the land has been converted to more natural methods.

People reach for that can of spray when something else would work just as well, if not better. Pesticides are being used too much, too often. They are being poured into drains, flushed down toilets, and running off lawns. They are ending up in water systems, ground water, streams, and rivers. Water-treatment plants are not designed to handle this additional burden.

TYPES OF INSECTICIDES & PESTICIDES

Pesticides include herbicides, fungicides, pesticides, and miticides. They are biochemical and contact poisons used to destroy, prevent or control insects, vegetation, rodents, and other pests. Pesticides also include substances used to regulate plant or insect growth and to attract or to repel insect and animal pests. Many different poisons are used and may be found on the grains, fruits, and vegetables that we eat, as well as in products derived from animals. Our air, water, and soil also contain these poisons.

Many insecticides are dispensed in kerosene or other solvents. Rugs are often moth-proofed, especially if put in storage. Rug shampoos may contain insecticides as well. Moth-proofed blankets need to be dry-cleaned to remove the smell because washing often doesn't work. Peelings on fresh fruits and vegetables often contain insecticide and herbicide residues. Tap water can contain these chemicals, too. Insecticides and weed killers can remain in the drinking water if the water-filter unit does not remove them.

Pesticides fall into one of the following source groups: minerals, plants, man-made, or living organisms. Pesticides derived from minerals generally contain heavy metals as the toxic ingredient. Zinc compounds control moss on roofs, sidewalks, and other surfaces. Sulfur and copper-containing compounds, as well as cadmium, are effective against fungi. Most pesticides used today are man-made. They contain carbon, hydrogen, and often include other elements like chlorine, sulfur, phosphorus, or nitrogen. Examples are malathion for controlling insects; diphacinone for controlling rodents; and 2,4-D for controlling vegetation. Exterminators typically use dieldrin, chlordane, and pentachlorphenol. Balls, cakes, and crystals used to repel moths contain naphthalene para-dichlorabenzene. The following contains information on the most commonly used insecticides/pesticides.

CHLORINATED HYDROCARBON INSECTICIDES

Some of these insecticides are Endrin, DDT, Endosolfan (Thiodan), Chlordane, Dicofol (Kelthane), and Lindane. This group plays a major role in combating insect-borne diseases and destroying insects. They are characterized by the presence of chlorine, hydrogen, and carbon. Before 1972, the insecticide DDT was commonly found in meat and dairy products. The body stores this toxic chemical for decades so most older Americans still carry residues of it.

DDT was phased out in the United States in 1972, but we continue to import foods into this country that have been sprayed with DDT. Chemical companies still sell it to Mexico and other countries. With the approval of the General Agreement on Tariffs and Trade (GATT), more pesticide residues will enter this country. Levels of DDT that are much higher than previous standards will come in on imported peaches and bananas, as well as grapes, strawberries, broccoli, and carrots.

Recent evidence strongly supports the relationship between high tissue levels of organochlorines such as DDT and the incidence of breast cancer. DDT is 50 to 60 percent higher in breast-cancer specimens compared with controls. This year, 180,000 American women will be diagnosed with breast cancer and one third will die from it. In the past twenty years, more American women have died of breast cancer than all the fatalities of World War I and II, the Korean War, and the Vietnam War. When these pesticides were banned in Israel in 1978, there was a decline in this type of cancer, even though the consumption of dietary animal fats also rose in the diet. Because of chlorinated hydrocarbon insecticides' association with fat tissues, breast milk may be contaminated as well.

Poisoning symptoms may vary depending upon the particular chlorinated hydrocarbon insecticide used. In general, they interfere with the proper functioning of the central nervous system, the brain being the pri-

330 Allergies and Holistic Healing

mary target organ. Symptoms include lack of coordination, tremors, convulsions, apprehension, excitability, twitching, disorientation, nausea, and weakness. Endrin and related compounds may cause convulsions without any preliminary symptoms. Some animal studies have indicated that these insecticides can make significant changes in the liver, and in some cases result in tumor formation.

Other known effects of the toxic hydrocarbons pentachlorophenol and lindane are fetal malformation, growth retardation, stillbirths, changes in the menstrual cycle, and immune disorders. During the past forty years, wood coated with polychlorinated organic compounds was used for ceilings and wall panels in homes. Carpets and leather upholstery impregnated with moth repellents may contain these compounds. The steady emission of these vapors can result in constant exposure to these chemicals. Studies prove that chemicals commonly found in the home can damage the hormonal and immune systems.

ORGANOPHOSPHATE INSECTICIDES

This group of insecticides includes Malathion, Acephate (Orthene), Parathion, Disulfoton (Di-Syston), Chlorpyrifos (Drusban), Diazinon, Ethion, Dimethoate (Cygon), and Dichlorvos (Vapona) and Systox. The most widely used pesticides and insecticides in the United States are organophosphates controlling a wide variety of insects. They are synthetic chemicals that kill insects by interfering with the normal operation of their nervous system, having the same action as nerve gases. They may kill insects on contact, cause systemic poisoning, or act as a stomach poison. Their toxicity to humans varies widely.

A commonly used pesticide, Diazinon, is turning up in the discharge water of many cities. This chemical is mostly coming from lawns and around homes. Approximately 70 million pounds of pesticides each year finds its way to turf areas in the United States alone. Because of the toxic overload on the water systems in many small towns, they are failing water-quality tests.

The primary target of organophosphate insecticides within the body is an important enzyme called acetylcholinesterase, required for normal functioning of the nervous system. If enough of this enzyme is inhibited, the nervous system cannot function normally and symptoms may appear. Neurological effects can begin within hours of exposure or two to three weeks later. It can and does cause behavior and learning deficits that may be irreversible. Even years after the poisoning, persistent symptoms can exist. Acetylcholinesterase and a similar enzyme, plasma cholinesterase, are present in the blood and can be measured to see if they have been inhibited. Monitoring these two enzymes can indicate exposure to organophosphate insecticides.

Organophosphate insecticides can affect brain, muscle, glandular, and respiratory functions. Typical symptoms are abdominal cramps, a reduced heart rate, salivation, pinpoint pupils, headache, muscle twitching, and blurred vision. Some exposures produce a temporary loss of feeling in both the arms and legs, impairments in simple motor skills, a loss of intellectual functioning, and a loss of abstract and flexible thinking.

The biggest offender causing "sick school syndrome" would have to be pesticides, especially organophosphates. Most school districts currently manage pests solely by using these neurotoxic chemicals in and around schools. One study conducted on the effects of pesticides on the nervous system concluded that it is possible that organophosphates may be a major factor in the disruption of the central nervous system in children. The resultant overstimulation can lead to many symptoms in children especially the behavior dysfunction so frequently demonstrated in our younger population. These can also be linked to allergic episodes as well.

CARBAMATE INSECTICIDES

Propoxur (Baygon), Aldicarb (Temik), Carbaryl (Sevin), and Methomyl (Lannate) are the names of common carbamate insecticides. There was hope that this group of insecticides would replace the more toxic organophosphate insecticides. As it turns out, many of the carbamate insecticides are more toxic.

PYRETHRUM, PYRETHRIN AND PYRETHROID INSECTICIDES

Pyrethrum is an insecticidal powder made from the flowers of a species of chrysanthemum plant. Some common names are Pyrethrin, Resmethrin, Permethrin, and Allethrin. They add other chemicals to pyrethrin formulations to protect against oxidation and decomposition from sunlight.

Pyrethroids are synthetic pyrethrins. They act by paralyzing the nervous system of the insect. Numerous synthetic pyrethrins are manufactured and many people are allergic to them. Pyrethroids are not usually as problematic as the pyrethrins. Symptoms commonly found with exposure are stuffy and runny noses, cough, skin and eye irritation, throat irritation, asthmatic wheezing, and other respiratory conditions.

A synergist is generally added to increase the toxicity of these chemicals, such as piperonyl butoxice. The primary health concern with this synergist is the possibility of allergies and tumor formation.

CHLOROPHENOXY HERBICIDES

The common names are 2,4-D, Dicamba, and MCPP. These herbicides are plant growth regulators that are selective for broadleaf plants. There have been a few reported cases of human poisonings from inhalation of 2,4-D. Symptoms of temporary loss of feeling in the arms and legs that lasted for several months are not common, but do occur. Other common symptoms are irritation of the mouth and throat, abdominal pain, diarrhea, hyperventilation, weakness, headache, nausea, and fever. Severe poisoning cases have led to convulsions, coma, and death.

ARSENIC-CONTAINING COMPOUNDS

These are effective insecticides, herbicides and rodent killers, but the recent use of arsenic compounds has decreased. Absorption of arsenic into the body through skin contact and breathing is minimal unless the individual has repeated or continuous skin exposure or inhalation of arsenic-laden dust. Early symptoms are headache, dizziness, abdominal pain, vomiting and bloody diarrhea. The more advanced symptoms of poisoning are liver damage, paralysis, respiratory depression, and death. Accidental poisonings have often involved children.

BORIC ACID

Boric acid is an insecticide for controlling cockroaches and ants. It seems to desiccate the insect and act as a stomach poison. The majority of human exposure is from ointments containing boric acid and from unintentional ingestion by infants. Some symptoms of poisoning are skin rash, flaky skin, vomiting, diarrhea, and convulsions.

HERBICIDES

Herbicides control vegetation. Dichlobenil (Casoron) does not seem to cause any major toxicological problems. The EPA has requested that additional studies be conducted to fill some data gaps. Its common use is for home and garden as a pre-emergency herbicide for controlling germination of grasses and broadleaf weed seeds among established plants.

Glyphosate (Roundup) is a non-selective herbicide used to control vegetation along driveways, fences, sidewalks, and around mature trees. It appears to be low in toxicity to mammals, but known adverse effects are gastrointestinal disturbances, irritation to eyes, skin, and respiratory tract.

ORGANIC FUNGICIDES

Two fungicides are Captan and Captafol. They control a variety of mildew and fungus diseases on fruits, vegetables, and ornamental plants.

They are not likely causes of birth defects or genetic damage to humans. The symptoms most likely to be experienced by human exposure are skin and eye irritation and lung damage. Irritations can be very severe and eye damage can be irreversible. It is advisable to wear goggles and skin protection when using these chemicals.

Beware if you buy used furniture or bedding. By law any bedding for resale through a store must be fumigated. This would not apply to private sales such as garage sales. Mold and mildew cleaners usually contain pesticides.

MOLLUSCIDES

Metaldehyde, a common molluscide, controls slugs and snails around the yard and garden. It is generally formulated as pelleted bait. Use caution because of the possibility of serious illness to domestic animals occasionally leading to death. Poisonings in children usually occur because they mistake the bait for edible food. Symptoms include severe abdominal pain, retching, and convulsions.

SYNERGIST AND INERT INGREDIENTS

These chemicals are not active ingredients, but may contribute to health problems. Synergists are chemicals that can increase the toxic effect of insecticides. Those most commonly used are related to compounds found in black pepper and sesame seeds. One of these, piperonyl butoxice, is added to pyrethrin and pyrethroid formulations. The primary health concern with these compounds is the possibility of tumor formation and allergies.

Inert ingredients are also in solvents, carriers, and diluents. They are not considered pesticides when used this way. Inert ingredients can be in the form of a gas, solid, or liquid. It is common to find them in petroleum products used as an aerosol and liquid formulations. A powder or dust formulation may contain products such as talc, silicates, diatomaceous earth, or clays. On inhalation, these products may cause headaches and respiratory distress. When they contact the eyes, mucous membranes, or sensitive skin areas, they may cause irritation.

EXPOSURE TO PESTICIDES

Petroleum-derived chemicals do not occur naturally so most microorganisms cannot break them down. Pesticides are designed to attack a pest's nervous system, and when humans are exposed to these toxins they can suffer nervous system damage as well. Pesticides contain some of the most toxic synthetic chemicals ever created by humans. The accumulation of such compounds find their way into storage in the fatty parts of each cell. The human body has no previous experience with these chemicals and there is no natural mechanism to break them down, much less eliminate them. The effects may be magnified in the developing nervous systems of children.

The average child now receives more exposure to pesticides than ever before. In 1993, a landmark study by the National Academy of Sciences discovered that children are at far greater health risk than was ever realized from the exposure to pesticides in the food supply. The EPA estimates that pesticides contaminate the ground water in at least thirty-eight states. They pollute the drinking water of millions of people. Many of the pesticides approved by the EPA were registered before extensive research was done linking these chemicals to illnesses.

Many pesticides are on our fruits and vegetables, but it is also shocking to learn that most of the pesticides ingested in this country come from animal products. Animals are regularly and repeatedly fed pesticide-laden products that they absorb and store in their tissues. The flesh of a large fish will accumulate the total amount of pesticides or toxins stored in the flesh of the thousands of smaller fish it has eaten. Each of those smaller fish will collect in its tissues all the pesticides ingested by thousands of even smaller fish it eat.

In the same way, farm animals retain in their flesh and fat all the pesticides that they absorb from their feed. They build up extremely high levels of chemical pesticides and toxins because their food consists exclusively of pesticide-laden fish meal and feed grown on lands sprayed repeatedly with many more dangerous chemicals. They dip and spray these animals with extremely toxic compounds and feed them massive doses of toxic drugs never given to animals raised naturally. Other drugs fed to animals, such as hormones and antibiotics, may also be dangerous for humans. When you eat products derived from these animals, you consume concentrated doses in uncontrolled combinations of many of the most deadly chemicals ever known. The desire to reduce the ingestion of deadly chemicals is just one more good reason to reduce your intake of animal products or buy chemical- and pesticide-free meats.

The home is another principal place of exposure to pesticides in the United States. Studies show that about 90 percent of all households in this country use pesticides. A wide variety of products are available for home use, including preparations for insects within the home, flea and tick sprays, shampoos for pets, and products used on house plants. Most homemakers routinely use disinfectants such as bathroom cleaners, room deodorizers, or laundry aids classified as pesticides. Other commonly used products are no-pest strips, pesticides to control termites, Kwell shampoo for head lice and scabies, flea collars on pets, pesticides in the garden, and herbicides to control weeds in the yard. Rugs are often moth-proofed, especially if they've ever been put in storage. Rug shampoos may contain insecticides as well. Peelings on fresh fruits and vegetables often contain insecticide and herbicide residues. Tap water can contain these chemicals, too. Insecticides and weed killers can remain in the drinking water if the water-filter unit does not remove these contaminants.

Ninety percent of all manufactured pesticides are used to exterminate common household garden and agricultural pests. We would all do well to investigate the natural alternatives. Severe pesticide poisonings number more than three million worldwide each year with 220,000 deaths. The U.S. figures are somewhere between 150,000 to 300,000 pesticide-related illnesses each year.

Symptoms and Illnesses Associated with Pesticide/Insecticide Poisoning

Insecticides can enter the body through the skin, eyes, mouth and nose. Absorption and onset of symptoms by ingestion and inhalation are typically rapid, occurring within a few minutes to a few hours after exposure. Symptoms from skin absorption are generally slower, but can still be dangerous. A brief, low-dose exposure may not necessarily cause symptoms, but severe exposures can lead to severe symptoms and even death. Long-term occupational exposures, below those that produce obvious symptoms, can still result in a chronic but mild flu-like condition.

The organs most affected are the brain and the nervous system. The symptoms are certainly varied, but common symptoms of pesticide poisoning include the inability to think, impaired memory, poor concentration, poor coordination, and drowsiness. Other possible symptoms are anxiety, diarrhea, itching and rash, restlessness, headaches, blurred vision, convulsions, pinpoint pupils, dizziness, weakness, nausea, vomiting, muscle pains or twitching, chest pains, disorientation, increased heart rate, loss of feeling, excessive sweating, stomachaches and cramps, increased salivation, breathing difficulties, impaired intellectual functioning, simple motor skills, and irritation of the eyes, throat, and skin.

Most school districts currently manage pests solely by using neurotoxic chemicals, especially organophosphates, in and around schools. The resulting symptoms could include hyperactivity, difficulty in focusing attention, impaired verbal ability, difficulty doing math, memory deficits, numbness, tingling, hoarseness, flu-like symptoms, and multiple chemical sensitivities. Less toxic methods of controlling pests need our attention, for the sake of our children.

Pesticides harm children more then adults. Their early exposure to these chemicals can cause permanent structural and functional damage to a growing body. They affect the child's immune system making it harder to fight disease. If a nursing mother has pesticide exposure, she can pass these toxins to her baby. Residues on a parent's clothing can be transferred to the child.

It has to be more than coincidental that the present epidemic of hyperactivity and behavioral problems among school children has coincided with steadily increasing levels of volatile organic chemicals found in modern buildings. Behavioral problems may be the earliest sign of chemical toxins. The potential of these substances for causing brain and neurologic damage is well documented in the medical literature.

Most organic solvents and pesticides in use today are fat-soluble and have an affinity for the fatty tissues of the body. The brain and nervous system are more than 25 percent fat in content and are especially vulnerable because of a rich blood supply to these areas. Children and developing fetuses are much more vulnerable to the damaging effects of these toxins because of their rapidly growing tissues and because of the immaturity of their detoxification systems.

Foods contaminated with even low levels of pesticides are known to cause learning and memory impairment, hyperactivity, and aggressive behavior. The possible effects of pesticide residues found in human milk surely deserve investigation. Repeated exposure to organophosphate pesticides by children, even at low doses, should cause concern because numerous studies show personality changes and learning disabilities after pesticide exposure. This fact is all the more important when we realize that pesticides may persist in indoor air up to twenty-one days following indoor application and they may persist for months in the fatty tissues of the body. Sadly, the EPA has not yet required testing of pesticides for brain toxicity or to detect neurological defects. Hopefully they will in the near future.

The primary target of organophosphate insecticides within the body is an important enzyme required for normal functioning of the nervous system. If enough of this enzyme is inhibited, the nervous system cannot function normally and symptoms may appear. Neurological effects can begin within hours of exposure, or two to three weeks later. They can and do cause behavior and learning deficits that may be irreversible. Even years after the poisoning, persistent symptoms can exist. Nervous system enzymes present in the blood can be measured by lab tests indicating exposure to organophosphate insecticides.

There is a known link between pesticides and pollutants and the "feminization" of male birds, turtles, alligators, and fish. Animal studies show that minute exposure to pesticides, far less than the amount needed to cause cancer, affects reproduction. The embryo appears especially sensitive to these environmental hormones.

Sperm counts and semen volume in humans have fallen sharply since 1940, and more newborn males have undescended testicles leading to infertility. In 1950, only 0.5 percent of male college students were sterile. In 1978, the sperm count was down 25 percent. Today, the sperm count of the average American male is down another 30 percent. The major contributor to sterility and sperm-count reduction in this country is chlorinated hydrocarbon pesticides, including Dioxin and DDT, according to Dr. Ralph Dougherty of Florida State University.

Ninety women went to a specialist because of habitual abortion, unexplained infertility, menstrual disorders, or menopausal symptoms. Twenty-two of these women had elevated blood levels of a polychlorinated organic compound called pentachlorophenol or Lindane, or both. The levels of these chemicals were highest in women with infertility. The source of the toxic vapors was present in the home of each patient. With the removal of the toxin their symptoms stopped. Most of the women who had continued exposure to the chemicals, even with medical treatment for the hormonal disorder, did not improve until the removal of the toxic chemical from their environment.

Individuals plagued by chronic illnesses of the autoimmune system such as arthritis, multiple sclerosis, and colitis are significantly more sensitive to pesticides. Around 16 million people experience some degree of immune system reactions to pesticides. Symptoms can range from runny eyes and itchy skin to shock and death. A recent National Cancer Institute sponsored study says garden or household pesticides can increase the risk of childhood leukemia by seven times. Pregnant women should be especially wary.

Pesticides are designed to attack a pest's nervous system. When humans are exposed to these toxins they can suffer nervous system damage as well. Pesticides contain some of the most toxic synthetic chemicals ever created by humans. The accumulation of such compounds find their way into storage in the fatty parts of each cell, especially in breast tissue. As the use of pesticides increases, the incident of breast cancer in women also increases. Studies are continuing to report the link between this type of cancer and the use of pesticides. The human body does not have enough previous experience with these chemicals and there is not any natural mechanism to break them down, much less eliminate them.

Another study indicated that children had a much greater risk of developing childhood leukemia if exposed to pesticides in the home. The effects may be magnified because of the developing nervous systems of children. It could be possible that organophosphate exposure may be another factor in the production of brain dysfunction found in the younger population. The Natural Resources Defense Council published a study called "Intolerable Risk: Pesticides in Our Children's Food." According to that study, pesticides in foods eaten before the age of six accounts for at least 55 percent of a person's lifetime cancer risk. Another study was done in 1993 by the National Academy of Sciences, called "Pesticides in the Diets of Infants and Children," concluded that pesticides posed a significant threat to health. Hopefully, these conclusions will cause people to seek pesticide-free food, especially for young children.

The National Coalition Against the Misuse of Pesticides says that there are no safe pesticides, only acceptable poisons. They claim that many of the gardening pesticides on the market affect the nervous system, harm the skin, cause birth defects, are carcinogenic, affect reproduction and hurt the kidneys and liver. Instead of using chemically-laden sprays, seek healthy alternatives and all-natural products for removing pests. Most natural products leave no toxic after-effect or lingering odors in buildings or homes.

Farming Practices

The government encourages the use of pesticides by not allowing farmers to rotate their crops if they want to qualify for government crop-support programs. Some banks and insurance companies require farmers who seek their services to use pesticides. Farmers using natural alternatives such as crop rotation and integrated pest management instead of toxic chemicals to control pests do not have significantly reduce yields.

Today, more than 2.5 billion pounds of pesticides are applied every year in the United States alone. The effects of pesticides remain even after their use is stopped. Pesticides such as DDT and Chlordane have remained in the food chain for more than 20 years.

The pesticides we use may be more obnoxious than the pest we are trying to discourage. After four decades of chemical pesticide use, the pest problems are not any better, and if anything they are worse. Before World War II, farmers lost about one third of their drops to pests. Today, the amount is about the same even with of all the chemicals in use. Over the last 40 years, nearly 600 species of insects have become resistant to major classes of insecticides and pesticides. What about all the beneficial insects that are killed by these poisons?

Commercial farming techniques have stripped our soils of vital trace minerals and left residues of dangerous chemicals in our fruits and vegetables, as well as in our meats. The meat industry claims that Dioxin and other pesticides in beef are not a concern because the quantities are so small. This doesn't seem to be true either. We are just beginning to see the profound effects on reproduction as well as other problems these chemicals are causing. Your body is a by-product of the soil that grows your food. It can only be as healthful as the source. Bugs and disease are nature's cleanup crew to eliminate the weak and defective. Pesticides kill pests, but also kill helpful bugs and the soil. Remember, pesticides are poison. They are not tested for their interactivity or for cumulative damage in humans. The use of pesticides is profit based, not health based. Our bodies were never intended for such large exposures to toxic chemicals. It is resulting in ailments that physicians can't even identify.

How are Pesticides Tested?

Many of the pesticides that are approved today by the EPA were registered before extensive research was done linking these chemicals to illnesses. When the FDA determines whether to legalize pesticides, each one is tested in isolation. No one ever tests what happens when a combination of pesticides are used and what effect this might have on the body. Over 500 foods analyzed in a pesticide test had as many as five pesticide residues on them. Why are there so many pesticides on one food? One reason may be that spray drift can average a distance of 25 miles. Another reason is that some farmers are spraying with illegal pesticides.

Most people believe that the U.S. Department of Agriculture protects our health through inspections. That doesn't seem to be true either. The USDA's sloppy job has been the recent subject of several television news specials. They tested fresh peaches for pesticide residue and over half of them contained more than one. Thirty percent of all samples contained Dicloran residues, and 20 percent of the FDA samples detected Captan residues. Dicloran has not been sufficiently tested for safety. Captan is a probable human carcinogen and most of the residues remain primarily on the produce's surface, but may enter the edible tissue.

When you poison things you are just asking for trouble. Petroleum-derived chemicals do not occur naturally in nature, so most microorganisms can't break them down. Besides poisoning us, these chemicals appear to be a major source of food allergies or sensitivities. It may be beneficial to allergy test for common insecticides such as Diazinon because of its common use on crops.

Protect Yourself from Pesticide Poisoning

Protect yourself when using pesticides. They can make you sick, hurt your eyes, cause skin rashes, and even kill you. Pesticides residues are small amounts of pesticides that remain on plants, soil, and in irrigation systems after the treatment of a field. It is important to avoid exposure to these residues. Wait until it is safe to go back into a pesticide-treated area because some pesticides are very poisonous. Signs warning of a treated field that cannot be entered must be clearly posted at the edge of the field and orchard. The following recommendations are important:

- Always read, understand, and follow the safety precautions on the label of any pesticide you are using.
- Use proper equipment when in contact with pesticides. Wear any protective equipment required on the pesticide label such as respiratory protection.
- Wear eye protection. Use safety glasses or chemical goggles if the pesticide is in a liquid or powdered form.
- Don't put your hands in your mouth or rub your eyes when you have been in contact with pesticides or when handling plants or soil in a treated area.
- Wear protective clothing such as long-sleeved shirts, long pants, a hat, socks, and rubber boots. If necessary, wear washable rubber gloves.
- After handling any toxic substance, wash your hands before eating, drinking, smoking, or going to the bathroom.
- Wash your clothes before wearing them again. Keep them in a separate plastic bag until you can wash them. Then wash clothing in a separate load from the rest of your other laundry.
- After using pesticides, wash yourself with soap and water, shampoo your hair, and put on clean clothes.
- Keep your children and pets out of a sprayed area.
- Do not eat fruits or vegetables sprayed with pesticides.
- Avoid water that has been exposed to pesticides.
- Do not take pesticides home from work. They are not safe for home use and can poison you and your family.

People living in rural areas are in a unique situation because they often live close to sprayed fields. The following are a few simple precautions to help prevent illness from pesticide drift:

- Close car and house windows if you are situated near a spray operation.

- Keep children, pets, and toys indoors when an application is being sprayed on the property next to your home.
- Hose down play equipment or outdoor furniture with water if it receives pesticide spray or drift.
- Do not hang laundry out to dry when pesticides are being applied.
- Observe re-entry times before entering a treated field. This should be on the pesticide label and usually ranges from 24 to 96 hours.
- Do not enter treated fields without protective clothing for at least four days if you do not know which pesticides were applied.
- If necessary, cover all livestock water and feed supplies to protect from drift.
- If you suspect pesticide poisoning, take the label, or copy it, and give this information to your doctor. Place any contaminated clothing in a plastic bag for testing.
- Be careful when handling pesticides. They can make you very sick.

RIGHTS ON THE JOB

You have the right to safety and protection on the job if you are being exposed to toxic chemicals. By law your employer must give you the training and equipment needed to work with pesticides. You have the right to know about hazardous chemicals used in your work area. If you think you are not being adequately protected or trained about pesticide dangers on the job, contact your state Department of Labor and Industries. You can complain about pesticide exposure or other unsafe or unhealthy working conditions to government agencies without having your name revealed to your employer.

The chance that a pesticide will affect you depends on your understanding of the hazards and how well you protect yourself. You have the right to know about hazardous chemicals used in your neighborhood under the community right-to-know law. For additional information or help with pesticides contact the following:

- The State Department of Health if you are suffering from pesticide poisoning.
- The State Department of Agriculture if you are concerned about the use of pesticides.
- The State Department of Labor and Industries if you think you are not being adequately protected or trained about pesticide dangers on the job.
- The County Health Department who is responsible for enforcing sanitation standards. They will inform you where to go for prenatal care. Look

for their number in your phone book under County Agencies-Health Services.
• Contact your local poison center.

Symptoms of pesticide poisoning may mimic other common illnesses, often making it difficult to determine the relationship of the exposure to the symptoms. The Department of Health believes that about half of last year's reported poisoning cases were probably related to pesticide exposure. One third of the time the exposure was from agricultural activities, but occurrences are common in and around commercial or residential settings.

CHAPTER 42

Water and Environmental Toxins

The purity and quality of the water you drink is vital to your body's well-being. Water is the key to all bodily functions: circulation, digestion, assimilation, elimination, temperature control, and lubrication. It flows through every artery and vein. Water makes up 60-70 percent of your body weight and is needed in all of your tissues. By weight, the brain and heart are 75 percent water, the lungs and liver are 86 percent, and the blood and kidneys are 83 percent water.

CHEMICALS, PESTICIDES, & CONTAMINANTS IN THE WATER

Consider that about 66,000 chemicals are used in the United States and close to 50,000 pesticides are currently being sold in the marketplace. At least 1,200 ingredients in pesticides are labeled as inert, but only 300 are considered safe, and at least 100 are known to be dangerous. Add to these contaminants the incredible amount of hazardous waste dumps, landfills, underground storage tanks and septic tanks and this adds up to at least 400 billion pounds of toxins being dumped into our air, water, water sources, and soil every year.

This contamination includes both ground and surface water. Ground water includes underground aquifers, wells or springs. These ground sources provide water to about one half the population. Surface water, such as ponds, rivers, and lakes serve as the water source for the rest of the population. Dumping contaminants onto the soil affects both types of water sources. Toxins will run down through the soil to the underground water sources or run off into lakes and rivers. The rivers, ponds, and lakes are also contaminated by pollutants carried by air and rain. Some sources of these problems are:

- Gasoline stations
- Coal strip-mine runoff
- Oil well leakage
- Highway de-icing salts
- Septic tank or cesspool leakage
- Sewer leakage
- Using pesticides, fertilizers, herbicides, etc.
- Accidental toxic spills
- Industrial disposal well leakage
- Waste lagoons or ponds
- Rusting underground tanks that are leaking
- Homeowners dumping chemicals down drains

These contaminants from industrial wastes, mining, agriculture, and other sources of modern living certainly contribute to hazards in our drinking water. This includes nitrates and other nitrogen compounds that are the result of chemical fertilizers, sewage, and feed-lot runoff. What are the effects of consuming these contaminants in small amounts over long periods of time? It is hard to diagnose health problems that develop over the span of many years, but there is genuine concern that prolonged exposure to certain elements, even at levels as low as a few parts per billion or trillion, may be increasing the incidence of cancer and heart disease. One part per billion is equivalent to one pound in 500,000 tons. Since the Safe Drinking Water Act was passed in 1974, over two thousand organic and inorganic contaminants have been identified in drinking water in this country. In 1988, Ralph Nader reported that this country is faced with a burgeoning water contamination crisis that local, state, and federal officials have been unwilling or unable to manage.

Water Systems

Millions of people may be needlessly exposed to unhealthy drinking water. In one of the most comprehensive drinking water studies ever, the Natural Resources Defense Council analyzed EPA records and found in 1991-1992 that 43 percent of all water suppliers violated federal health standards. At least 250,000 violations affected more than 120 million people, but only 3,900 of the 250,000 violations were acted on. Noncommunity water systems (hospitals, hotels, and schools, etc.) had an additional 10,000 violations affecting 1.4 million people.

A report also warned that most of the nation's water treatment plants are grossly inadequate. Less than 40 percent of U.S. water treatment plants effectively remove organisms such as cryptosporidium. The water supply infrastructure does not seem to be capable of providing safe water consistently in many areas of this country.

Developing standards and enforcing them are two different issues. Usually, the larger, municipal water-treatment systems that supply more than 100,000 customers have the resources to keep up with EPA standards. Small water systems serving less than 3,500 people have neither the technology nor the resources to keep pace. In a recent study, 92 percent of the small water systems were in violation of EPA standards.

The standart system used to treat contaminated ground and surface water involves the following process:

- The water is moved from surface and ground water sources to a storage area.
- Copper sulfate is sometimes used to control the growth of algae.
- Chemicals such as chlorine, lime, and alum, are added to clump particles together, disinfect, and sometimes to soften water.
- Water sits in sedimentation basins until solid particles sink to the bottom. The basins are then strained to remove debris.
- For final filtering, the water then flows through beds of gravel and sand.
- Chlorine or other disinfectants are added as a final treatment to kill bacteria.
- They test the water to ensure that it does not contain any quantities of pollutants in excess of the Environmental Protection Agency's or the State's maximum contaminant levels.

We are at the mercy of the EPA. If they do not test for a substance, or do not consider that substance harmful, it is possible to find it in the water. Unfortunately, most of the health risks present in drinking water today are the result of contaminants finding a way into the water after it leaves the treatment and distribution plant. Some of these contaminants are: lead and asbestos entering the water as it flows through the pipes to your tap; trihalomethanes forming as chlorine acts on debris in the water; and back flow into the water line from air conditioners, stopped-up toilets and sinks. Water staying in the pipes for periods of time have higher levels of trihalomethane, a suspected cancer-causing agent.

Most water delivery systems in the United States include cement-asbestos pipes that can pollute water with asbestos fibers, especially at points of repair and alteration. The fibers are virtually undetected, but they are a serious health hazard. Even changes in water pressure within the pipes can cause high levels of asbestos to enter the water. The gray pipe commonly used in water distribution systems in this country is porous to gaso-

346 Allergies and Holistic Healing

line and paint thinner, as well as many herbicides and pesticides. Lead, cadmium, and other toxic metals leach out of valves and pipe couplings between the water-treatment plant and your home faucet.

Illness from Water

From the years 1971 to 1985, the Center for Disease Control, Atlanta, says an average of 7,400 cases of illness in the United States can be linked to drinking water. From 1971 to 1990, according to the Environmental Protection Agency, over 140,000 people in the United States became ill as a result of 570 documented cases of contaminated water. For each illness reported, it is thought that at least 25 probably go unreported.

Water contaminants such as pesticides and herbicides can cause adverse effects in the liver, kidney, nervous system, reproductive system, and play a role in several types of cancer. Contaminated drinking water is thought to contribute to low fertility in American males.

Chlorine does not rid the water supply of many harmful organisms. Microorganisms such as protozoa, fungi, viruses, and coliform bacteria have been found alive in chlorinated tap water. These organisms are potentially dangerous to anyone who consumes them. They are especially dangerous to people with weakened immune systems such as in the cases of people receiving chemotherapy, radiation therapy, and those who have AIDS. Chlorine also does not kill other pathogens, including the one that causes the pneumonia known as Legionnaires' disease. Almost all recent outbreaks of Legionnaires' disease were traced to water-distribution systems.

The protozoa *Giardia lamblia* is found in many areas, even previously pristine ones. Tap water, mountain streams, and well water are prime sources of contamination. Outbreaks of giardia can hospitalize hundreds of people because of severe gastrointestinal symptoms. The protozoa *Cryptosporidium muris* is transmitted via contaiminated ground water, farm animals, and the fecal-oral route. These organisms are especially difficult to eliminate. The usual dose of chlorine added to most water systems does not kill cryptosporidium and may not kill giardia. In April of 1993, over 370,000 residents of Milwaukee became ill, and at least 40 died from the contamination by cryptosporidium. It entered the water supply through fecal material from an upstream dairy farm, but the city's treatment system did not filter out this pathogen. It is hard to detect and harmful strains are not easily distinguishable from the harmless.

Tap Water

Tap water may contain arsenic, asbestos, or toxic metals such as aluminum, copper, cadmium, and lead. It may also contain organic chemicals such as pesticides and nitrites, as well as other microorganisms such as parasites and bacteria. Most city water supplies are chlorinated to kill bacteria, but chlorine itself is not that healthful to drink. Some studies have isolated about 700 different chemicals from supposedly safe tap water.

Be aware of copper toxicity that can develop from tap water being exposed to copper pipes. If you notice any bluish color around drains and shower heads then you probably have copper pipes. Even newer plumbing may be toxic because it contains plastic called polyvinyl chloride (PVC). Cadmium may be leached from these new PVC pipes. It does leach less as the pipe ages. To avoid the build up of these toxins, leave your water running for approximately 2-3 minutes before drinking if you do not have any type of filtering system.

Chlorine

There are other chlorine-based products found in our environment. That industry produces 12 million tons of chlorine a year for use in paper products, plastics, pharmaceuticals, pesticides, water treatments, and bleach. There is cause for concern about the potential health risks associated with chlorine by-products. Chlorinating our water sources can produce trihalomethanes that produces two by-products, chloroform and carbon tetrachloride. These toxins can enter the water after leaving the processing plant and may even increase during transit to the storage facilities. They are cancer-causing substances, especially of the bladder and rectal area.

There may be a relationship between birth defects and the by-products of chlorine in our water. Researchers from the Federal Centers for Disease Control and Prevention teamed up with the New Jersey's Department of Health to examine birth records and tests of drinking water. Birth defects and lower birth weights increased in areas where mothers were exposed to higher levels of trihalomethanes.

According to the National Institutes of Health, 20 percent of bladder cancer in nonsmokers can be attributed to drinking chlorinated water. Some authorities believe virtually no water in the world is safe for drinking the way it is delivered to the water taps in homes. An interesting fact is that the EPA has set 100 parts per billion (ppb) as a safe level for trihalomethanes in drinking water in the United States. The Environmental Council of the European Economic Community has set only one part per billion as a safe level for trihalomethanes in drinking water. This vast difference should make one wonder if anyone really knows what safe levels for trihalmethanes are.

A United States and Canadian advisory commission blames chlorine-based chemicals for "startling" health problems and is calling on the governments of both countries to ban them from the marketplace. This commission believes enough scientific evidence warrants dealing with the problem. Other health problems linked to chlorine-based toxins include breast cancer in women, prostate and testicular cancer among men, learning disabilities and other behavioral problems among children, and an increase in male reproductive-tract disorders.

Fluoridated Water

It is common to find fluoride added to drinking water. Chlorine and fluoride are powerful enzyme poisons to the body. Excessive fluoride may cause a dark brown spotting of the teeth causing the teeth to become chalky in appearance. There are reasons not to swallow calcium supplements with fluoridated tap water. If you consume calcium and fluoride at the same time, the fluoride in the water will render the calcium insoluble. Calcium is useless to the bones if it can't be absorbed. If the body does not eliminate the additional calcium out through the urine or feces, then it can build up as deposits in other areas. Drinking chlorinated and fluoridated tap water also puts additional stress on the kidneys of the elderly.

Lead

The most abundant metallic toxin in drinking water today is lead. Over 42 million Americans probably drink toxic amounts of lead each day. Most U.S. apartments and older houses still have lead plumbing. Some iron pipes are galvanized with a zinc-cadmium coating, and most iron pipes are soldered with a lead compound. This may contaminate your water supply, especially if the water sits in the pipe for any length of time.

The EPA found lead above what it considers a safe level in 819 water systems that serve 30 million people. Most of the faulty systems are on the east coast and in older communities with lead pipes. A subsequent problem resulted from lead solder on copper pipes installed in the 1980s. Lead pipes are now banned in newer construction, but contamination could be coming from brand new brass fixtures that are leaching lead into the water.

Lead exposure can be especially dangerous to children. It can impair a child's mental and physical development and reduce birth weight and cause premature birth. In adults, excessive lead can increase blood pressure and damage hearing. At very high levels it can cause anemia, kidney damage, and mental retardation.

If you are concerned about lead or other heavy metals in your water supply you could contact your state or local Department of Health or Environment Protection Agency and ask them to recommend an EPA-certified laboratory in your area that can test your water. It is best not to test your water just once, but conduct many tests over an extended time.

You can find reliable and inexpensive lead test kits at most hardware stores. Stores or companies offering in-home water tests are often expensive and some may even be scams. Reducing your family's exposure to these environmental risks require that you find out what toxins may be in your water. To rid your house of toxins, you may have to buy some filtration equipment. Even the most expensive systems are not that expensive and can provide your family with a reassuring margin of safety.

Wells

Some people believe that they are safe because their water comes from a well or from the lake where they live. You couldn't be more wrong. The surrounding land at your well site may have toxic chemicals or metals leaching into your water supply. Contaminated ground water from any source can affect rural area wells. Lake water is also subject to parasites and bacteria. These hazards add to the dangers of toxic and corroding pipes between your water supply and your kitchen faucet.

Radon and Other Gases

Radon is a radioactive gas that comes from the breakdown products of uranium. Water-processing plants that draw on underground water supplies maintain the water in a reservoir. If the radon does not completely outgas during this time, it can reach homes. This is especially dangerous in homes or rooms that are poorly ventilated or completely air conditioned. Inhaled radon can damage the cells of the lung and possibly cause cancer. The contamination of water supply systems varies in different parts of the country, but no safe level of radon outgassing has been established. Radon contamination is more prevalent in Appalachia, New England, and the Midwest; uranium contamination is more prevalent in the West; whereas radium is more common in the Midwest and Southeast.

Other Toxic Metals

Measure your water's pH—the level of acidity or alkalinity. Excessive acidity increases the leaching of toxic metals from your water pipes. The total hardness of your drinking water is another piece of information that is important to know because heart disease is generally lower in areas with hard water. Hard water is a measure of the amount of calcium and magnesium present in the water. Hard water tends to form a protective lining in water pipes that prevents leaching of toxic metals from the pipes.

Testing

The EPA only tests for a small number of the contaminants found in our water. If their standards are met, the water is considered safe, but they do not test for many other contaminants. The most hazardous contaminants, including asbestos and lead, enter the water after leaving the water treatment plant.

You can often avoid expensive water testing by asking utility officials for an analysis of water-quality. It will list the names and the levels of contaminants affecting your region. Lead is the exception; because lead usually contaminates the water through the household's pipes and fixtures, you must test the water at your tap. If you get your water from a private well, contact your region's public health office for test guidance.

If you want to be sure that you will have water that is safe to drink, then add a good filtration system. The best of these will remove virtually any health hazards from your drinking water. There are many inadequate systems on the market that remove little of the unhealthy substances. Buying the best system that you can is a small price to pay when considering the alternative. Filtering your water is far more advantageous than the price you pay for bottled water.

Before buying any method of water purification, test your drinking water to find out what undesirable or toxic agents are present. Then acquire the particular type of purification device that removes those substances. It is important to buy a filtration or purification system for your home that best fits your needs. To guarantee clean, contaminant-free water, you will have to take matters into your own hands, and you easily can. Water filtration systems that combine several features are often necessary. The following is a list of the most common equipment choices:

CARBON FILTERS

Most of the home water-treatment devices found on today's market are simple carbon filters. They come in sizes that can be mounted at the faucet or under the counter. In general, carbon filters work best at removing odors, chlorine, bad taste, organic chemicals, and pesticides. It may be more effective when used in conjunction with reverse osmosis or distillation. Carbon filters are less effective against microorganism contamination, lead and other heavy metals. They will not remove most minerals.

The simplest and least expensive way to filter your water is to use activated charcoal. It will remove organic chemicals, pesticides, some heavy metals, and improve the taste of the water. Activated charcoal filters are inexpensive and do not require electricity to filter the water. All you have to do is just turn on the tap. Activated charcoal filters do not remove many toxic metals, including lead, mercury, cadmium, and fluoride. They also must be replaced regularly to maintain good water quality. If you do not frequently change the filters, bacteria will grow on the carbon. Cheap faucet-mounted carbon filters may become contaminated within days of use. Higher volume models that are used under the counter cost a lot more.

Some charcoal units are impregnated with silver to inhibit bacteria growth. The addition of silver does not improve the ability of the unit to physically remove bacteria or other contaminants, especially chemicals. Studies on the effectiveness of bacteriostatic filters have not shown promising results regarding their ability to control bacterial growth.

Bone carbon or hydroxyapatite charcoal is better at absorbing heavy metals and toxic minerals from the water. In order for the carbon filter to remain effective and not further contaminate the water, clean the filters of the algae, mildew, and other life forms that collect on it.

CARBON BLOCK FILTER

The carbon block filter is better than just using a simple carbon filter. It is more densely packed with a finer carbon that traps even smaller particles and some toxic metals. It removes most bacteria, organic chemicals, and some toxic metals, but allows some minerals to pass through the carbon block. Different stages of carbon remove different size particles.

The nationally recognized standards established for the drinking water treatment industry confirm that the most effective systems for removing contaminants are those that utilize solid carbon block filtering technology. This type of filter does a better job, but is more expensive than simple carbon. It must still be changed often, can grow bacteria, and does not remove all the toxic metals. If you do not replace the filter often enough, it can dump the accumulated toxic organic matter back into your water.

DISTILLATION METHOD

If your purpose is to remove lead and other heavy metals, distillers offer the best choice. You'll pay approximately $200 to $600. This method involves boiling water and then recondensing it. This produces a very pure, mineral-free, bacteria-free water. A problem with this method is that organic chemicals boil at a lower temperature than water. When the water recondenses, the organic chemicals can return to the purified water. Solve this problem with a fractional distilling system or use a carbon block filter. Some systems double boil to remove the organic chemicals. One of the main disadvantages of the distillation method is that it leaves a flat taste unless a little air is mixed with the water. It also uses electricity and so has a higher cost than some other systems.

Not everyone wants to remove all the minerals from their drinking water because they are beneficial when in reasonable balance. At least no toxic substances exist in distilled water. If you choose to drink distilled water to the exclusion of all other liquids, then you should supplement your diet or water with extra minerals to make up for the poor supply. Otherwise, this may produce serious health hazards. For short-term, detoxification purposes, distilled water is usually not a problem.

REVERSE OSMOSIS METHOD

Reverse osmosis involves forcing water through a semipermeable plastic membrane that allows only the water to pass through. The purified water is then passed through a carbon filter to eliminate any gases and other volatile chemicals. It removes minerals and organic compounds. Combined with a charcoal filter, the reverse osmosis method provides one of the best filtering systems available today. Reverse osmosis is now the industry standard for water purification. They are available in under-the-sink units and counter top ones. They produce almost distilled quality water without using extra electricity. The filters operate as long as there is adequate water pressure.

Reverse osmosis systems require that you change the membrane and carbon filters regularly. Since the membrane is back-washed to prevent clogging, some water is wasted. It uses three to six gallons of water for every gallon of drinking water produced and requires an hour or more to produce a gallon of water. These systems cost more, usually, than carbon filters and other simple devices. Some reverse osmosis devices may be ineffective at removing high levels of hard minerals such as calcium and magnesium.

Of all the water-purification systems available, reverse osmosis furnishes the purest and best-tasting liquid product, without the flat taste of distilled wate. If you are drinking reverse osmosis filtered water you will need to supplement your diet or the water with extra minerals, since it has a poor supply. One brand, Multi-Pure, does not remove the natural minerals and does not waste water.

BOTTLED AND SPRING WATER

You can buy a variety of water from worldwide sources in your local supermarkets. The water quality varies depending on the source. They are often high in minerals. This is fine as long as they don't include toxic metals. You can't tell from the label what type of filtration has been used so you don't really know how pure the water is. Hopefully, it doesn't contain any pesticides, nitrates, or high levels of bacteria, but how do you know? Some food markets have facilities to buy some type of purified or filtered drinking water. It is usually inexpensive, but how do you know when the filters were last changed, or what kinds of filters are being used? Some bottled drinking water has fluoride added.

The economics of filtering your own water is far more advantageous than buying bottled water. The latest information suggests that some bottled water may have higher than acceptable levels of bacteria. With a home filter, you can bottle your own water and know that it is safe. It is always best to take care of yourself, because the general water supply may not be as healthy as you want.

How to Choose a Water Filtration System

You may choose from many drinking water systems. With more than 500 companies selling treatment products, it is hard to compare one product to another. The EPA does not establish standards or testing protocol for devices used to treat drinking water. They refer consumers seeking information to NSF International. This is an organization devoted to developing and administering programs related to public health. These are international standards for consumer products and services, including drinking water treatment units. They provide assurance to the consumer that these filtering devices certified by them will perform according to the claims made by the manufacturer or distributor. NSF has two standards that apply to devices used to filter drinking water:

Aesthetic Effects (NSF Standard No. 42)

NSF Standard No. 42 includes claims for taste, odor, color, and other aesthetic effects, including the reduction of chlorine and particulate matter. The different classes that define the level of chlorine and particulate reduction are:

• TASTE, ODOR AND CHLORINE REDUCTION
Class I   Reduces chlorine by 75 to 100%
Class II   Reduces chlorine by 50 to 74%

Class III   Reduces chlorine by 25 to 49%

• PARTICULATE REDUCTION
Class I   0.5 to 1 micrometers (sub micron)
Class II   1 to 5 micrometers (extra fine)
Class III   5 to 15 micrometers (medium fine)
Class IV   15 to 30 micrometers (fine)
Class V   30 to 50 micrometers (medium coarse)
Class VI   50 micrometers and larger (coarse)

Health Effects (NSF Standard No. 53)

NSF Standard No. 53 includs claims for the reduction of specific contaminants from drinking water (public or private). These contaminants are considered potential health hazards. Such hazardous contaminants may be microbiological, chemical, or particulate (including filterable cysts) in nature. A unit may be effective in controlling one or more of these contaminants, but it is not a requirement that it control all of them. Included under this standard are:

• Chemicals and heavy metals: This includes contaminants such as lead, trihalomethanes, lindane, 2,4-D, asbestos, trichloroethylene, and others.
• Volatile organic chemicals: This includes twenty volatile organic contaminants.
• Turbidity: A condition caused by the presence of suspended particulate matter.
• Cysts: Tests determine the effectiveness of the unit in removing microscopic organisms such as *Giardia lamblia*.

When choosing a drinking-water system, you can use the NSF standards and listings to compare one device to another. In addition, the NSF standards also provide the basis for comparing the service life of the units and/or their replacement filters, as well as the flow rate of the device. The following important questions can help to evaluate any drinking water system:

1. Ask for the NSF listing for the specific product(s) you are evaluating. Is the product listed under NSF Standard No. 53 or No. 42?
2. Ask for the product Performance Data Sheet. Many states require that data sheets be provided to all prospective customers of drinking water treatment devices.
3. Ask about the service cycle (stated in gallons of water treated) of the

device. How often will you need to change the filter and what will replacement filters cost?

4. Ask about the range of contaminants that the unit can reduce under Standard No. 53. Be sure that the contaminants concerning you can be removed by the device you are considering. Most units certified under NSF Standard No. 53 are listed for turbidity and cyst reduction only. Fewer units also reduce chemicals, lead, VOCs, and trihalomethanes.

5. Ask about the product's flow rate.

6. Ask if the manufacturer or distributor provides a customer satisfaction guarantee or warranty.

Consumers are often deceived by manufacturer's claims and the information, or lack of it, given by sales people. This makes it more important than ever to refer to industry standards and state regulation. You need to know if the effectiveness of the drinking-water systems has been certified or registered in reducing the substances and/or contaminants that you are paying for. To receive more information on drinking water and equipment, you can contact the following:

National Sanitation Foundation
3475 Plymouth Road
P.O. Box 1468
Ann Arbor, MI 48105

Water Quality Association
4151 Naperville Road
Lisle, IL 60160
(708) 505-0160

EPA Drinking Water Hotline
(800) 426-4791
call (202) 382-5533 in Alaska
and the District of Columbia

The following mail order laboratories offer a variety of home water-testing options and prices:

National Testing Laboratories
6151 Wilson Mills Road
Cleveland, OH 44143
(800) 458-3330

Suburban Water Testing Labs
4600 Kutxtown Road
Temple, PA 19560
(800) 433-6595

Water Test
33 South Commercial St.
Manchester, NH 03101
(800) 426-8378

CHAPTER 43

Hay Fever

The common symptoms of hay fever usually include sneezing, runny nose, irritated eyes, and nasal congestion. The primary part of the body affected is the membrane lining of the nasal passages that become swollen and uncomfortable. Hay fever is often the result of an over-burdened immune system triggered by exposure to the pollens of grasses, trees, and flowers in the spring; ragweed and molds cause problems in the late summer and fall.

There are many herbal and homeopathic medicines that benefit hay fever and allergy sufferers. Numerous herbal decongestants and naturally derived supplements support adrenal function and the immune response that becomes compromised from prolonged allergic reactions. They can also clear out toxic metabolites from the body that result from the allergic response. Supplements such as vitamin C and bioflavonoids are particularly effective for inflammation. The following are helpful hints to decrease hay fever symptoms:

1. TIME TO COOL DOWN

Seek air conditioning to escape the outdoor allergen load; central air systems are best. Keep window units off during the day if you are not home. After arriving home, turn on the unit and close the vent to the outside, but get out of the room when the unit is first turned on. Come back in a half-hour or so when the mold and dust have settled.

2. NOSE CHILL

Set any air conditioning at the highest comfortable setting; no lower than 70 degrees. A nose that is too cold can trigger nasal symptoms.

3. SEA BREEZE

Wind blowing off the ocean is great, providing it's not passing over a land mass before it reaches you. Air blowing out to sea can cause intense allergy symptoms. If the wind is blowing in the right direction, sea air is as pollen-free as you'll find.

4. SEEK SHELTER FROM WINDS

The worst weather for pollen and mold exposure is the kind of summertime climate that sends families down to the beach. A hot sun and a strong breeze ensure that you'll be breathing in any allergens present in the air. Avoid outdoor activities in the early morning and late evening because pollen loads in the air are heaviest at these times. Minimize your outdoor activities on dry, windy days. Pollen is released and spread widely under these conditions. Symptoms can be even worse when mold blows off the plants themselves. When the wind blows, air conditioned places can help reduce your exposure.

5. BAD WEATHER IS GOOD FOR YOU

Enjoy those rainy days. Showers wash pollen right out of the air and create a chance for hay fever sufferers to step outside. However, if mold is your problem, symptoms may be worse for several days after a rain shower.

6. RESIST THE ALCOHOLIC DRINK

Alcoholic beverages increase symptoms in some people, especially when the air is thick with allergens. Wine is the worst offender with beer a close second. Turning down a drink may turn down your symptoms.

7. USE YOUR HOMEOPATHIC MEDICATIONS AHEAD OF TIME

If you know there will be exposure to allergens, take your homeopathic remedy before symptoms begin.

8. BEWARE OF BEE POLLEN

Many people must avoid bee pollen at any time of the year. Capsules and powders containing bee pollen usually contain high levels of ragweed and other high-allergy pollens. The risk of such a reaction is even greater when there are also high levels of pollen in the air. Yet, there are some people who benefit from bee pollen to decrease their hay fever symptoms. It can be helpful, not only in allergies and hay fever, but in asthma, sinus, and chronic pulmonary diseases. Be cautious when starting bee pollen and begin with low doses in case you are sensitive. Honey can have suspended solids in it with pollen being one of them. The label on the bottle may say clover honey, but how do you know that the bee did not stop off at a ragweed blossom?

9. CLEAN YOUR FILTERS

Air conditioner filters can trap some pollen and other stuff you'd rather not breathe. If you haven't cleaned yours lately, it is probably full of tree and grass pollen and mold. Wash or change it at least once a month from now on.

10. STAY CLEAR OF CORNFIELDS

Ragweed and other pollens grow around grains such as corn and soybeans.

11. LOWER MOISTURE LEVELS

Lowering your indoor humidity may prevent late fall and early winter indoor allergies. It also keeps dust mites to a minimum. The mites need humidity to thrive and multiply. They depend on a moist summer for their annual population explosion. Air conditioning and dehumidifiers can really reduce their numbers.

12. IS IT THE WATERMELON?

If you are sensitive to ragweed, you can have a cross-reaction with a variety of similar plant species such as watermelon. It is common to develop an itchy mouth after eating a piece of watermelon when ragweed pollen is in the air. Beware of mangoes and watch those fruity ingredients in summertime tropical drinks.

13. SNEEZE-FREE MOUNTAINS

Mountains are often the most allergy-free areas in the Americas (unless the dampness causes a problem). A sea cruise certainly will get you away from pollens, but avoid the tropical drinks.

14. NATURAL INSECTICIDES

Many natural insecticides are derived from flowers such as chrysanthemums. Inhaling even the tiniest bit of the powder can make people with hay fever miserable.

15. MEDICATION IN THE CAR

Don't keep medication in the car, glove compartment or car trunk. Cars get very hot in the summer. This can ruin homeopathic remedies as well as other medications. If you are traveling, you need to store medications in a cooler or take them with you.

16. WATCH THE HIGH DIVE

Swelling inside the ears is a fairly common allergy symptom. The pressure changes that occur when someone dives into water can greatly aggravate ears that get plugged up because of allergen exposure. This condition can lead to water being trapped inside the ear resulting in a painful condition called swimmer's ear.

17. TAKE A LONG RIDE

One way to get out and enjoy nature is to drive around in an air-conditioned car. It can keep your symptoms at a tolerable level.

18. PETS

Pets can carry allergesn in their fur; these include pollen, dust, and mold. Your pet's fur and dander can shed indoors along with the allergen. Keep pets away from your favorite areas.

19. THE YARD

Plant nonallergenic ground covers in place of grass. Remove any plants that release a lot of pollen. This will reduce your hay fever exposure.

20. CLOTHING

During pollen season remove your outer clothing and shoes when coming indoors. Leave them outdoors in a protected area or put the clothes immediately into the washing machine. Shower and rinse your hair, particularly before going to bed. While you are outdoors pollen attaches to clothing and hair and, once indoors, can trigger allergy symptoms.

21. AVOID CEREALS

Sometimes certain foods are in the same family as certain pollens. Avoid eating foods related to grasses such as wheat, rice, oats, etc. Eating these foods can aggravate airborne allergies.

22. NO COWS ALLOWED

A good reason not to drink milk is that pasteurized and raw cow's milk contain enough antibodies of rye grass pollen, house dust mites, *Aspergillus* mold, and wheat proteins to cause allergic reactions in someone sensitive to these substances. Ina recent study, antibodies were detected in every sample of milk tested, including all samples of commercially pasteurized milk. When they are absorbed in the intestinal tract, antibodies can result in allergic reactions. They can even affect people who are not usually sensitive to pollen, dust, mold, or wheat.

23.CARS AND YOUR NOSE

As pollutants increase in the air, hay fever symptoms also increase. Car exhaust contains nitrogen dioxide that can kill the cilia (hairs) in the nasal passages and respiratory tract. Cilia help move mucus and foreign objects to the mouth and nose and then out of the body. When nitrogen dioxide exposure kills the cilia, the body cannot rid itself of these allergens.

24. FOOD SENSITIVITIES AND POLLEN

Reducing food sensitivities and balancing the body's biochemistry can decrease your seasonal hay fever symptoms. It is possible to decrease hay fever symptoms when you also reduce the total burden on the immune system and the digestive tract.

CHAPTER 44

Additional Treatments for Allergies and Sensitivities

T he following pages provide additional material covering those treatments for allergies and sensitivities that may not be as prominent, or not as fully understood as those discussed in the previous chapters. Hopefully they can be of use to you. Please note that

Allopathic Treatment

Most traditional over-the-counter antihistamines can offer some temporary relief, but they usually cause fatigue and sleepiness as a side effect. Cortisone therapy can provide dramatic temporary relief, but a person can become dependent upon this medication. After stopping the use of cortisone, the symptoms often return worse than before treatment. There may be an association between the long-term use of cortisone and osteoporosis, diabetes, immune system suppression, and other health problems. The adrenal glands also lose their ability to function adequately after cortisone is withdrawn. Since cortisone greatly reduces immunity and weakens the bones, try to stay away from it. Natural antihistamines or substances that support the body's allergy defense system would be a better choice.

Alkalization for Acute Allergic Reactions

If you have a severe reaction to foods or if you don't want a reaction to run its course, consider the following information to stop the reaction. There is a caution, however. If you have kidney or heart disease, do not take any of the products listed below without medical advice. They often contain high amounts of sodium and other alkaline salts.

• Mix two heaping tablespoons of baking soda (sodium bicarbonate) with one heaping tablespoon of potassium bicarbonate. Add a heaping teaspoon of this mixture to sixteen ounces of spring water and drink.

- Aspirin-free Alka Seltzer Gold is helpful and has a pleasant taste. Place one tablet in a glass of water and take two successive doses, if needed.
- Unflavored milk of magnesia may be taken (one to four tablespoons) for additional relief.
- Most allergic people have a very high systemic acid level. To avoid this, take lemon juice because it is a systemic alkalizer. Mix one ounce of fresh lemon juice with nine ounces of water. Drink in morning and evening.

The chronic use of antacids causes permanent atrophy of the stomach's parietal cells thus affecting digestion. Usually, the cause of an over acid system is the excessive use of acidic foods. See the chapter on "Acid-Alkaline Balance" for more information.

Body Cleansing

As you begin a program of improved nutrition and lifestyle changes, expect your body to undergo changes. It may go through a "house cleaning" to rebuild strong, healthy cells. House cleaning is the body's way of ridding itself of as many toxins as it can. Symptoms reflect the toxic burden that has been dragging you down for years. Expect periodic ups and downs on the path back to optimal health. As you reach new levels of wellness, your body will use this new-found energy to clear out old deposits and release them for elimination. You may briefly experience again some of the discomforting symptoms that plagued you in the past such as skin rashes and eruptions. Colds, fevers, nervousness, frequent urination, fatigue, bowel sluggishness, or occasional diarrhea may also be part of the housecleaning process. It is not unusual to have headaches at this time, but such symptoms are temporary. You need to support your body with good nutrition and good bowel elimination. It is not advisable to stop this cleansing process by introducing symptom-suppressing drugs or massive doses of vitamins. It will only keep the toxins from leaving your body while adding more toxins at the same time. Instead, help the body along by drinking ample filtered water and eating lightly. Some people experience this cleansing process without any unpleasant symptoms because of an efficient detoxification system.

Botanical Medicine

Botanical medication is much more difficult to use wisely at home without some in-depth knowledge about herbs and their individual properties. To use herbs safely, it is best to educate yourself about each herb prior to their use. I have found the following ones to be helpful with allergies:

- *Achillea millefolium* (Yarrow): Some allergy sufferers claim that drinking a cup of yarrow tea when an attack of hay fever is coming on will ease all their symptoms.
- *Angelica sinensis* (Dong Quai): This herb has shown to be effective in people sensitive to a variety of substances such as pollens, animal dander, dust, and food. Angelica has been long used in Chinese herbology for the prevention and treatment of allergic symptoms. It inhibits the production of allergic antibodies (IgE). For people who have higher than normal levels of these antibodies, angelica reduces them.
- *Ephedra sinica* (Ma Huang): As a tea Ma Huang is especially good for asthma. The Chinese have used this herb for the symptoms of allergies, asthma, and hay fever for thousands of years. The crude plant also contains other components that contain anti-inflammatory and antihistamine properties.
- *Euphrasia officinalis* (Eyebright): Use as a tea for itchy eyes and as an eyewash. Eyebright, along with vitamin A and C, promotes cell membrane stability. This reduces histamine thus reducing allergic reactions. It helps with symptoms such as inflammation of the eyes, nose, throat, and upper respiratory tract, as well as with sneezing, itching, and an abundant flow of mucus. Drink several cups of this herb a day.
- *Ginkgo biloba* (Ginkgo): Perhaps because of its high bioflavonoid content, this herb has shown clinical effects in asthma, inflammation, and allergies. Ginkgo also protects the lining of the intestinal tract from damage.
- *Glycyrrhiza glabra* (Deglycyrrhizinated Licorice Root): Licorice root exhibits anti-inflammatory and anti-allergic action. Licorice inhibits antibody formation, stress reactions, and inflammation. This herb has been helpful in the treatment of allergic skin conditions. It also supports the adrenal glands.
- *Grindelia squarrose* or *G. camporum* (Gum weed): Use gum weed for allergic dermatitis (rashes and itching). Mix one ounce of the herbal fluid extract with one to two ounces water and apply to the itching area. It is also a good herb to use for allergic asthmatic symptoms.
- *Hydrastis canadensis* (Goldenseal): Goldenseal has been found to be of some help in inhibiting some of the microbial damage of the intestinal lining. This decreases intestinal permeability that in turn reduces allergies. Don't take goldenseal for more than a week without the advice of a health professional trained in herbal medicine.
- *Ligusticum porteri* (Osha): Use for milk or milk-product allergies, especially if there is also an increase in mucus production. Take five to ten drops in 1/4 glass of water three times a day. Osha is best if taken twenty or thirty minutes before meals.

- *Piper longum* (Long Pepper): This herb is a classic Ayurvedic remedy in India. It has the ability to block histamine and decrease the symptoms of chemical irritants in the airway.
- *Scutellaria baicalensis* (Chinese Skullcap): Scutellaria can be used like quercetin to block some inflammatory reactions. Its therapeutic action appears to be related to its high content of bioflavonoid molecules that inhibit the formation of compounds that cause the allergic reactions.
- *Silybum marianum* (Milk Thistle): Milk thistle blocks allergic and inflammatory reactions. It helps to clean the liver and improve liver function that may be impaired when allergies are a problem. It can greatly decrease the histamine response.
- *Trifolium pratense* (Red Clover): This herb helps to build up the body's resistance to allergies. Use one teaspoon red clover blossoms to one cup boiling water and steep for five to ten minutes. Drink three or four cups a day before exposing yourself to the causes of your allergy or hay fever. During the season, or if an attack occurs, double your intake of the tea. Also take large amounts of vitamin C every hour. Rosehips supply the most easily assimilated source of vitamin C.
- *Urtica dioica* (Stinging Nettles): Nettles is a standard over-the-counter remedy for allergic rhinitis and sinusitis throughout Europe. A standardized, freeze-dried extract of this plant is effective in the treatment of seasonal allergic rhinitis. For inhalant sensitivities take two tablespoons of stinging nettles and one tablespoon mint; infuse in two cups of water; drink one cup in the morning and one in the evening during the time you are having symptoms, or three or four cups if needed. Another way is to buy the tincture of stinging nettles and take five to sixty drops daily in a little water three times a day. Stinging nettles is usually helpful for alleviating allergic reactions, especially allergic skin reactions. If taken in the form of capsules, take one to three capsules per dose, or as needed. Also consider these formulations:
- Mix this herbal tincture: Nettles (*Urtica dioica* or *U. urens*), echinacea (*Echinacea angustifolia*), and licorice root (*Glycyrrhiza glabra*) together in equal amounts. Take thirty to sixty drops three times a day until symptoms stop. Then take only as much as needed to keep your symptoms from returning. They can also be prepared as a tea. Take 1/2 ounce of mixed herbs and put in one pint of water. Make a decoction with the lid on, and drink two or three cups a day for several days, or until symptoms stop.
- Make a tea from the equal combination of each of the following herbs: ma huang (*Ephedra sinica*), eyebright (*Euphrasia officinalis*), and goldenseal (*Hydrastis canadensis*). Use one teaspoon of this mix per cup of

boiling water and let it steep for ten to fifteen minutes. Drink this combination two or three times a day.
- Expectorants are herbs that modify the quality and quantity of respiratory tract secretions, resulting in the expulsion of excess mucus and an improvement in respiratory tract function. Commonly used expectorants include: licorice root, gum weed (*Grindelia camporum*), euphorbia (*Euphorbia hirta*), sundew (*Drosera rotundifolia*), and senega (*Polygala senega*).
- For swollen runny eyes and classic allergic reactions mix together a tincture of eyebright (2.5 parts), goldenseal (1.5 parts), *Achillea millafolium* (2.5 parts), and *Cochlearia armoracia* (1.5 parts). The dosage is thirty drops in a small amount of water three times a day.

Desensitization

If you can't eliminate the offending allergen and symptoms persist, then desensitization therapy may be necessary. Conventional physicians usually use a lengthy series of weekly or twice-weekly injections in a method called isotherapy. The procedure is invasive and expensive. Allergy shots offer temporary relief, but most people must continue receiving the desensitization shots since they do not address the real cause of the allergy. Because of the poor results and undesirable side effects so common with antihistamines and antiallergy drugs, a more natural approach is desirable here as well.

You can become desensitized to an offending substance with homeopathic drops. They are available for sensitivities to foods, pollens, additives, animal dander, dust mites, dust and mold, and other allergic substances. Homeopathic desensitization stimulates the immune system to produce antibodies stimulating the body's defense system. This desensitizes the body and neutralizes the allergic reaction. It involves introducing small amounts of the allergens into the body sublingually (under the tongue) in homeopathic drops. This oral administration is convenient, comfortable, nonirritating, and particularly advantageous in the treatment of children.

Many people are less sensitive to trees, grasses, weeds, dust, molds, and other inhalants if the homeopathic treatment continues all year. Reduce the seasonal offenders by taking a low dosage homeopathic remedy in the allergen off-season and resume to full dosage as the season approaches. Each allergy season usually requires less medication as the body becomes less sensitive to the allergen. You may not need to start over each season as is common with antihistamines. If the allergen is not seasonal, daily treatment may be required, at least temporarily.

Detoxification

It is amazing that our bodies function as well as they do considering all the toxins, pollutions, and dietary abuses that we subject them to. Healthy digestion requires the efficient elimination of waste. A sluggish digestive system leads to a body that cannot detoxify itself properly. This is often the results of slow digestive functions, inadequate exercise, and poor eating habits. Some diets support detoxification, but they don't eliminate food allergies or intolerances. It is important to lower the total allergic load on the intestinal tract by digesting all foods properly, especially proteins. The intestinal bowel flora must be balanced, and leaky gut syndrome must be prevented.

Avoid constipation. Keep the bowels moving smoothly with the aid of colonic irrigation, fiber, or a natural laxative. A formula containing water-soluble fibers such as oat bran and psyllium helps to bind to poisons, heavy metals, and fats to move them through the system. Adequate and proper fiber sweeps waste material through the system and speeds up the bowel's transit time. On a diet of red meat, dairy products, and sugar the transit time is usually very slow. This food can remain in the intestinal tract for a week or more, just sitting there rotting. Colon cleansers remove pathogens and long-standing feces from the colon. These cleansers usually contain psyllium seed with bentonite and herbs. Charcoal, besides binding and removing toxins, helps to absorb and destroy many toxic chemicals. Other ingredients in bowel cleaners usually include the following ingredients to prevent reabsorption of toxic chemicals in the intestinal tract: guar gum, karaya gum, apple pectin, oat bran, and dandelion root. Take the fiber supplement at night before bedtime.

Saunas or sweat baths are often useful in ridding the body of released toxins. Rest and do not overtax your body with vigorous exercise. Eat organically grown foods from local sources, if possible. It defeats the whole purpose of cleansing your body if you continue to introduce residues of herbicides and pesticides. The vitamin, mineral and enzyme levels of fresh, local, organically grown produce are better for the body. For a basic detoxification program you need to:

- Support the liver. Always include vitamin C to help the liver remove toxic compounds from the blood.
- Drink at least two quarts of distilled or purified water daily.
- Take a high-potency multiple vitamin and mineral formula.
- Take a lipotropic formula containing choline and L-methionine. This will help to digest fats and eliminate toxins.

- Reduce total carbohydrates. Studies indicate that a diet high in carbohydrates may reduce the body's ability to detoxify effectively.
- Take essential fatty acids and medium chain triglycerides to provide energy for cell function.
- Take antioxidants such as bioflavonoids, vitamin C or E, or selenium to quench free radicals produced during the detoxification process.
- Take the amino acids glutathione and glutamine because they play an important role in detoxification. The amino acids methionine and cysteine provide sulfur that is used in part of the detoxification process.
- Improve your diet with lightly steamed, nonstarchy vegetables, fresh fruits, salads, and adequate amounts of high-quality protein. These foods nourish the system without burdening it.
- Increase good bowel flora by taking *Lactobacillus acidophilus* and *bifidus.* Include a product that contains fructo-oligosaccharides (FOS) to stimulate the growth of these good bacteria in the intestinal tract. Always take on an empty stomach only with water unless directed otherwise.

Fasting is the avoidance of all food and drink, except water, for a specific period of time. Fasting is often used as a detoxification method, because it is one of the quickest ways to increase the elimination of wastes from the body. Because the body's detoxification pathway needs energy to function properly, methods such as this may do more harm than good. A water fast deprives the body of protein, fat, and micronutrients and may suppress detoxification rather than enhance it. Never require a child to fast. Even adults should not fast for any extended period of time without professional help.

Substances applied to the skin, scalp, nose, mouth, and vagina can enter the bloodstream and act as toxins. Avoid the use of toothpaste, mouthwashes, deodorants, cosmetics, and cleansers with undesirable ingredients. The skin has a tremendous ability to absorb substances and is also the largest organ of elimination.

Digestive Enzymes

Hypersensitive people often need digestive enzymes. Some indications may be excessive gas, bloating, belching, burning, flatulence immediately after meals, undigested food in the stool, uncomfortable fullness, and other signs of indigestion. Digestion function usually slows down, along with the decrease in some digestive enzymes because of poor dietary habits over a long period, not just because of aging. You may need to experiment with different types of enzymes until you find the best one for your particular needs.

Digestive enzymes called proteases are vital to the breakdown of protein and are of benefit in treating food allergies. Typically, individuals who are also short on stomach acid (hydrochloric acid) will suffer from multiple food allergies. Other digestive enzyme deficiencies may be involved, such as pepsin, pancreatin, etc.

L-histidine, 500 milligrams twice a day, improves gastric acid production in allergic patients with low hydrochloric acid. The addition of apple cider vinegar fortifies stomach hydrochloric acid and adds flavor to food. Dietary supplements containing betaine hydrochloride may be helpful. Since there is a danger of gastric irritation when using hydrochloric acid supplements, consult with a health practitioner trained in their use. Stop or reduce the dosage if you have any digestive symptoms such as burning.

Food allergies and sensitivities often improve when using the appropriate digestive enzymes. Plant enzymes can help a wide variety of conditions including celiac disease, maldigestion, malabsorption, lactose intolerance, and fatty stool. Enzymes derived from *Aspergillus oryzae* can digest food antigens that leak into the blood stream because of inadequate protein digestion. It is advisable to consult a health practitioner to determine the type of digestive enzyme necessary for your particular problem.

Many people confuse milk allergies and a lactose intolerance, but they are two different conditions. The enzyme lactase is needed to digest lactose (milk sugar), but some people do not produce this enzyme If the lactase levels are too low or missing, milk will not digest and ferments instead. Drinking milk containing acidophilus does not correct this problem. Many people benefit from the addition of an enzyme to their milk to break down lactose or by buying lactose-reduced milk.

Dosage

It is important to take the correct dosages of vitamins, minerals, herbal preparations, homeopathic remedies, glandular, or other supplements. This is why it is important that you have a well-trained health professional guide you when using these products. This is essential to attaining the maximum benefit from your supplements. An adult dosage is different than what a child would take. All references to dosages in this book apply to adults unless stated it is for a child.

Dysbiosis

Dysbiosis means abnormal intestinal flora. Some individuals with food intolerances and gastrointestinal symptoms have too many aerobic bacteria in the stool. It seems that if there is a high concentration of the wrong bacteria in the gut, it can cause increased intestinal permeability (leaky gut syndrome) leading to food allergies and sensitivities. An imbalance of intestinal flora, rather than being the primary cause of food intolerances, may in fact be a result of ingesting allergic foods. The amount of fiber in the diet influences the intestinal micro-environment. Including probiotics such as *Lactobacillus acidophilus* and *L. bifidus* can be very helpful, but don't forget the role of diet for keeping the bowels healthy.

Even with abnormal intestinal microflora pathogens don't have to be present. It may be a disorder of bacterial fermentation in the colon such as *E. coli*. It is present in the stool in higher percentages when people have a variety of food-related autoimmune problems such as Crohn's disease.

Under normal conditions, good bacteria produce a variety of vitamins in the digestive tract. Due to poor diet, broad-spectrum antibiotics, corticosteroids, and birth control pills, the internal environment can become polluted. The excessive uptake of toxic food and bacterial, fungal, and viral antigens causes a continued immune response and contributes to increasingly adverse reactions. Toxins can also be produced during an infection by organisms such as bacteria. The antibiotics may kill the bacteria, but the bacteria's toxic contents are still liberated into the body.

Histamine Release

Histamines are chemicals found in foods that often cause allergic reactions. It is a good idea to avoid foods that may contain histamines: sausage, sauerkraut, tuna, wine, preserves, spinach and tomatoes. It might also be necessary to avoid foods that cause an excessive release of histamines from white blood cells: eggs, milk, shellfish, strawberries, chocolate, bananas, papayas, pineapples, certain nuts, and alcohol.

Exercise

Exercise every day, especially a good brisk aerobic walk to oxygenate the blood. Walk for at least thirty minutes every day. When you are experiencing congestion and nasal stuffiness, three minutes of vigorous exercise is often sufficient to reverse this condition.

Immune System

With allergies and sensitivities to substances such as dust, dander, pollen, etc., the immune system needs support. Be aware of the following:

• Adrenal and thymus glandular preparations further enhance the immune response.

- B-complex vitamins are also called the stress vitamins and help to support the adrenal glands.
- Bioflavonoids are immune stimulating, especially quercetin and catechin.
- Chromium may be needed if there is hypoglycemia (low blood sugar). Being excessively stressed can decrease immune function and make hypoglycemia worse.
- Herbs such as astragalus root (*Astragalus canadensis*), echinacea (*Echinacea angustifolia*), cayenne (*Capsicum frutescens*), and goldenseal (*Hydrastis canadensis*) help strengthen the immune system.
- Vitamin A reduces stress on the thymus gland.
- Vitamin C is especially effective in activating a type of white blood cell needed for immune defense, but this vitamin is usually needed in higher amounts to accomplish this action.
- Vitamin B6 is helpful in maintaining a healthy immune response.
- Zinc is needed when someone is under prolonged stress.

Leaky Gut Syndrome

The increase in intestinal permeability is often caused by the overgrowth of intestinal yeast, but other things can create such a condition. Viral, bacterial, and protozoan infections may contribute, as well as the excessive use of alcohol, nonsteroidal anti-inflammatory drugs, elevated levels of toxins, or food-borne reactions. The solution includes building up the intestinal flora and the immune system. It may be necessary to eliminate the organisms, but natural means should be used if possible.

Physiotherapy

- Using a nasal lavage with a 20cc bulb syringe can relieve nasal hay fever symptoms. Fill a large container with hot water (100-105 degrees) and mix approximately one tablespoon salt to 1/2 gallon water. This solution is administered with a bulb syringe by expelling all the air and filling it completely. The irrigation of the nasal passages is carried out over a basin with the head tilted to one side. Place the syringe into one nostril and squeeze the bulb. Allow the solution to escape through the opposite nostril into the sink. This should be continued for five to ten minutes with equal attention paid to both nostrils.
- Cold applications are effective in relieving hay fever symptoms for some people. Wring cold cloths from ice water and apply to the forehead. Replace as soon as they begin to warm up. Relief occurs in about 45 minutes, but continue treatment for three hours, then intermittently for another six hours.

- A colon cleanse can reduce the total toxic burden often reducing the allergy symptoms.
- A hot foot bath is very helpful in relieving nasal congestion. Guard against chilling since it constricts blood vessels.

Sulphur

Sulphur, an indispensable element in human nutrition, binds with a variety of toxins in the body, and together they are excreted. Proper sulphur oxidation requires molybdenum for enzyme activation and enough dietary sulphur levels to ensure that the pathway can be completed. The body needs a constant intake of assimilable sulphur to perform these functions. If this process is defective, it is possible that symptoms might result from an overburden of toxins. This is common in nearly all "universal reactors" and the majority of those highly sensitive to foods, inhalants, and chemicals.

Psychology for Allergies

Stress and anger can bring on an allergic attack. Find ways to relax; be as unhurried as possible. Adequate rest and relaxation is important. Consider the following treatments to reduce stress: hypnotherapy, imagery, visualization, lifestyle modification counseling, affirmations, meditation and relaxation exercises.

Supplements

Make sure that all supplements taken are hypoallergenic. Many allergens are used as preservatives, fillers, and binders in medications. Even pills that are white often contain dyes. Check the labels and inserts for ingredients that might be harmful or could cause a reaction. All references to dosages in this book apply to adults unless stated otherwise.

Adrenal Glandulars: The state of the adrenal glands is often the difference between an allergic individual and one who doesn't experience allergies or sensitivities. Adrenal glandulars are known to be helpful in allergies and build immunity. They buffer the reactions to specific allergens. The dosage for these glandulars is usually one tablet three times a day for adults.

Amino Acids: They often improve digestive enzyme production and brain allergies. Tyrosine helps many people during hay fever season when the problem is grass pollen. There seems to be few side effects.

Antioxidants: Antioxidants are thought to provide important defenses against allergies and sensitivities. Exposure to contaminants in the air, water, food, as well as household and occupational contaminants, all increase the need for the various antioxidant nutrients that help to neutralize these toxins in the body. Antioxidants such as the vitamins C, E, and A, as well as selenium and other nutrients, help prevent free radical damage. Other natural antioxidants are beta carotene, ascorbic acid, zinc, and superoxide dismutase. Pycnogenol, another free radical scavenger, is being prescribed for a very wide spectrum of conditions including hay fever, chronic allergic rhinitis and asthma. It seems that pycnogenol inhibits tissue levels of histamine. Grape seed extract at a dose of 100-300 milligrams also has antihistamine effects. Some people also respond to cat's claw. It seems that the quality of different brands can have different effects.

Bentonite Clay: This is a well-known intestinal absorbent. It absorbs numerous toxins and bacteria. It may help by decreasing the toxin load in the intestinal lumen, allowing the body to repair itself.

Bioflavonoids: Citrus fruits such as oranges, grapes, plums, strawberries, prunes, grapefruit, cherries, and blackberries contain bioflavonoids. Still other bioflavonoids have remarkable antiallergic compounds helping reduce the inflammatory process that often characterizes allergic reactions. Taking two to three grams a day decreases histamine release. During the height of symptoms, you may need to take up to six grams. They work especially well when combined with vitamin C and A, but high doses may be required.

Natural bioflavonoids are a healthier choice to avoid an allergic reaction than many other antihistamines. Bioflavonoids function by strengthening the walls of the cells that are involved in the allergic response (basophils, eosinophils and mast cells), as well as the capillary beds. As a result, histamine is not released from the cells and the capillary beds become less permeable to any histamine already circulating. The liver is spared the strain of having to clear both the drug used as an antihistamine and large levels of circulating histamine. An example of an antiallergy flavonoid is quercetin. It has a strong affinity for mast cells which release histamine and other inflammatory molecules in the gastrointestinal and respiratory tract and the skin.

Bromelain: Bromelain has been shown to be effective in treating many conditions, including allergies. Bromelain gets high marks for its anti-inflammatory activity. It seems to enhance the anti-inflammatory action of hesperidin, quercetin, and other bioflavonoids, as well as improve absorption. All forms of bromelain are not equal. There are different grades of bromelain and an activity of 1,800 m.c.u. or higher is considered a very high quality. Copper and iron in the same tablet taken at the same time tend to inactivate bromelain, whereas magnesium and cysteine enhance its therapeutic effect. Enteric-coated tablets also tend to decrease bromelain's absorption. Bromelain is best taken between meals for the symptoms of hay fever.

Catechin: This bioflavonoid can inhibit the enzyme that causes histamine release. Histamine increases significantly in response to an allergen, especially in people with skin rashes, itching, and food sensitivities. Catechin can help prevent food reactions when about fifteen minutes before eating the foods.

DHEA (dehydroepioandrosterone): DHEA levels are often low in highly allergic individuals. The starting dose for men is 100-400 milligrams spread over the day, for women three to five milligrams twice a day. Start the dosage at a low level and observe any side effects for a period of time before increasing the dose. For both men and women it is important to follow testosterone and estrogen levels at intervals to guard against over dosing. Testosterone appears to be adversely affected by high doses of DHEA. This substance needs to be monitored by a physician.

Essential Fatty Acids: Aspirin may contribute to deficiencies of gamma linolenic acid (GLA), an important EFA. People who suffer from allergic disorders may benefit from avoiding aspirin and other NSAIDs. Fatty acids are important mediators of allergies. GLA may be blocked in people with atopic dermatitis. It seems that these people cannot convert their fatty acids into the proper pathways that would help to eliminate many skin conditions. Increasing healthy fatty acid intake can significantly increase or decrease allergies and inflammation, depending on the type of oils being increased. Take about 190 milligrams of GLA daily in the form of flaxseed oil or evening primrose oil, along with 500 milligrams of pantothenic acid.

EPA (eicosapentanoic acid) and *DHA (docosahexaenoic acid):* EPA and DHA may be helpful in inflammatory processes and hypersensitivity reactions such as asthma and other allergic conditions.

Glutamine: Glutamine increases alkali reserves. Taking two grams of glutamine daily might have positive implications for the treatment of allergies. Since allergic individuals tend to have decreased alkali reserve, taking alkali salts are an effective treatment for acute allergic reactions. Long-term treatment with glutamine may not have the same effect as short-term use. Since glutamine is relatively safe at therapeutic doses, these possibilities warrant investigation. Glutamine is the principal fuel used by the upper intestinal tract and has been shown to prevent and reverse intestinal lining damage.

Hesperidin: Hesperidin inhibits histamine release from cells called basophils. The antiallergy actions of hesperidin can be significantly increased by taking catechin at the same time. Bromelain may also enhance the anti-inflammatory action of hesperidin and other bioflavonoids, as well as improve absorption.

Lactobacillus acidophilus/ bifidus: Lactobacillus helps to correct *Candida albicans* overgrowth and other imbalances in the intestinal microflora community. Take on an empty stomach and only with water. Foods and drinks taken at the same time as the lactobacillus interfere with its effectiveness.

MSM (Methylsulfonylmethane): Sulphur in the form of MSM appears to have beneficial effects in relieving allergies and hypersensitivities to foods, chemical and environmental substances such as pollen, house dust, wool, animal hair, feathers, and other allergens. Some sufferers report complete relief of allergic symptoms after daily doses of 50 to 1000 milligrams per day. Even if MSM does not eliminate all allergic responses, a significant reduction in symptoms is often possible. Individuals with allergic asthma usually report an improvement in their symptoms.

People with allergic responses to drugs, including aspirin, nonsteroid antiarthritic agents, and oral antibiotics, report an improved or complete tolerance to these substances when ingesting 100-1000 milligrams of MSM at the same time. MSM appears not to have any side affects. Extremely high doses in animal studies did not produce adverse results, but had a broad and profound beneficial effect in improving allergic reactions to many kinds of allergens.

There is a direct correlation between the concentration of MSM used and resistance to the allergen. The recommended maintenance dose of MSM is 500-2000 milligrams per day. Some people need anywhere from 1000 milligrams up to 10,000 milligrams (10 grams) before gaining symptom relief. The effective dosage depends to some extent on the nature and severity of symptoms. A single dose is usually not effective. Taking MSM periodically throughout the day ensures an adequate daily supply of available sulphur. Noticeable results usually occur within two to twenty-one days. Continue a maintenance dose after you obtain the initial relief of symptoms.

To derive the maximum benefit of MSM, take 25 micrograms of molybdenum at the same time and 100 milligrams of ascorbic acid. Supplying adequate dietary molybdenum may play an important role in preventing an insufficiency concerning this important sulphur pathway. Today, there are usually inadequate amounts of the sulphur-containing amino acids—methionine and cysteine—in our food supply. All other nutritionally important sulphur compounds can be made from these compounds. Most raw and unprocessed foods contain sufficient amounts, but they are easily lost due to sulphur's volatile nature. This is why is may be important to supplement with MSM.

Minerals: Minerals can decrease histamine levels and play many important roles in regulating body chemistry. They are required for glandular activity and serve to regulate the nervous system, as well as every other system of the body. Minerals are essential to health and for all body functions.

Quercetin: This compound is the most active of the many bioflavonoids for its anti-allergic effects. Quercetin and many other bioflavonoids, but not rutin, are potent inhibitors of histamine release from mast cell and basophils, preventing the spilling of histamine into the blood stream. This release of histamine and other inflammatory substances is involved in allergic and inflammatory responses. Quercetin may offer significant effects including those involved with the lungs, large intestine, and skin.

About 1000 to 2000 milligrams of quercetin a day, divided into three to six doses, is usually sufficient to control most allergy cases and many cases of asthma. It can take several weeks to a month before quercetin becomes effective. Enhance quercetin's action by taking catechin at the same time. Since quercetin is not absorbed that well, combine it with an equal amount of bromelain, the anti-inflammatory enzyme from pineapple, to increase absorption and effectiveness. Bromelain and quercetin each demonstrate remarkable effects on their own, but used in combination greatly increases their therapeutic activity. To decrease the effects of food reactions take 250 to 500 milligrams of quercetin fifteen to twenty minutes before meals along with bromelain.

Another formulation that should be helpful to take for food allergies is the combination of 125 milligrams bromelain, 125 milligrams quercetin, 100 milligrams vitamin C, 100 milligrams mixed flavonoids, 75 milligrams L-cysteine, and about 25 milligrams magnesium. Take fifteen to twenty minutes before meals to reduce food reactions or between meals for other types of allergic reactions.

Selenium: Selenium's role is well established as an antioxidant and seems to affect all aspects of immunity. A deficiency suppresses many aspects of the immune response and leaves the person open to free radical attacks and disease. The body needs selenium for the normal production and function of white blood cells, and antibody production. Supplementing with even moderate doses of selenium restores some level of immune function. Selenium also helps to protect and maintain the circulatory, digestive, and reproductive systems, as well as protect us from the flood of toxins that invade the body every day. It is helpful in the treatment of chemical allergies and allergic toxins. The best form to take is selenomethionine. Take 100 to 200 micrograms per day.

Spirulina: Consuming spirulina lowers the levels of IgE allergens in the blood and normalizes allergic sensitivities in the body. A growing number of scientific studies have documented the immune enhancement benefits of spirulina. The recommended dosage for radiation exposure is 20 tablets (about five grams) per day in divided doses. For children who are constantly living in highly radioactive areas the dosage is: ages three to five, take five tablets twice a day; ages five to seven, take seven tablets twice a day.

Thymus Glandular: Thymus glandulars increase immune system support and assist in regulating excessive activity of the adrenal glands. The usual dosage is one tablet three times a day.

Tyrosine: The *British Medical Journal* and *Lancet* reported that there were good clinical results when a compound containing tyrosine was given to patients whose hay fever was directly linked to grass pollen. It took fewer doses and had a tendency to fewer side effects than less natural antihistamines.

Vitamin A: Vitamin A is an excellent antioxidant and prevents damage to the cell membranes. If an adequate supply is taken it can increase the body's ability to fight off allergies. It also decreases cellular membrane permeability that decreases leaky gut syndrome. Doses of vitamin A can be toxic, especially to the fetus of pregnant women. Do not take any dose over 50,000 IU per day without medical supervision. Taking beta carotene is a better choice unless you have low thyroid function or diabetes.

Vitamin B Complex: A good B-complex supplement helps the mucous membranes, reduces stress, aids in the digestion process, and supports adrenal function. A complete B-complex supplement is a mixture of the B vitamins that tend to occur together in foods of animal, plant, and microorganism origin. They consist of eight members: thiamine (B1), riboflavin (B2) nicotinic acid (B3), pantothenic acid (B5), pyridoxine (B6), biotin, folic acid, and B12. These are the vitamins that the body cannot make. Some authorities include choline and inositol, but they can be synthesized by the body.

Vitamin B2 (riboflavin) is used by the adrenal glands and needed for the proper utilization of protein. Sixty milligrams of vitamin B2 before meals is recommended. Vitamin B6 (Pyridoxine) may be helpful for MSG sensitivity. It may also help if you eat meat or have a very heavy protein diet. The usual dosage is 25-100 milligrams daily, but it may take 200 milligrams of B6 (about 1/2 hour before meals) to reduce allergic reactions. Vitamin B6 is often overlooked when treating the hypersensitive person, even though low levels are usually present in the allergic individual. The dosage of 1000 micrograms of vitamin B12 injected once weekly for four weeks has helped people with asthma and various skin reactions.

Vitamin B5 (pantothenic acid) is essential for adrenal support and prevention of adrenal exhaustion during any type of stress. In large doses pantothenic acid helps to reduce allergic reactions because of its antihistamine effect. Almost instant relief occurs in some people when taking about 100 to 250 milligrams after breakfast, after lunch, and following dinner. Some people do fine on a dosage of 500 milligrams two times per day. Even high doses of approximately 4000 milligrams daily are very beneficial for some allergy suffers. If you take too much pantothenic acid, you will get a dry and uncomfortable nose. Results may be better if you use a B-complex supplement at the same time. Start slowly and gradually increase the dosage of pantothenic acid.

Vitamin C: Vitamin C is an effective antioxidant and antihistamine (especially if taken with bioflavonoids). It helps adrenal and immune function and helps the liver detoxify histamine. Since vitamin C reduces the blood levels of histamine, increasing the dosage during an allergic attack may help. It is also helpful in MSG sensitivity. Magnesium ascorbate, the preferred form, has immune, antihistamine, and anti-inflammatory effects. The buffering magnesium ion helps to stabilize the mast cells, the cells involved in allergies. Magnesium aids in the stabilization of the inflammatory response.

Take 2000 milligrams (two grams) daily and increase if needed to 3000 to 5000 milligrams, or up to bowel tolerance. Vitamin C may have to exceed twelve grams per day to be effective in some people. If you begin to have loose stools, reduce the amount you are taking. Others have a better response to about two grams of sodium ascorbate. With continuous sodium ascorbate treatment some asthmatics, especially those with seasonal hay fever, remain symptom free. It seems that sodium ascorbate is more effective than ascorbic acid for some people. Unfortunately, sodium ascorbate causes increased urinary output.

Vitamin E: Take 200-400 I.U. one to two times per day. As an antioxidant, use vitamin E to decrease tissue damage. It also has antihistamine properties. Its ability to enhance the function of the immune system increases with the addition of selenium, especially in the form of selenomethionine. It is best to increase the dosage of vitamin E gradually.

Zinc: Zinc plus vitamin E prevents the release of histamine from mast cells. This is why people with low zinc levels often have more allergies. Zinc also helps with immune and enzyme system support. The amount most commonly used is sixty milligrams daily. Don't take high doses of zinc long term without taking small amounts of copper.

Homeopathy

Allergies commonly affect the skin, resulting in symptoms such as eczema or hives. Many foods, especially milk, wheat, and eggs bring on these symptoms. If it is hard to avoid your food allergens, then desensitization with homeopathic remedies may offer a desirable alternative. Using homeopathic remedies of the specific allergens (animal hair, mold, foods, etc.) allows your immune system to be gently and gradually exposed to the substance that is offending you. The dose is small enough to allow your natural defenses to properly adapt to the allergen without reacting to it adversely.

Homeopathy uses the same mechanism involved with conventional allergy injections, causing your naturally occurring antibodies not to react to the allergen as foreign. Histamine and other allergy-activating compounds are no longer released so your allergic symptoms resolve and your natural defenses are strengthened. When used as directed, homeopathic formulas reduce the severity and frequency of future allergic reactions, as well as controlling the symptoms during an allergic reaction.

This mode of treatment is based on the theory of "like cures like." Homeopathic medications are preparations of potentized dilutions of scientifically formulated substances such as foods, airborne material, and chemical antigens. These remedies should not produce any harmful side effects and do not produce drowsiness or a medicated feeling. This is an advantage when treating children. Homeopathic formulas offer a combination of symptomatic relief without the side effects of prescription antihistamines and drugs like cortisone. The advantages of using homeopathy are numerous; no hypodermic injections, no continued office visits, and homeopathic prepared remedies are inexpensive.

When symptoms are acute, it may be necessary to take the drops more than three times a day; sometimes as often as every 15 minutes to 1/2 hour. The best dosages for home use are 6X to 6C or 30X to 30C. If you are using drops for desensitization therapy, the adult recommended dose is 10-fifteen drops, three times a day. Children under twelve usually need five to seven drops twice a day. Place these drops under the tongue and hold. If you are using pellets, the usual dose is two to three pellets at the same frequency as the drops.

The person's mouth should be clean, meaning free of food and beverages. Avoid garlic and other strong odors, strong drinks, tobacco, smoke, toothpaste, mouthwash, gum, mints, or other foods and drinks at least fifteen minutes before and after taking the homeopathic medication. Substances with strong odors can neutralize the action of the homeopathic remedy. If the food was particularly spicy, then wait for thirty minutes before taking your medication.

There may be homeopathic products available at health food stores for acute hay fever and environmental allergies. Allergy treatments can be very complicated and should be supervised by a professional health care expert. Since homeopathic medications must be prescribed correctly before they will work, you may need to consult a health practitioner trained in homeopathy that can provide you with the correct remedy or remedies, especially for serious or chronic ailments. To find a qualified physician in your area see your phone book yellow pages or contact the American Association of Naturopathic Physicians for more information (see the Resources section at the end of this book).

Homeopathic formulations can greatly reduce or entirely eliminate allergies and sensitivities. Find the one that fits your symptoms the closest and take in the 30C potency. If your initial prescription fails, this is not to be regarded as a failure of homeopathic medicine, but a failure by the prescriber to determine the appropriate remedy. Don't give up, but try again. The following are the names of specific homeopathic remedies used for allergies, accompanied by specific symptoms that correlate to the remedy.

ALLIUM CEPA

Eyes: sensitive to light; better in open air and waters profusely, but the discharge is bland and non-irritating

Eyelids: sore and burn

Nose: nose and eyes stream; nose becomes red and sore with burning, smarting discharge; sensation of a lump at the root of nose; discharge is copious, watery, and extremely acrid

Throat: hoarseness

Discharge: bland from eyes, but burning from nose

Sneezing: severe with increasing frequency or may not sneeze

Misc: cough; thirsty; lip becomes sore from acid discharge from the nose; hoarseness

Worse: indoors, warm room; in the morning; from contact with flowers and peach bloom

Better: open air and cool room

AMBROSIA

Eyes: much watering from the eyes

Eyelids: intolerable itching

Nose: nose and head feel stuffed up; watery discharge

Throat: irritation in trachea

Cough: wheezy

Sneezing: occurs

Misc: typical hay fever symptoms; sensitivity to rag weed; asthma attacks

ANTIMODIUM CRUDUM

Eyes: red, itch, inflamed

Ears: pain in Eustachian tubes

Throat: increased thick yellow mucus from posterior part of the nose: hawking in open air

Tongue: coated white tongue

Misc: thirst; desire for acid foods

ARSENICUM ALBUM

Eyes: burn with acrid tears, painful inflammation; intense photophobia edema around eyes; better external warmth

Eyelids: lids red, ulcerated, granulated, scaly

Nose: violent tickle at one particular spot inside nose, not relieved by scratching; feels stopped up; may bleed; discharge is profuse, thin, watery, burning, and burns the upper lip

Sneezing: violent and painful; sneezing without relief

Misc: sensitive to smells, odor of food, sight or thinking of food; burning thirst for cold drinks; drinks in sips; headache is dull and throbbing; remedy especially good for food, grain, and dust allergies; feels restless, worried, chilly.

Worse: change in weather, wet weather, seashore; every 14 days; after midnight, food especially watery fruit; exertion; right side, lying on affected part; all symptoms are worse in open air

Better: hot application, wrapped up; motion, head elevated, sitting erect; with company; sweating

ARSENICUM IODATUM

Eyes: itching, red

Nose: irritation in nose with constant desire to sneeze; red, swollen, burning, sore, itching; ulcers of nose; aggravated by sneezing; nose drips water

Ears: itching

Throat: burning

Discharge: when symptoms are acute the discharge may be thin; with chronic symptoms the discharge may be thick, irritating, burning; chronic mucus may be profuse, thick, yellow

Sneezing: aggravates symptoms; sneezing is at night

Misc: thirsty, chilly

Worse: dry, cold weather, windy weather, foggy weather; exertion; tobacco smoke; apples

Better: open air

ARUM TRIPHYLLUM

Eyes: smarting of eyes; rest of eye symptoms are not severe

Nose: much pricking in nose with desire to bore into nostril until it bleeds; stuffed up on left side or runs profusely making nostril raw and sore; breathes through mouth; pain at root of nose; scabs high up on right side of nose

Throat: hoarseness of voice

Discharge: acrid, burning, blood streaked

Face: feels chapped

Sneezing: worse at night, without relief

Misc: throbbing headache; lips raw, cracked; thirst, but drinking causes pain; excessively cross, stubborn, nervous; drowsiness; asthmatic breathing

Worse: overuse of voice, talking; left side, lying down; wet, cold, winds, heat; sneezing is worse at night

ARUNDO

Nose: burning and itching; loss of smell; discharge excessive and watery

Mouth: roof burns and itches

Ears: burns and itch in auditory canals; eczema behind ears

Sneezing: occurs

DULCAMARA

Eyes: swell and water, then nose runs, then eyes water again; profuse watery tears; worse open air

Eyelids: granular

Nose: stuffed up especially with a cold rain, or nose and eyes stream; nose completely stopped up; aching in nose

Discharge: thick mucus, bloody crusts; excessive/watery discharge

Sneezing: constant

Misc: summer colds with diarrhea; frequent urination; thirst; chilly

Worse: open air, before storms, autumn, dampness, being cold and wet, or chilled, when hot, sudden temperature changes; rest; contact with newly cut hay; night; suppressed sweat; discharges or eruptions

Better: moving about; external warmth

EUPHRASIA

Eyes: eye symptoms predominate; frequent inclination to blink; water constantly; discharge is acrid, thick, burning, yellow; intense aversion to light; sticky mucus on cornea; pressure in eyes; chronic sore eyes

Eyelids: burn and swell constantly

Nose: discharge is bland, watery and profuse; sore and painful inside nose
Throat: often involved
Cough: hard dry cough
Sneezing: much sneezing
Misc: headache with nasal discharge; diarrhea
Worse: open air, wind, sunlight; lying down; warm room
Better: winking; wiping eyes; coffee; in the dark

GELSEMIUM

Eyes: feel hot and heavy; double vision
Eyelids: heavy, drooping
Nose: streams in morning; thin discharge, watery, and burns; feels as if hot
    water is flowing from nose; much tingling in nose; edges of nostrils red
    and sore; fullness at root of nose; dryness of nasal passages; swollen
    inside nose; stuffy nose; the remedy of choice for the delicate little
    nerves that are irritated and causing the sneezing; both have action on
    tiny hair-like nerve endings in the nose
Ears: deafness
Throat: throat dry and burning; swallowing causes pain in ears
Face: hot
Sneezing: violent; in the a.m.
Misc: headache is concurrent, dull and feverish; with profuse urination;
    thirstless; body aching all over, limbs feel heavy; hands and feet are cold;
    chills runs up and down spine; good remedy at the beginning of allergy
    season and for summer colds
Worse: emotions, dread, surprises, shock, bad news, thinking of ailments;
    spring weather, when humid, foggy weather, heat of summer, before
    thunderstorms; teething; tobacco
Better: profuse urination; sweating; open air; alcohol use; mental effort;
    bending forward; stimulants

KALI BICHROMICUM

Eyelids: swollen
Nose: dry, stuffy; pinching pain across bridge of nose; worse with hard
    pressure; pressure and pain at root of nose; ulcerated septum; tough elas-
    tic plugs in nose; loss of smell
Discharge: fluid, acrid; burning mucous membrane from nose to throat
    thick, ropy, greenish yellow discharge or yellow discharge
Sneezing: violent
Misc: snuffles in children; chronic inflammation of frontal sinuses; aching
    and fullness in forehead; thirsty; chilly

KALI IODATUM

Eyes: puffy; aching and heavy pressure between eyes
Discharge: copious and watery, acrid, salty, hot, green; foul odor with difficulty breathing
Sneezing: incessant for an hour or more every a.m.
Misc: colds from damp days; thirsty

MEZEREUM

Nose: interior of nose burns
Discharge: watery and excessive
Sneezing: may occur

NAPHTHALINE

Eyes: inflamed, painful, and burn
Eyelids: often swollen
Sneezing: frequent
Misc: often used in combination with other remedies; head feels hot

NATRUM MURIATICUM (NAT MUR)

Eyes: tearing from the affected side; burning, acrid discharge
Eyelids: swollen
Nose: loss of smell; thin, fluent, watery discharge; alternates between fluent and dry; may last 1-3 days then stops; sore internally; discharge violent
Sneezing: early in a.m.
Misc: headache hammering, heavy, bursting over eyes; thirsty; chilly; breathing difficulty; loss of smell and taste; least exposure to sun brings on most violent attack of watery discharge
Worse: 9-11 a.m., alternate days; warm room, heat; exertion; mental, violent emotions, sympathy; music; noise
Better: open air; cool bathing; perspiration; rest; deep breathing; before breakfast; lying on right side; tight clothes; pressure in back

POLLENTINUM

Use when pollens are the main allergens. Use high potencies over a period of several months at least.

PSORINUM

Eyes: acrid secretion
Eyelids: red
Nose: boring, stinging in right nostril followed by excessive sneezing; dry watery discharge with stoppage of nose

Throat: chronic post-nasal drip

Discharge: burning followed by increased discharge which relieves

Misc: hungry or feel unusually well before an attack; anxiety; profuse sweating; sensitive to drafts about head; chilly; if the hay fever returns every year on the same day of the month and there is a previous history of asthma or eczema; also helpful in preventing hay fever if given a number of months before the season begins

Worse: cold, cold air, weather changes, storms, winter, heat, warmth of bed, draft; bathing; exertion; suppression; coffee

Better: lying with head low, lying quietly; washing; nosebleeds; hard pressure; profuse sweating, heat, warm clothing

PULSATILLA

Eyes: thick, profuse, yellow, non-acrid discharge; itch and burn; profuse tearing and watering; in general the condition of the eyes is worse from warmth

Eyelids: lids are inflamed; eyelids are matted shut by a sticky mucus

Nose: stoppage of right nostril; pressing pain at root of nose; loss of smell; large green fetid scales in nose; stoppage in evening; yellow mucus abundant in morning

Discharge: excessive watery discharge from nose

Misc: chilly, changeable symptoms; thirstless; can't tolerate pork and fats in general

Worse: from heat, warm room; towards evening; lying on left side

Better: open air; motion; cold applications; cool food & drinks

SABADILLA

Eyes: red, tearing; tearing in open air and with bright lights

Eyelids: red

Nose: either stuffed up or running freely with a copious, watery discharge; much itching inside nose; tickling in nose spreads over entire body; very sensitive to the smell of flowers, fruit, garlic, and other odors

Mouth: dry without thirst

Discharge: copious watery discharge from nose and eyes

Face: mottled

Cough: muffled especially with grass-seed allergies

Sneezing: frequent spasms of severe sneezing

Misc: itching of soft palate; thirstless; craves hot things, sweets, milk; typical; symptoms of hay fever; extremely chilly; possible associated with severe frontal headache or with bleeding from nose; children may have problems with worms, tonsils, and adenoids

Worse: cold air; drinks; periodically, forenoon, same hour; new moon, full moon; odors
Better: heat, wrapped up, being outdoors, walking in the open air; eating; swallowing

SILICA

Eyes: swelling of lachrymal duct; aversion to daylight; eyes tender to touch
Nose: itching, tingling; dry hard crust that bleed; obstruction with loss of smell; itching irritation of posterior nares or Eustachian tube; swallowing relieves
Discharge: frothy; excessive watery discharge with nose bleed; burning discharge from nose
Sneezing: violent; morning
Misc: chilly, thirsty
Worse: eyes when closed

SOLIDAGO VIRGA

Eyes: watery, burning, stinging, injected
Nose: irritated with increased mucus
Sneezing: paroxysms
Misc: hay fever leads to asthma

STICTA

Eyelids: burning and soreness of eyelids
Nose: feeling of fullness or pinching sensation at root of nose; extreme nasal dryness and obstruction; may not have discharge; constant need to blow nose but no discharge; scabs in a.m. and p.m.
Throat: raw
Cough: dry hacking especially at night, worse on inspiration
Sneezing: persistent
Misc: hay fever symptoms; headache before discharge appears
Worse: nose fullness is worse when discharge appears
Better: nose fullness is better when discharge disappears

ZINCUM METALLICUM

Eyes: smarting, tearing, itching; pressure if pressed into head
Eyelids: soreness, itching
Nose: nasal obstruction accompanied by sensation of pressure at the root of nose as if the nose is being pushed into the skull; sore
Throat: dry; constant inclination to hawk up mucus
Cough: spasmodic; accompanied by burning and oppression in the chest

made worse at night on lying down; great difficulty in coughing up phlegm

Misc: asthma is worse in the evening after a meal; general weakness; don't give with the remedies *Chamomilla* and *Nux vomica*

Worse: from jarring or noise; evening; exertion (physical or mental)

Better: bringing up phlegm

The following remedies are the ones most commonly used when treating allergy symptoms in acute situations. The potency may vary from a 30X to a much higher potency:

- Acute allergic reactions to foods in general—give *Urtica urens* when *Apis mellifica* and carbolic acid are not indicated, especially to foods such as strawberries, cheese, goat's milk, citrus, shellfish.
- Acute allergic reactions to drugs or shellfish—give Apis mellifica for reactions to penicillin or other drug-related reactions or to shellfish.
- Acute air hunger, swelling, and edema—give carbolic acid (*Carbolicum acidum*) or *Carbo vegetabilis*.
- Allergic shock—give Apis mellifica, *Carbo vegetabilis*, carbolic acid (*Carbolicum acidum*), or epinephrine.
- Bread allergy—give *Dioscorea villosa*.
- Contact allergies—give *Rhus toxicodendron* or *Urtica urens*
- Fine dust—give Ipecacuanha. Use Hydrastis or Aralia racemosa if Ipecacuanha doesn't work. Use for fine dust-like pollen or fine wood dust.
- Fish allergy—give Medusa.
- Grass allergy—give Sabadilla.
- Ill effects of foods—give Nux vomica or Carbo vegetabilis, especially for coffee, alcohol, spices, or just food in general. The person is worse with cold food or drinks.
- Itchy patches of skin—give Sepia, Selenium, Glonoine, or Lithium.
- Meat allergy—give Glonoine.
- Milk and cheese allergy—give Lactic acid, Calcaria carbonicum, Pancreatin, or Dioscorea villosa.
- Mixed pollens or mixed grasses can be taken orally in homeopathic dosage.
- Poison Oak or Ivy—giving Rhus toxicodendron or Rhus diversiloba can be very effective for people reacting to these plants or for contact dermatitis to other substances.
- Pork and fat intolerance—give Pulsatilla or Carbo vegetabilis.

- Rash comes on suddenly—give Belladonna, Arsenicum album, Hydrastis, or Urtica urens.
- Pine tree allergy—give Terebinth.
- Sugar allergy—give Syzygium jambolanum or Hydrastis.
- Tobacco and cigarette smoke—give Tabacum 6C. Take when allergic to tobacco smoke. It will ease the ill effects of inhaling tobacco and cigarette smoke.

CHAPTER 45

Naturopathic Medicine and Naturopathic Physicians

WHAT IS NATUROPATHIC MEDICINE?

Naturopathic medicine is founded on the healing power of nature. Within every person there is an innate ability for healing and maintaining health. The results of poor nutrition and lifestyle choices can lead to the breakdown of our bodies. This leads to a decrease in resistance and the onset of disease. The symptoms of disease indicate improper functioning of organs and tissues. Our bodies can be restored to normal function, effectively and naturally. This is possible with treatments that support and stimulate, rather than disrupt or suppress the body's innate ability to heal itself.

The holistic approach to health includes the physical, mental, emotional, and spiritual aspects of each individual. These aspects are inseparably connected to the well-being of the body. Therapies treat the whole person by supporting each of these areas throughout the healing process. The practice of naturopathic medicine prefers non-invasive treatments that minimize the risks of harmful side effects. Naturopathic treatment corrects the fundamental imbalances and restores proper function and health by safe, effective, and natural methods. Treatment includes showing ways to support the healing process and maintain renewed health. Our approach to health care can prevent minor illnesses from developing into more serious or chronic degenerative diseases.

Naturopathic physicians (N.D.) are educated and trained as primary-care providers. We are trained as general practitioners specializing in natural medicine. We treat a wide range of ailments and aim to restore health using an array of therapies that can include nutrition, herbal medicine, homeopathy, physical medicine (including hydrotherapy, exercise, and manipulation), natural childbirth, minor surgery, counseling techniques, and Oriental medicine. When you come to us for your medical care our objective is to determine the underlying cause of your condition or disease. We will also advise you if there are any nutritional and lifestyle imbalances.

Nutritional Counseling

Nutrition has always been a major therapeutic tool of the naturopathic physician. Improper dietary choices and problems with digestion and the assimilation of foods play a major role in the disease process. Making proper choices in what, when, and how we eat helps to bring us to a place of optimum health. Individuals may also need vitamins, minerals and other nutritional supplements to strengthen the body.

Botanical Medicine

Herbs are nature's gift for healing. All cultures around the world use the healing powers of leaves, bark, roots, flowers, seeds, and the oils of plants that grow around them. Certain herbs strengthen and tonify specific conditions. Plant formulations, capsules, extracts, tinctures, and teas can treat or assist in the treatment of a variety of acute or chronic illness.

Homeopathy

Many naturopathic physicians use homeopathic medications in their treatment plans. Homeopathy is a highly systematic method of directly and naturally stimulating the body's innate healing power to cure disease. For this reason, homeopathy effectively treats many conditions, including some diseases that do not respond to conventional medicine. Homeopathy treats the whole person and increases one's resistance rather than simply suppressing symptoms. By stimulating the body's healing power, homeopathy gently brings the patient to a greater state of health and vitality, thus helping to prevent future health problems.

Other Services That May Be Available

Physical Medicine: the therapeutic use of water (hydrotherapy), light, electricity, ultrasound, massage, and exercise. Many naturopathic physicians also do spinal and extremity manipulation. This type of treatment often corrects stress or trauma-induced misalignments of muscles, connective tissue, and the skeletal system.

Natural Childbirth: prenatal and postnatal care and natural childbirth care in an out-of-hospital setting.

Minor Surgery: the repair of superficial wounds and the removal of superficial foreign bodies, cysts and other superficial masses.

Counseling Techniques: counseling, hypnotherapy, emotional support, and biofeedback.

Oriental Medicine: includes the use of acupressure and Chinese herbology. Some naturopathic physicians also seek training in acupuncture.

Naturopathic Training

At the turn of the century there were thousands of naturopathic physicians and nearly two dozen naturopathic medical colleges spanned the United States. When pharmaceutical and technical medicine came along, and the idea swept the nation that drugs could eliminate most diseases, naturopathic doctors and colleges became rare. Today, they are making a comeback. Thousands of licensed naturopathic physicians are located in most states. Currently, there are five naturopathic colleges in North America. The accrediting agency for naturopathic medical programs has been recognized by the United States Department of Education.

Someone seeking the degree of Doctor of Naturopathic Medicine must first complete pre-admission requirements at an accredited college or university. These requirements are equivalent to those for entrance to other medical schools. Then they must complete four years of post-graduate study at an approved naturopathic medical college. The first two years focus on standard medical science and is modeled after traditional medical colleges. The following two years focus on a wide range of natural and holistic therapeutics. Graduating students receive a doctoral degree, Doctor of Naturopathic Medicine (or N.D). Naturopathic doctors are the only licensed primary health-care providers with extensive training in therapeutic diets and preventive medicine.

To be licensed, practitioners must possess a Doctor of Naturopathic Medicine degree from one of the recognized four-year graduate-level Naturopathic medical colleges. Each licensing state requires a Naturopathic physician to pass state board licensing exams and maintain their license through continuing education. They can then practice medicine as a primary health-care provider with the same patient care responsibilities of any licensed physician.

How Do I Locate a Naturopathic Physician?

Check the yellow pages under the heading "Physicians, Naturopathic" for a local listing. Since naturopathic medicine is new to many people, it is usually helpful to ask some questions before beginning treatment. Most physicians offer a brief consultation at no charge to the patient for this purpose. Please feel free to contact your state's Association of Naturopathic

Physicians for a list of physicians. You may also contact the American Association of Naturopathic Physicians (AANP) in Seattle, Washington, for more information.

Does Health Insurance Cover Naturopathic Care?

Many health insurance companies cover naturopathic services, but not all insured patients have such policies. This inconsistency occurs when the patient or the employer does not specifically request naturopathic services included in their health plan. We encourage all insured patients to contact their employer, or individual insurance agent, and request that their policy include naturopathic services. In most instances this change can be made easily. If not, please contact your naturopathic state association for the names of insurers who cover all licensed physicians. You can also contact the American Association of Naturopathic Physicians in Seattle, Washington.

Advantages of Naturopathic Care

The goal of naturopathic physicians is to understand the needs of the patient. This approach reflects the naturopathic concern with treating the underlying source of illness and applying treatments that work with the body's natural healing mechanism instead of against it. It is believed that, given the right tools, the body can heal itself. Treatments are highly individualized to each patient. Although synthetic drugs can produce seemingly dramatic improvements, their use is avoided. They may mask underlying causes or result in serious side effects.

The cost of naturopathic care is also an advantage, since it frequently eliminates the need for more costly surgery and hospitalization. In addition, the patient learns to make effective decisions that may prevent future health problems. Teaching people to take responsibility for their own health and how to prevent disease is a basic naturopathic principle.

Naturopathic medicine offers a viable alternative for people who suffer from minor discomforts, chronic pain, and diseases of the respiratory or digestive tract. It is especially good for people who have been diagnosed and treated with conventional medicine with little success. Naturopathic physicians typically treat people with colds, minor infections, allergies, muscle and joint problems, gynecological disorders, fatigue, and other poorly defined disorders. Often, these people have already gone the drug route and want something more than harsh medication with side effects.

A well-educated and licensed naturopathic physician can give you the type of primary health care needed to solve many health concerns. Our goal is to use therapies that support the body's own healing processes and avoid treatments that suppress or replace the body's own ability to function normally. Naturopathic medicine integrates the latest advances of scientific research with the ancient healing wisdom of traditional cultures—it is this philosophy that guides naturopathic medicine and that can guide you to optimum wellness.

Naturopathic Schools and Organizations

Bastyr University
14500 Juanita Dr, NE
Bothell, WA 98011
(206) 523-9585

Canadian College of Naturopathic Medicine
60 Berl Avenue
Etobicoke, Ontario
Canada M8Y 3C7

National College of Naturopathic Medicine
049 SW Porter
Portland, OR 97201
(503) 499-4343

Southwest College of Naturopathic Medicine
6535 East Osborn Road, Suite 703
Scottsdale, AZ 85251
(602) 990-7424

University of Bridgeport
College of Naturopathic Medicine
221 University Ave, Bridgeport, CT 06601
(203) 576-4109

American Association of Naturopathic Medicine
601 Valley Street, Suite 105
Seattle, WA 98109
Phone: (206) 298-0126 Fax: (206) 298-0125

Resources

Allergen-Proof Encasings, Inc.
450 E. 363 St.
Eastlake, OH 44094
Carries all types of encasings and other products for the dust-sensitive person.

Allergy Control Products, Inc.
96 Danbury Rd.
Ridgefield, CT 06877
(800) 422-DUST
Carries air cleaners, vacuums, allergy-control products, and much more; catalog available.

Allergy Health Shopper
P.O. Box 239
Tate, TX 75132
(800) 447-1100
Sells air purifiers and vacuums; catalog available.

Allergy Relief Shop
2932 Middlebrook Pk.
Knoxville, TN 37921
(615) 522-2795
Sells products for the chemically sensitive and environmentally aware.

Allergy Resources, Inc.
P.O. Box 444
Guffey, CO 80820
(800) USE-FLAX or (719) 488-3630
Has products for the chemically sensitive, including water filters, ultra-pure bedding, and nontoxic cleaning supplies. A free catalog is available full of unique foods and beverages.

Alpine Industries
9199 Central Avenue N.E.
Blaine, MN 55434
(612) 780-9388
Makers of the Living Air units for air purification and the reduction of bacteria, mold, allergens, and smells in the home and office.

Basically Natural
109 East G St.
Brunswick, MD 21716
(800) 352-7099
Natural personal-care products, household cleaners, and pet care; free catalog.

Blue Sky Labs
8655 39th Ave. S.
Seattle, WA 98118
(206) 721-2583
Home testing kit for detecting formaldehyde. This type of kit can help you find out if formaldehyde poisoning is a problem in your home.

Bob's Red Mill Natural Foods, Inc.
5209 S.E. International Way
Milwaukie, OR 97222
(800) 553-2258 or in Oregon call (503) 654-3215
Send for a catalog. They are millers, manufacturers, and distributors of whole-grain natural foods. They have bread mixes for bread machines as well as a fat replacer for all baked goods. They also have a wide selection of books on beans, grains, flours, and gluten-free and wheat-free cooking and baking.

Chemtrec
24-hour emergency number is (800) 424-9300
This is a hotline of the Chemical Manufacturers Association in Washington, D.C. Call for information on spills, leaks, fires, and exposure to chemical products.

Cotton Place
P.O. Box 59721
Dallas, TX 75229
(800) 451-8866 or in Dallas call 243-1491
Provides cotton products for chemically sensitive people.

Community Re-Hope House, Inc.
25492 Westborn
Dana Point, CA 92629
(714) 240-6167
A place where psychiatric patients can receive total care. They receive adequate food high in nutrition, but not the major allergen foods. Foods low in nutrition are not served and sugar, milk, salt, and coffee are not used at the facility.
(CSA) Community supported agriculture is an idea developed about twenty-five years ago in Europe. CSA is a way for each of us to become directly involved in the food system that

nourishes us. This program provides people with a direct connection to organic farmers. It provides high quality food at a reasonable price by establishing a direct link between those who grow the food and those who eat it. This program works because the individuals and families who associate with a CSA farm pledge to support it annually. This is done by buying shares in the harvest at the beginning of each year. The income from these shares covers the operating expenses of the farm. In return, the farm provides the shareholders with fresh food throughout the season. Some CSA farm shareholders can work on the farm a few hours during the season as part of their support.

CSA farms have certified organically grown crops. They are dedicated to preserving the health of the soil, to ecological balance, and diversity. Goals are to rediscover, develop, and use sustainable methods and practices for growing a variety of nutritious and healthful foods for local consumption. The farmers strive to restore and maintain the vitality of the earth through the use of composts, cover cropping, crop rotation, and natural methods of fertilization, disease and pest control. Look for a CSA farm in your area and please become a shareholder. Our individual well-being is dependent on the health of the world around us. Farms who practice food production that mirrors the natural laws of living organisms and emphasizes respect for all life need your support. Become a customer in the movement to organic agriculture.

Dietary Specialties
P.O. Box 227
Rochester, NY 14601
(716) 263-2787
Sells a wide selection of pre-packaged gluten-free muffins, cookies, and bread mixes.

Ener-G Foods, Inc.
5960 1st Ave. S.
Seattle, WA 98124-5788
(800) 331-5222 or in Washington call (206) 767-6660
Write for a list of alternative food products including gluten-free and wheat-free foods; catalog available. They have mixes for short cut baking that contain no artificial flavoring or coloring and no preservatives. They also sell prepared foods such as breads, cookies, doughnuts, pizza shells, hamburger buns, crackers, etc. that are wheat-free and can be delivered to your home by UPS.

Environmental Construction Outfitters
44 Crosby St.
New York, NY 10012
(800) 238-5008
A building-supply store with environment-friendly products.

Environmental Health Center
1500 Marrilla
Dallas, TX 75201
(214) 744-1000
Dr. Rea's health center for the treatment of multiple environmental sensitivities.

Environmentally Sound Products, Inc.
8845 Orchard Tree Lane
Towson, MD 21286
(800) 886-5432
Home environmental test kits, recycled school and office supplies, rechargeable batteries, and more; catalog available.

Feingold Association of the United States
Box 6550
Alexandria, VA 22306
(800) 321-3287 or (516) 369-9340

First Alert
(800) 323-9005
The company that invented the smoke detector now has a carbon monoxide detector. It detects this deadly gas at .01 percent levels. It is battery operated and has a suggested price of $60. It can usually be found at stores that sell smoke detectors.

Food-Allergy Hot Lines:
General Mills: (800) 231-0308
Nabisco Foods Group: (800) 932-7800
Pillsbury Company: (800) 767-4466

Food Allergy Network
4744 Holly Avenue
Fairfax, VA 22030
(703) 691-3179
A study in the August 6, 1992 *New England Journal of Medicine* on food allergies shows how difficult it can be for kids to avoid foods that trigger allergies. The consequences of a dietary slip can be serious. At fault were hidden provokers such as chopped nuts in cookies, and peanut butter in cake icing. Only a small percentage of children with allergies suffer life-threatening problems, but the number with potentially deadly allergies seems to be growing. The first contact with a problematic food can cause hives or swelling. Repeated encounters result in more severe reactions. Parents seeking advice on handling children with food allergies can send a stamped, self-addressed envelope to the Food Allergy Network.

Food and Drug Administration (FDA)
Parklawn Bldg.
5600 Fisher's Ln., #14-71
Rockville, MD 20857
Write to the FDA Commissioner with your concerns about foods and drugs.

Friends of the Earth–Groundwater Protection Project
218 D St., SE
Washington, DC 20003
(800) 426-4791 is the Safe Drinking Water Phone Hot-line
If you have a concern about lead in your water supply, or other water contaminants, get a copy of their fact sheets. They have "Do You Have Lead in Your Drinking Water?" and "Preventing Drinking Water Contamination."

Gardens Alive!
5100 Schenley Place
Lawrenceburg, IN 47025
(812) 537-8650
Safer pest control, organic fertilizers, beneficial insects, composting aids, etc.

Gluten-Free Pantry
P.O. Box 840
Glastonbury, CT 06033
(800) 291-8386 or fax them at (860) 633-6853
Glurmet, gluten-free baking mixes as well as cookbooks.

Gluten Intolerance Group of North America
P.O. Box 23053
Seattle, WA 98102

Green Earth
2545 Prairie Ave.
Evanston, IL 60201
(708) 475-0205
A source of organic natural foods, nuts, dried fruits, meats and poultry.

HRI & Health Information Network
4213 Montgomery Dr.
Santa Rosa, CA 95405
(800) 743-6996 or (707) 539-3966
This is a service providing customized computer searches on virtually any health or med-

ical concern or therapy, from Lyme's disease to antioxidants. Search results usually include references, summaries, abstracts, or full text articles. It costs from $25 to $120 depending on the complexity of the search.

Health Resource
Attn: Janice R. Guthrie (Health Information Specialist)
209 Katherine Drive
Conway, AK 72032
(501) 329-5272
The Health Resource, Inc., established in 1984 by Janice Guthrie, is a pioneer in the medical-information industry. You are provided with individualized, comprehensive research reports on your specific medical problems. Information is gleaned from international computer databases, medical conferences, interviews with medical researchers and clinicians, studies as yet unpublished, and feedback from other clients. A typical report contains information on treatment options, both conventional and alternative, as well as other research, self-help measures, specialists, and resource organizations.

Healthful Hardware
P.O. 3217
Prescott, AZ 86302
(520) 445-8225
Natural linoleum and carpeting, testing kits, non-radioactive smoke detectors, etc.

Heart of Vermont
P.O. Box 183
Sharon, VT 05065
(800) 639-4123
Natural furniture, bedding, and other organic items for the chemically sensitive.

Human Ecology Action League
Box 49126
Atlanta, GA 30359
(404) 248-1898
Publishes a quarterly journal, the *Human Ecologist*, for $20.00 yearly. It is for those whose health has been adversely affected by environmental exposures and provides information to those who want to understand the health effects of chemical toxins.

JANICES
(800) JANICES
Providers of cotton mattresses.

Karen's Nontoxic Products
1839 Dr. Jake Rd.
Conowingo, MD 21918
(410) 378-4621
Natural products for the family home and health; a charge for the catalog.

Livos Plant Chemistry
1365 Rufina Circle
Santa Fe, NM 87501
(505) 998-9111
Suppliers of natural finishes, preservative, stains, waxes, paints, cleaners, and art materials.

Memtec Corp.
19-B Keewaydin Dr.
Salem, NH 03079
(603) 893-8080
Sell gaussmeters to measure electromagnetic fields.

National Center for Environmental Health Strategies
1100 Rural Ave.
Voorhees, NJ 08043
(609) 429-5358
This is a clearinghouse of information. There is a newsletter available called *Delicate Balance,* and there are discounts on subscriptions to *Chemical Exposures* magazine.

National Allergy Supply, Inc.
4400 Ga. Hwy. 120, P.O. Box 1658
Duluth, GA 30136
(800) 522-1448
Send for their catalog that includes mattress encasings, mite-proof pillow encasings, HEPA air cleaner, vent-filtration kits, vacuum-replacement bags that are almost dust-free, mold and mildew sprays, HEPA vacuum cleaners, dust and pollen masks, dust cloths, and a humidity gauge.

National Coalition Against Misuse of Pesticides
530 Seventh St.
Washington, DC 20003
(202) 543-5450
For more information about organic food.

National Pesticide Telecommunication Network (NPTN)
Oregon State University-Agriculture Extention
Weniger Hall Room 333
Corvalis, OR 97331
(800) 858-7378
Funded by the Environmental Protection Agency and Texas Tech University, this 24-hour
hot-line provides technical chemical and regulatory information, toxicity and health data,
and resources and referrals. Hours are 6:30 a.m. to 4:30 p.m.

Natural Baby Company
816 Silvia St. 800 B-S
Trenton, NJ 08628-3299
(800) 388-BABY or (609) 771-9233
Organic cotton diapers, acupressure bands for morning sickness, and other supplies for the
youngest members of the natural household; catalog available.

Natural Bedroom by Jantz Design
P.O. Box 3071
Santa Rosa, CA 95402
(800) 365-6563
Natural-fiber bedding products as well as towels and sleepware; free catalog.

Natural Choice
1365 Rufina Circle
Santa Fe, NM 87501
(800) 621-2591 or (505) 438-3448
Specializes in natural paints and finishes, hypoallergenic body-care products and more.

The Natural Gardening Co.
217 San Anselmo Ave
San Anselmo, CA 94960
(707) 766-9303
Seedlings, gardening clogs, organic pest control, and more; catalog available.

The Natural Grocer Radio Show
This radio show features expert guests discussing all aspects of alternative health and nat-
ural healting. The show is now heard weekly in:
• Phoenix, AZ, KRDS 1190 a.m., Sat., 12-1:30 p.m.
• Miami/Ft. Lauderdale, FL, WWNN 980 a.m., Mon.-Fri., 3-4 p.m.
• Chicago, IL, WYLL 106.7 FM, Sat., 12-1 p.m.
• Los Angeles, CA, KRBT 740 a.m., Sat., 12:30-1:30 p.m.

Natural Resources/Allergy Resources, Inc.
745 Powderhorn
Monument, CO 80132
(800) USE-FLAX or (719) 488-3630
Products for the allergic and environmentally sensitive person; catalog available.

New Hope
Upper Marlboro, MA
(301) 946-6395
A center for the treatment of the mentally ill using fasting and nutritional treatments. This
is being run by a couple who saw their daughter make a remarkable improvement after such
care. They also witnessed dozens of other patients with serious mental symptoms improve
under a fasting and nutritional treatment. They were motivated to open a project with similar intent as the Community Re-Hope House in Dana Point, California.

Non-Toxic Environment
Contact Barbara Jenkenson or David Greenspan
Canby, OR 97013
(800) 789-4348
Catalog of products for aware and chemically sensitive individuals.

Non-Toxic Network: Connecting Health and Home
P.O. Box 174, Route 175
Holderness, NH 03245
(603) 536-0171   Fax 603-968-9670
The purpose of the Non-Toxic Network is to provide a national database linking the health-
conscious consumer with health, design and building professionals, and the products needed to create an appropriate living environment.

ONN
P.O. Box 510504
Melbourne Beach, FL 32951
(407) 724-6475
ONN's Non-Toxic Network supplies products for the home and personal care that are envi-
ronmentally sensitive, biodegradable, nontoxic, made with no animal testing, and packaged
in recyclable containers. They are more effective than store brands and far less expensive.
You can call direct, order, and have the products delivered at your door in two to three days.

Peaceful Valley Farm Supply
P.O. Box 2209
Grass Valley, CA 95945

(916) 272-4769
Organic gardening supplies; catalog available.

Plants for Clean Air Council
10210 Bald Hill Rd.
Mitchellville, MD 20721
Send a large self-addressed stamped envelope and $1.00 to receive their information.

Practical Allergy Research Foundation
P.O. Box 60
Buffalo, NY 14223-0060
(726) 875-0398
Books, audio tapes and educational videos for the public and physicians on environmental-related health and emotional illnesses in children. Doris Rapp, M.D., founder, has compiled a comprehensive library on environmental illness and its impact on children. They also offer her best-selling book *Is This Your Child?*

Preconception Care Foundation
5724 Clymer Road
Quakertown, Penn 18951
A guidebook for preconception care is being prepared and should be available.

Safe Technologies
145 Rosemary St. Suite F
Needham, MA 02194-3258
(800) 638-9121 or (617) 444-7778
Safe computing sells a couple of products for both IBM and Macintosh computers that partially or completely eliminate electromagnetic pollution for about $300 to $1000. A cheaper route is to have Safe "retrofit" your existing monitor for about $200.

Special Foods
9207 Shotgun Court
Springfield, VA 22150
(703) 644-0991
Offer unusual bread, flours, and infant formulas that are milk- and gluten-free.

Spectrum Naturals of Petaluma, California
Manufacturer of Spectrum Spread, a non-hydrogenated, non-dairy spread. It is made by using a patented process that mixes canola oil and water together without hydrogenation. The product is a spread that stays solid enough to be spreadable. It is made from canola oil, water, xanthan and guar gums, soy protein isolate, annatto, citric acid, sorbic acid, natural

flavor, and turmeric. The texture and taste is different from both butter and margarine and may take some getting used to. Spectrum Spread is best used as a cold spread on bread or muffins, as an ingredient in baked goods, or in low-heat sauteing. Frying at high heat can cause it to break down and should be avoided. It is available in natural-foods stores nationwide.

The Teff Company (208) 455-0375
Call for more information on the nutritious grain teff.

Well Mind Association
4649 Sunnyside North
Seattle, WA 98103
(206) 547-6167
A non-profit organization dedicated to helping victims of brain dysfunction and environmental sensitivities. Publishes a newsletter and has a resource library.

Wilde Temptings
4760 Lucerne Lakes Blvd.West, Suite 401
Lake Worth, FL 33467
(800) 434-4846
Gourmet catalog for the food allergic and health-conscious gourmet. Flours, brownie, pancake, pizza mixes, yeast-free, wheat-free bread mixes, etc.

World Research Foundation
15300 Ventura Blvd., Suite 405
Sherman Oaks, CA 91403
(818) 907-5483
According to the World Research Foundation, there are many healing techniques used elsewhere in the world that are overlooked or unavailable in the United States. They draw from more than 500 computer data bases that access important medical, scientific, and environmental information. This is from more than 100 countries (as well as books and periodicals). The foundation provides information on the most up-to-date treatments for a wide variety of medical conditions. Two medical search options are available for an average cost of $45 each. The library search primarily contains information on alternative and natural treatments. The computer search focuses on the latest allopathic information.

Organic Food Products available by mail order

You can bring organic farmers' products to your doorstep year-round. By phone you can order almost everything you need. Mail-order organic foods often come directly from the producers and may be fresher than from the supermarket. Most of the growers will sell in bulk. These sources are from *Green Groceries: A Mail Order Guide to Organic Foods* (Harper-Collins, 1992). If you live in an area that encourages and promotes organic foods, then get to know your local organic growers and businesses that sell organic foods. Give them as much business as you can. If you don't live close to organic products, then the following mail order companies may be more convenient. They sell organic produce and products in many categories and order from a variety of suppliers. This offers you a one-stop shopping advantage. The *Organic National Directory* provides information and resources for organic meat and produce throughout the U.S. Write CAFF, P.O. box 464, Davis, CA 95617 or call them at (916) 756-8518. The following are companies that sell organic foods by mail:

Allergy Resources, Inc.
195 Huntington Beach Dr.
Colorado Springs, CO 80921
(719) 488-3630

Organic Foods Express
11003 Emack Rd.
Beltsville, MD 20705
(301) 937-8608

Specialty Organic Source
Champaign, IL 61824-1628
(217) 687-4730

Rising Sun Organic Food
P.O. Box 627, PA 150 & I-80
Milesburg, PA 16853
(814) 355-9850

Pacific Bakery
P.O. Box 950
Oceanside, CA 92049
(800) 585-1980
Ready-made yeast-free, fat-free, 100% organic breads, bagels & buns. Rapid delivery available. Delicious baked goods.

The Green Earth
2545 Prairie Ave.
Evanston, IL 60201
(800) 322-3662

Walnut Acres Organic Farms
Walnut Acres Rd.
Penns Creek, PA 17862
(800) 344-9025

Mr. Ark Trading Co.
120 South East Ave.
Fayetteville, AR 72701
(501) 442-7191

Starr Organic Produce
P.O. Box 561502 Miami, FL 33256-1502
(305) 262-1242
Organically grown tropical fruits as well as dried fruit

Morningland Dairy
Rt. 1, Box 188B, Mt. View, MO 65548
Organic raw milk and cheeses

Diamond Organics
P.O. Box 2159, Freedom, CA 95019
(800) 922-2396
Organic varieties of lettuce, fresh herbs, vegetables, and fruits

D'Artagnan
399-419 St. Paul Ave Jersey City, NJ 07306
(800) DAR-TAGN
Organic meat and poultry

Eagle Organic and Natural Food
407 Church Ave., Huntsville, AR 72703
(501) 738-2203
Organic whole grain flour, hot cereals, mixes, grits, beans, coffee

The Meat Shop
13419 Vickery Road, Tacoma, WA 98446
(206) 537-4490
Organic meat and poultry.

Community Mill & Bean
267 Rt 89 South Savannah, NY 13146
(800) 755-0554
Organic baking mixes, whole grains, beans

Windy River Farm
P.O. Box 312 Merlin, OR 97532
(503) 476-8979
Organic culinary herbs, dried fruits, vegetables

Stevia Products

Stevia Products—The Body Ecology Catalog
(800) 4 STEVIA
A stevia "starter kit" that includes a 10 gram jar of powdered stevia extract, a dropper bottle, and an information booklet. Refills are available.

Wisdom of the Ancients
(800) 947-6417
Sells whole-leaf liquid stevia for use as a dietary supplement for skin care. (Liquid stevia is also available in some health food stores.)

Jeans' Greens
(518) 239-8327.
Supplier of cut stevia leaf. You can request an article about the history and use of stevia in other countries.

The Herbal Advantage
(417) 753-3999
Offers 100 percent powdered stevia leaf with a minimum purchase of four ounces.

Sunrider International
(310) 781-3808
Sells a dietary supplement of stevia extract and other ingredients called Sunectar. Call to find a distributor near you.

Bibliography

Billman, Al. *Guidelines: A Compilation of Products and Resources for the Chemically Sensitive.* Dallas: Human Ecology Research Foundation, 1981.

Bland, J. *Lectures of Dr. Jeffrey Bland,* selected papers.

Bodman, FH. "The Homeopathic Treatment of Allergic Condition," *British Homeopathic Journal* (3) 1991.

Braly, J. *Food Allergy and Nutrition Revolution.* Connecticut: Keats Publishing, 1992.

Braverman, E. *The Healing Nutrients Within* Connecticut: Keats Publishing, 1987.

Broad, F.E. "Early Feeding History of Children with Learning Diosorders," *Developmental Medicine and Child Neurology* 21 (1979):822.

California State Dept.of Consumer Affairs. *Clean Your Room!* California State Dept. of Consumer Affairs Compendium, Sacramento, 1982.

Crook, W.G. "Can What a Child Eats Make Him Dull, Stupid, or Hyperactive?" *Journal of Learning Disabilities* 13 (1980): 53-58.

Crook, W. *Detecting Your Hidden Allergies.* Tennessee: Professional Books, 1988.

Davies, G. *Overcoming Food Allergies.* London: Ashgrove Press, 1985.

Davis, J.R.; Brownson, R.C.; Garcia, R.; Bentz, B. *Family Pesticide Use and Childhood Brain Cancer.* Archive Environmental Contamination Toxicology, 1993.

Diamond, H.; Diamond, M. *Fit for Life.* New York: Warner Books, 1985.

Feingold, B.F. *Why Your Child is Hyperactive.* New York: Random House, 1975.

Frompovich, C. *Understanding Body Chemistry and Hair Mineral Analysis.* Pennsylvania: CJ Frompovich, 1982.

Gerrard, J.W. "Allergy in Infancy," *Pediatric Annals* 3 (1974): 9.

Green, N.S. *Poisoning Our Children.* Chicago: Noble Press, 1991.

Griffin, L. *Is Any Sick Among You?* Orem, Ut: Bi-World Pub, 1974.

Horvilleur, A. *The Family Guide to Homeopathy.* VA: Health & Homeopathy Pub Co, 1986.

Hughes, M.C., Goldman, B., Snyder, N. "Hyperactivity and the Attention Deficit Disorder," *American Family Physician* 27 (1983):119-126.

Jackson, M., Teague, T. *The Handbook of Alternatives to Chemical Medicine.* CA: Lawton-Teague Pub, 1975.

Kraus, B. *Calories and Carbohydrates.* NY: Times/Mirror, 1981.

Kridl, J.C., Shewmaker C.K. "Food for thought: improvement of food quality and composition through genetic engineering," *Proc NY Acad Sci* (1996): 1-11.

Krohn, J., Taylor F., Larson, E.M. *The Whole Way to Allergy Relief and Prevention.* (Hartley & Marks Pub, 1991).

Kuzemko, J. *Is Your Child Allergic?* London: Thorsons Publishers, 1988.

Lindlahr, H. *Natural Therapeutics* Vol. III Dietetics. London: The C.W. Daniel Co, Ltd, 1914.

Lindlahr, H. *Natural Therapeutics* Vol. II Practice. London: The C.W. Daniel Co, Ltd, 1919.

Marcarness, R. *Eating Dangerously; the Hazards of Hidden Allergies.* New York: Harcourt, Brace, Javanovich, 1986.

Martin, C. *Low Blood Sugar—The Hidden Menace of Hypoglycemia.* New York: ARC Books, 1971.

Matsen, J. *Eating Alive—Prevention Thru Good Digestion.* Canada: Crompton Books, 1987.

Miller, I., Schwartz, C. "An Olfactory-Limbic Model of Multiple Chemical Sensitivity Syndrome: Possible Relationships to Kindling and Affective Spectrum Disorders," *Biological Psychiatry* 32 (1992): 218-242.

Mitchell, J.W. *Help for the Hyperactive Child.* VA: Betterway Pub., 1984.

Monheit and Luke. "Pesticides in Breast Milk—A Public Health Perspective," *Community Health Studies* 14 (1990): 3.

Morgan, D.P. *Recognition and Management of Pesticide Poisonings (4th ed).* Washington, D.C.: U.S. Environmental Protection Agency, 1989.

Murray, M., Pizzorno, J. *Encyclopedia of Natural Medicine.* CA: Prima Publishing, 1990.

Netzer, C. *The Complete Book of Food Counts.* New York: Dell Book, 1991.

Null, G., Null, S. *The Complete Handbook of Nutrition.* New York: Dell Pub, 1972.

Null, Gary. *No More Allergies.* New York: Villard Books, 1992.

Percival, M. *Infant Nutrition.* Canada: Dynamic Essentials, 1991.

Rapp, D. *Allergies and the Hyperactive Child.* New York: Simon & Schuster, 1979.

Rapp, D. *Allergies and Your Family.* New York: Sterling Pub, 1980.

Rapp, D. *The Impossible Child.* Washington: Life Sciences Press, 1986.

Rapp, D. *Is This Your Child?* New York: William Morrow & Co, 1991.

Reed, B. *Food, Teens, and Behavior.* Manitowoc, WI: Natural Press, 1983.

Remington, D., Higa, B. *Back To Health—A Comprehensive Medical and Nutritional Yeast Control Program.* UT: Vitality House International, 1989.

Roberts, H.J. "Reactions attributed to aspartame-containing products: 551 Cases," *Journal of Applied Nutrition* 40 (1988): 85-94.

Roberts, H.J. *Astartame (NutraSweet): Is It Safe?* PA: The Charles Press, 1989.

Roberts, H.J. "The Hazards of Very-Low-Calorie Dieting," *American Journal of Clinical Nutrition* 41 (1985): 171.

Rogers, S. *The E.I. Syndrome: An Rx for Environmental Illness, Are You Allergic to the 21st Century?* New York: Prestige Pub, 1986.

Rogers, S. *Tired or Toxic.* New York: Prestige Pub, 1990.

Schauss, A. *Diet, Crime, and Delinquency.* Parker House, 1981.

Shannon, I. *Brand Name Guide to Sugar.* ILL: Nelson-Hall, 1977.

Simon, G.E., Daniell, W., Stockbridge, H., et al. "Immunologic Psychological and Neuropsychological Factors in Multiple Chemical Sensitivity: A Controlled Study," *Annals of Internal Medicine* 119 (1993):97-103.

Sonberg, L. *The Complete Nutrition Counter.* New York: Berkley Books, 1993.

Smith, L.H. *Feed Your Kids Right.* New York: M.Evans and Co, Inc. 1993.

Smith, L.H. *Improving Your Child's Behavior Chemistry.* New York: Prentice-Hall, 1976.

Steinman, D. *Diet For A Poisoned Planet.* New York: Ballantine Books, 1992.

Thatcher, R.W., Lester, M.D. "Effects of Low Levels of Cadmium and Lead on Cognitive Functioning in Children," *Arch Environmental Health* 37 (1982):159-166.

Townslend Letter for Doctors, selected articles.

Trattler, R. *Better Health through Natural Healing.* New York: McGraw-Hill, 1985.

Verrett, J., Carper, J. *Eating May Be Hazardous to Your Health.* New York: Anchor Press/Doubleday, 1975.

Weiss, B. "Food Additives and Environmental Chemicals as Sources of Childhood Behavior Disorders," *Journal American Academy Child Psychiatry.* 1982; 21:144-152.

Wender, P.H., Wender, Esther, *The Hyperactive Child and the Learning Disabled Child.* New York: Crown Co, 1978.

Weintraub, S. *Natural Healing with Cell Salts.* Pleasant Grove, UT.: Woodland Publishing, 1996.

Winter, R. *A Consumer's Dictionary of Food Additives.* New York: Crown Pub, 1984.

Wright, J. *Guide to Healing with Nutrition.* CN: Keats Pub, 1990.

Wunderlich, R.D. *Nourishing Your Child.* CN: Keats Pub, 1984.

Index